HEAD, FACE, AND NECK TRAUMA

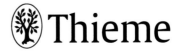

HEAD, FACE, AND NECK TRAUMA

COMPREHENSIVE MANAGEMENT

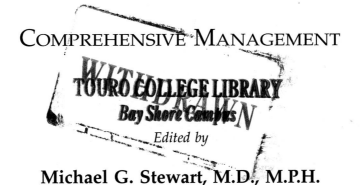

Edited by

Michael G. Stewart, M.D., M.P.H.

Associate Professor
Director of Resident Education
Bobby R. Alford Department of Otorhinolaryngology and Communicative Sciences

Associate Dean of Clinical Affairs
Baylor College of Medicine

Chief of Otolaryngology – Head and Neck Surgery
Ben Taub General Hospital
Texas Medical Center
Houston, Texas

Thieme
New York ● Stuttgart

BS

Thieme New York
333 Seventh Avenue
New York, NY 10001

Consulting Medical Editor: Esther Gumpert
Associate Editor: Owen Zurhellen
Director, Production and Manufacturing: Anne Vinnicombe
Senior Production Editor: David R. Stewart
Marketing Director: Phyllis Gold
Director of Sales: Ross Lumpkin
Chief Financial Officer: Peter van Woerden
President: Brian D. Scanlan
Medical Illustrator: Joel Herring
Compositor: Datapage International Limited
Printer: The Maple-Vail Book Manufacturing Group

Library of Congress Cataloging in Publication Data is available from the publisher

Important note: Medical knowledge is ever-changing. As new research and clinical experience broaden our knowledge, changes in treatment and drug therapy may be required. The authors and editors of the material herein have consulted sources believed to be reliable in their efforts to provide information that is complete and in accord with the standards accepted at the time of publication. However, in view of the possibility of human error by the authors, editors, or publisher of the work herein, or changes in medical knowledge, neither the authors, editors, or publisher, nor any other party who has been involved in the preparation of this work, warrants that the information contained herein is in every respect accurate or complete, and they are not responsible for any errors or omissions or for the results obtained from use of such information. Readers are encouraged to confirm the information contained herein with other sources. For example, readers are advised to check the product information sheet included in the package of each drug they plan to administer to be certain that the information contained in this publication is accurate and that changes have not been made in the recommended dose or in the contraindications for administration. This recommendation is of particular importance in connection with new or infrequently used drugs.

Some of the product names, patents, and registered designs referred to in this book are in fact registered trademarks or proprietary names even though specific reference to this fact is not always made in the text. Therefore, the appearance of a name without designation as proprietary is not to be construed as a representation by the publisher that it is in the public domain.

Printed in the United States of America

5 4 3 2 1

TNY ISBN 1-58890-308-7
GTV ISBN 3-13-140331-4

This book is dedicated to my family

CONTENTS

PREFACE

Trauma is unfortunately a consistent presence in contemporary society, whether accidental or intentional, or blunt or penetrating. In recent decades, advances in trauma research, education, and certification have resulted in the development of a large number of state-of-the-art trauma centers, staffed with well-trained experts. However, not every patient is fortunate enough to reside near a trauma center, and many injured patients are treated at other sites. Therefore, the staffs of these sites must be well versed in the management of injured patients.

In addition, even in sophisticated trauma centers, care of the trauma patient has become increasingly multidisciplinary, as new technologies and areas of special expertise have blossomed within different medical subspecialties. In particular, trauma to the head and neck region is perhaps unique in its multispecialty involvement because of the close proximity of many critical anatomic structures.

This book provides a contemporary overview of head and neck trauma care. Some of the topics that are covered in a mere chapter in this book could fill a book, if the entire spectrum were to be exhaustively covered. Instead, we have included a wide range of interrelated topics, with sufficient depth and detail for the treating physician. Therefore, this book is intended for three audiences: first, for the occasional trauma surgeon who does not see these injuries regularly, but nevertheless sometimes must treat injured patients; second, for the experienced trauma subspecialist, to provide a review of contemporary management from the perspective of multiple different subspecialties; and third, for the medical student, resident, or fellow in training who is exposed to patients with head and neck trauma.

This multidisciplinary text includes contributions from the specialties of general surgery, ophthalmology, oral and maxillofacial surgery, otolaryngology–head and neck surgery, neurotology, plastic surgery, radiology, and thoracic surgery. Many of the authors practice in the Texas Medical Center in Houston and at the two level I trauma centers located there: Ben Taub General Hospital and Memorial Hermann Hospital. Our collaboration and cooperation in those centers has resulted in high-quality trauma care, and we hope that the reader can benefit from our experience.

Michael G. Stewart, M.D., M.P.H.

ix

CONTRIBUTORS

Anthony J. Ascioti, M.D.
Clinical Instructor
Thoracic and Cardiovascular Surgery
University of Texas M.D. Anderson Cancer
Center
Houston, Texas

Eric T. Becken, M.D.
Department of Otolaryngology
University of Minnesota
Minneapolis, Minnesota

Anthony Edwin Brissett, M.D.
Assistant Professor
Director of Facial Plastic and Reconstructive
Surgery
Bobby R. Alford Department of
Otorhinolaryngology and Communicative
Sciences
Baylor College of Medicine
Houston, Texas

C.Y. Joseph Chang, M.D., F.A.C.S.
Associate Professor and Chairman
Otology, Neurotology, and Skull Base Surgery
Department of Otolaryngology–Head and
Neck Surgery
University of Texas–Houston Medical School
Houston, Texas

Newton Jasper Coker, M.D.
Bobby R. Alford Department of
Otorhinolaryngology and Communicative
Sciences
Baylor College of Medicine
Houston, Texas

Orlando Diaz-Daza, M.D.
Department of Radiology
Baylor College of Medicine
Houston, Texas

Pedro J. Diaz-Marchan, M.D.
Department of Radiology
Baylor College of Medicine
Houston, Texas

Paul J. Donald, M.D., F.R.C.S.(C).
Department of Otolaryngology
UC Davis Medical Center
Sacramento, California

Danny Jordan Enepekides, M.D.
Assistant Professor
Department of Otolaryngology
UC Davis Medical Center
Sacramento, California

Carlos A. Farinas, M.D.
Department of Radiology
Baylor College of Medicine
Houston, Texas

Jaime Gateno, D.D.S., M.D.
Associate Professor
Department of Oral and Maxillofacial Surgery
University of Texas–Houston Health Science
Center
Houston, Texas

Carla Marie Giannoni, M.D.
Assistant Professor
Bobby R. Alford Department of
Otorhinolaryngology and Communicative
Sciences
Director of Pediatric Otolarygology Fellowship
Education
Department of Pediatrics
Baylor College of Medicine
Houston, Texas

Peter A. Hilger, M.D.
Division of Facial Plastic Surgery

Department of Otolaryngology–Head and
Neck Surgery
University of Minnesota
Minneapolis, Minnesota

Larry Hollier, M.D.
Associate Professor
Division of Plastic Surgery
Chief of Plastic Surgery
Ben Taub General Hospital
Baylor College of Medicine
Houston, Texas

James V. Johnson, D.D.S., M.S.
Clinical Professor
Department of Oral and Maxillofacial Surgery
University of Texas Health Science Center
Houston, Texas

Zahid S. Lalani, D.D.S., Ph.D.
Private Practice
Houston, Texas

Jose M. Marchena, D.M.D., M.D.
Assistant Professor
Department of Oral and Maxillofacial Surgery
University of Texas Health Science Center
Houston, Texas;
Chief of Oral and Maxillofacial Surgery
Ben Taub General Hospital
Houston, Texas

Becky McGraw-Wall, M.D.
Clinical Associate Professor
Department of Otolaryngology
University of Texas–Houston Medical School
Houston, Texas

John C. Oeltjen, M.D., Ph.D.
Division of Plastic Surgery
Baylor College of Medicine
Houston, Texas

John S. Oghalai, M.D.
Assistant Professor
Bobby R. Alford Department of
Otorhinolaryngology and Communicative
Sciences
Baylor College of Medicine
Houston, Texas

Roberta Pileggi, D.D.S.
Department of Endodontics and Peridontics
University of Texas Dental Branch
Houston, Texas

Steven D. Schaefer, M.D.
Professor and Chairman
Department of Otolaryngology
New York Eye and Ear Infirmary
New York, New York

Bradford G. Scott, M.D., F.A.C.S.
Assistant Professor of Surgery
Baylor College of Medicine
Trauma Medical Director
Minimally Invasive Surgery Director
Ben Taub General Hospital
Houston, Texas

Charles N.S. Soparkar, M.D., Ph.D.
Plastic Eye Surgery Associates, PLLC
Houston, Texas

Michael G. Stewart, M.D., M.P.H.
Bobby R. Alford Department of
Otorhinolaryngology and Communicative
Sciences
Baylor College of Medicine
Houston, Texas

Richard A. Vickers, M.D., D.D.S.
Department of Oral and Maxillofacial Surgery
University of Texas Health Center Houston
Houston, Texas

Matthew J. Wall, Jr., M.D.
Professor
Department of Surgery
Baylor College of Medicine
Houston, Texas;
Deputy Chief of Surgery
Chief of Cardiothoracic Surgery
Ben Taub General Hospital
Houston, Texas

Mark Eu-Kien Wong, D.D.S.
Department of Oral and Maxillofacial Surgery
University of Texas Health Science Center
Houston, Texas

Chapter 1

GENERAL MANAGEMENT OF THE TRAUMA PATIENT

Michael G. Stewart

Trauma continues to be a major public health issue, and is a leading cause of death in adolescents and young adults in the United States. In addition to its mortality impact, the care of trauma patients consumes a huge amount of health care resources.

ADVANCED TRAUMA LIFE SUPPORT

There is a well-developed protocol from the American College of Surgeons for the management of the acutely injured patient: the Advanced Trauma Life Support (ATLS) protocol. This protocol is updated regularly as results from new studies become available, and it is taught to physicians who provide initial care for trauma patients. Because of its standardization, dissemination, and regular updating the ATLS course has become a model of continuing medical education. Frequent recertification is required, so all certified physicians remain up to date. The ATLS protocol is divided into four sections: (1) primary survey, (2) resuscitation, (3) secondary survey, and (4) definitive treatment.

PRIMARY SURVEY

The primary survey involves assessment of the ABCs of trauma: *airway*, *breathing*, and *circulation*. If needed, resuscitation is performed at the same time as the primary survey. First the upper airway is assessed for patency. In trauma the airway can be directly injured, as in a laryngeal fracture, or indirectly occluded due to tissue edema, bleeding, secretions, or tissue collapse. Even if patients are making respiratory effort, airway obstruction means they will be unable to breathe, so the first step is assessment of airway patency. If obstructed, then a patent airway needs to be established; this is discussed below.

Next, breathing effort is assessed. If the patient's breathing efforts are inadequate, despite a patent airway, efforts are made to assist the patient with ventilation, and techniques are discussed below. There are several reasons that a patient may have impaired breathing, and these should be assessed as part of the primary survey. The most common is loss of respiratory drive due to head injury. Other common reasons are chest injuries, either to the chest wall or to the intrathoracic structures. Common traumatic injuries resulting in poor ventilation are sucking pneumothorax, tension pneumothorax, and hemothorax. These should be identified quickly and treated to allow adequate ventilation to occur.

Finally, adequacy of circulation is evaluated, using the pulse rate and blood pressure. If circulation cannot be maintained, that is defined as *shock*. Shock can be due to loss of blood volume, loss of vascular resistance, decreased cardiac output, or increased venous capacity. There are four categories of shock—septic shock, cardiogenic shock, neurogenic shock, and hypovolemic shock—and the last three are all possible in patients with trauma; the most common is hypovolemic shock. The treatment of shock (inadequate circulation) is discussed below.

RESUSCITATION

Just as airway assessment is the first step in the primary survey, establishment of a patent airway is the first step in resuscitation. This can be performed by sweeping out a foreign body, or suctioning blood or secretions. Other important injuries that can cause loss of airway are neck trauma, maxillofacial trauma, and laryngeal trauma. Treatment of the airway is divided into airway maintenance, airway establishment, and supplemental ventilation. Simple and effective airway maintenance maneuvers are the chin lift, the anterior jaw thrust, placement of an oropharyngeal airway, and placement of a nasopharyngeal airway. In all trauma patients you must keep in mind the possibility of a cervical spine injury, so when that is a concern, the cervical spine must be kept immobilized during airway maneuvers. A common scenario in the patient with airway obstruction is head injury, loss of consciousness, and soft tissue collapse in or around the upper airway; in that situation, limited airway manipulation may establish airway patency. If the airway can be opened and the patient is breathing, then the airway can be maintained in that state. To maximize tissue perfusion, the ATLS protocol calls for supplemental oxygen in all trauma patients. If simple manipulations do not reestablish the airway, then a more invasive intervention—airway establishment—may be needed.

If the airway cannot be opened using external maneuvers, but the patient is making some respiratory effort, bag-mask ventilation can be attempted to assist ventilation, and, if successful, maintained for a period of time. However, definitive airway establishment requires placement of a tube in the trachea with the cuff inflated. There is no recommended preference for orotracheal versus nasotracheal intubation, all else being equal. However, orotracheal intubation can require neck extension, and is difficult if a cervical spine injury cannot be ruled out. In such patients, simultaneous in-line cervical traction can be maintained by one person while another performs oral intubation. Fiberoptic nasotracheal intubation can be performed in cases of suspected cervical spine injury, but requires some experience and skill by the intubation physician. Blind fiberoptic intubation is another option, but is contraindicated if the patient is not breathing spontaneously. Facial fractures and basilar skull fractures are relative contraindications for nasotracheal intubation. Another option to establish an airway is the laryngeal mask airway, which has gained increasing recent acceptance,[1] although it is still not recommended by the ATLS protocol for the trauma patient.

If the patient's airway cannot be established with some type of intubation, a surgical airway will be required. In a patient who needs an immediate airway, cricothyroidotomy performed rapidly is the preferred procedure; in that situation, there is no time for a "stat tracheotomy" because it is quite likely that bleeding vessels and the thyroid gland will be encountered, which means that the airway cannot be established fast enough. Another option is

needle cricothyroid membrane, in which a needle is placed through the cricothyroidotomy and a plastic catheter is threaded over the needle. Supplemental oxygen can be used, or jet ventilation can be performed through the catheter. An open surgical cricothyroidotomy is performed by making a skin incision to expose the cricothyroid membrane, followed by an incision into that membrane. That opening is widened using a blunt instrument, and a small endotracheal tube or tracheotomy tube is placed. The technique of cricothyroidotomy is depicted in Fig. 1–1.

Placement of the endotracheal tube in the airway can be confirmed by detecting end-tidal CO_2. A gas analyzer can be attached to the ventilation circuit, or a CO_2-detection valve with a color-changing filter can be attached into the circuit to confirm the presence of end-tidal CO_2. Although those filters confirm placement in the airway, they do not assess the optimal position for the endotracheal tube or the adequacy of ventilation. Bilateral breath sounds can also be auscultated over the chest to confirm placement of the tube into the airway, but in the case of pneumothorax or chest injury, breath sounds may not be normal despite the fact that the tube is correctly placed in the airway. Similarly, in patients with cardiac arrest, end-tidal CO_2 may not always be detected. The overall protocol for airway management, in patients with possible cervical spine injury, is shown in Fig. 1–2.

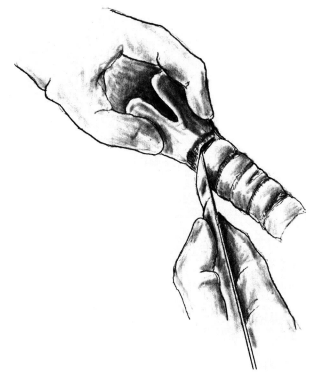

FIGURE 1–1 Technique of cricothyroidotomy.

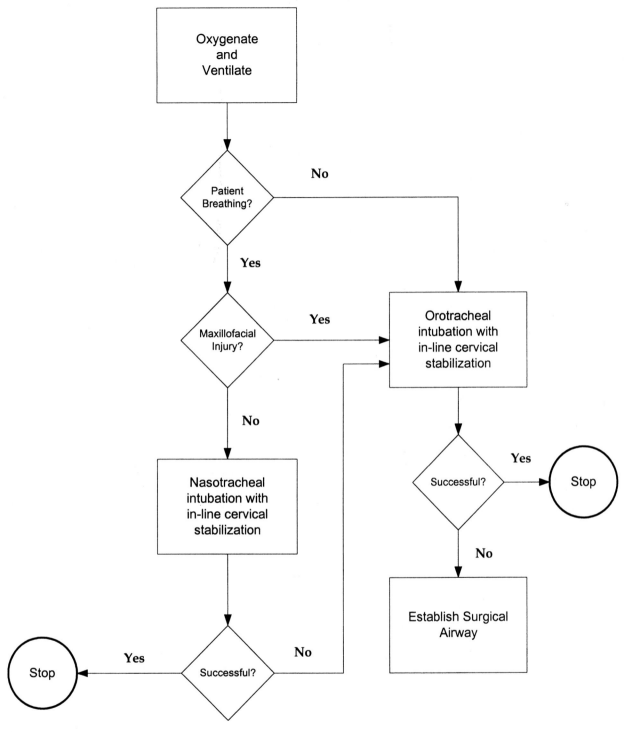

FIGURE I–2 Algorithm for airway management in the trauma patient.

Once the airway has been established, breathing is assisted using hand ventilation or the mechanical ventilator. If the patient has a significant thoracic injury resulting in decreased ventilation—tension pneumothorax, sucking pneumothorax, or hemothorax—that injury should be addressed. Definitive management may require a surgical procedure, but the immediate goal is stabilization. In a sucking pneumothorax, the problem is an open chest wound through which air is passing preferentially rather than through the airway; this injury is stabilized by placement of an occlusive dressing over the chest wall defect along with chest tube placement.

In a tension pneumothorax, air is leaking from the lung into the pleural space in a one-way valve mechanism increasing intrathoracic pressure and preventing lung expansion and ventilation; this injury is stabilized by evacuation and decompression of the pleural space. Unilateral tension pneumothorax is suspected when there are decreased or absent breath sounds on one side of the chest, hypoventilation, and tracheal deviation to the opposite side; the diagnosis can be confirmed with placement of a needle into the second intercostal interspace anteriorly in the midclavicular line. A rapid rush of air confirms the diagnosis, and the needle also temporarily decompresses the pleural space and allows ventilation; definitive treatment is obtained by placement of a chest tube. Tension pneumothorax can also impair circulation by shifting the mediastinum into the opposite chest cavity, with kinking and compression of veins and increased intrathoracic pressure leading to decreased venous return. Bilateral tension pneumothorax can cause decreased breath sounds, hypoventilation, and hypotension without tracheal deviation. Untreated, tension pneumothorax can be rapidly fatal, and if clinically suspected it should be addressed with rapid needle thoracostomy; there is often not enough time for chest x-ray evaluation.

Hemothorax should be treated initially by drainage of blood from the pleural space to allow lung expansion and ventilation. This is accomplished by placement of a large-bore chest tube through the fourth or fifth intercostal space laterally in the midaxillary line. Most patients with hemothorax eventually require operative thoracotomy for definitive hemorrhage control, but evacuation of a large volume of blood from the pleural space allows continued ventilation during the initial resuscitation.

Restoration of adequate circulation requires assessment of the underlying mechanism of shock. As mentioned previously, most trauma patients have hypovolemic shock from hemorrhage and loss of intravascular volume. The degree of hemorrhage and hypovolemic shock can be subclassified (e.g., class I hemorrhage means 15% of blood volume lost); however, at the time of injury the fundamental treatment principle is rapid replacement of intravascular volume until there is physiologic evidence of adequate intravascular volume. Crystalloid solutions, such as normal saline or Ringer's lactate, are preferred. Blood volume is ~7% of body weight, so a 160-pound person has about five L liters of blood volume (weighing ~11 pounds). Volume should be replaced at 3 mL of crystalloid for every 1 mL of blood lost, and it should be replaced rapidly until heart rate and blood pressure return to near-normal levels. If blood loss was massive, then blood—in the form of packed red blood cells—needs to be replaced along with crystalloid. If possible, cross-matched blood should be used, but in trauma patients that information is seldom available, so type O-negative (universal donor) blood should be used. If blood loss was significant, then coagulation factors were also lost, and with rapid volume replacement the remaining circulating clotting factors can become diluted and ineffective. So, in patients requiring significant crystalloid and blood replacement, replacement of fresh frozen plasma and platelets should be considered.

Cardiogenic shock in the trauma patient is usually caused by tension pneumothorax, cardiac tamponade, or myocardial contusion. Common features are distended jugular veins or adequate central venous pressure in the presence of hypotension. However, in patients with both hypovolemic and cardiogenic shock, the cardiogenic component may not become apparent until adequate intravascular volume has been restored. Cardiac tamponade can be difficult to distinguish from tension pneumothorax, but if tension pneumothorax is ruled out, then a diagnostic (and possibly therapeutic) pericardiocentesis can be performed. In some cases of tamponade, emergency thoracotomy with direct cardiac massage is necessary during resuscitation. A hemodynamically significant myocardial contusion is unusual, but when seen it is accompanied by significant chest wall trauma. Some sort of cardiac outflow assistance may become necessary to maintain vascular perfusion.

Neurogenic shock should be considered a diagnosis of last resort even in patients with obvious head trauma, because many patients with head trauma also have hypovolemic shock. Nevertheless, in patients with adequate volume and cardiac function and persistent systemic hypotension, decreased peripheral vascular resistance caused by central nervous system (CNS) injury should be considered. Classic signs are warm extremities and lack of tachycardia despite hypotension. Treatment involves maintenance of adequate volume and vasopressors, with reversal of the CNS injury if possible.

SECONDARY SURVEY

Continuing along the same mnemonic as "ABC" for the primary survey, the complete trauma evaluation has been dubbed "ABCDE," where D stands for *disability* as in neurologic evaluation, and E stands for *exposure* and *examination*. Both D and E are part of the secondary survey, which is performed after the critical lifesaving aspects of the primary survey and resuscitation are completed.

The secondary survey consists of a detailed head-to-toe physical examination. It is important to expose and examine the entire body for other injuries or sequelae, otherwise significant injuries, such as a gunshot wound to the back or buttock, or extremity fracture, can be easily overlooked. The secondary survey includes laboratory evaluation and radiographic evaluation, including assessment of the cervical spine. Laboratory evaluation should include toxicology when appropriate, and blood typing for cross-matching can also be performed.

The extent of the secondary survey is partially dependent on the mental status of the patient. In the conscious and coherent patient, asking about sites of pain, and palpation during examination can elicit sites of injury. Similarly, in an awake patient with a radiologically intact cervical spine, clinical evaluation for pain on movement can complete the "clinical clearance" of the cervical spine. However, in an unconscious or incoherent patient, the secondary evaluation and cervical spine evaluation require meticulous attention.

Mental status is assessed using the Glasgow Coma Scale, shown in Table 1–1. Lower scores are correlated with poorer neurologic outcome, and a score less than 8 indicates significant head injury. The scale is scored from 3 to 15, or 3 to 11 in the intubated patient. Neurologic evaluation, including deep tendon reflexes, pupil reflexes, and sphincter tone, can also indicate the severity of intracranial injury. Management of the head-injured patient is

TABLE 1–1   THE GLASGOW COMA SCALE: FUNCTION SCORES

Eye

Spontaneous opening 4

Opens to verbal stimuli 3

Opens to painful stimuli 2

None 1

Verbal

Alert and oriented 5

Confused 4

Inappropriate 3

Incomprehensible sounds 2

No response or intubated 1

Motor

Obeys commands 6

Localizes stimuli 5

Withdraws from pain only 4

Flexion response 3

Extension response 2

No movement 1

the subject of entire textbooks, and is not covered here.

In addition to evaluation of the cervical spine, the neck should be examined for signs of trauma, such as a penetrating injury, sucking wound, hematoma, and crepitance. The evaluation and treatment of neck trauma are discussed in Chapters 22 through 25.

Common injuries to the chest and thoracic cavity include pulmonary contusion, rib fracture, pneumothorax, hemothorax, flail chest, aortic injury, and tracheobronchial injury. Intrathoracic injuries in blunt trauma are often due to compression of soft tissue structures between the sternum and vertebral column, or to the acceleration/deceleration force applied to soft tissue structures. Traumatic rupture of the thoracic aorta is a common cause of immediate on-the-scene death in motor vehicle accidents, but patients with a partial aortic tear that is contained by the aortic lining might survive to make it to the emergency room. Careful physical examination of the chest, plain chest x-rays, computed tomography (CT) scans, bronchoscopy, and arteriography can be combined to assess the site and severity of intrathoracic injury.

Structures that can be injured in the abdomen include the gastrointestinal tract; the solid organs such as the liver, spleen, and kidneys; and intraabdominal vessels such as the aorta and vena cava. In addition to physical examination and radiologic assessment, the secondary evaluation of the abdominal often includes diagnostic peritoneal lavage, which involves surgical placement of a small flexible catheter to instill and then withdraw saline from the abdominal cavity. The cell counts in the saline are evaluated, and the presence of a significant amount of blood indicates a high probability of visceral injury that requires surgical repair. The uses of abdominal CT scanning and abdominal ultrasound are increasing in the trauma patient because of their high levels of diagnostic accuracy and their ability to image areas not well evaluated with lavage such as the retroperitoneum.[2,3] Ultrasound and CT scan have been used successfully in the evaluation of both blunt and penetrating trauma. In addition, management philosophy has been moving toward observation of selected solid organ injuries rather than mandatory exploration and repair, as it is recognized that many injuries do well with observation alone and surgery may be needed only if certain complications develop.

Extremity injuries can involve the musculoskeletal system, the neurologic system, and the vascular system. Significant injuries can cause a compartment syndrome, where edema or bleeding causes an increased pressure in a closed fascial space that does not permit adequate vascular perfusion. In addition to physical examination and radiologic evaluation, arteriography and venography can be useful in the secondary evaluation of the extremities.

DEFINITIVE TREATMENT

Once patients have been stabilized and the secondary survey completed, they are taken for definitive treatment, for example, for laparotomy if the patient has a bowel perforation. Traditional management principles held that once patients were stabilized, they should go to the operating room where all injuries would be repaired as rapidly as possible, to minimize continued blood loss, peritoneal contamination, and hypoperfusion. However, at some centers there is a recent trend toward patients undergoing a limited procedure with only certain injuries being addressed, followed by immediate transfer to the intensive care unit (ICU) for further stabilization and resuscitation with several subsequent trips back to the operating room for staged repairs of injuries, rather than putting a critically ill and unstable patient through an extensive initial procedure.[4] An example of the limited nature of initial repair might be placing a clamp or ligature on perforated bowel (rather than formal closure, or resection and reanastomosis), and clamps on bleeding sites, with towel-clip closure of the skin with the clamps still in the abdomen. This type of approach has been called "damage control" surgery, and its principles have been cited as follows[2]: only blood loss kills early; gastrointestinal (GI) injuries cause problems later; everything takes longer than you think; it's easy to miss an injury if you rush; hypothermia, acidosis, and coagulopathy only lead to more of the same; the best place for a sick person is the ICU. Regardless of the management philosophy relative to timing and extent of surgery, the definitive treatment phase includes repair of injuries identified in the primary and secondary surveys.

PEDIATRIC TRAUMA

In the injured child, many of the basic trauma treatment principles are the same, although there are some differences.[5,6] The primary survey and initial resuscitation are very similar, with minor modifications. Concerning airway stabilization, because of the relatively large head in pediatric patients, when lying supine even a seemingly neutral position may result in neck overextension and airway closure. Jaw thrust may open the airway, but in-line stabilization is important until the cervical spine is cleared. An oral airway may be used, but care should be taken in placement because it can actually displace the tongue posteriorly, or if too long it can cause gagging and aspiration. If bag-mask ventilation is used, cricoid pressure should be applied to prevent excessive inflation of the stomach, which is common in children. If a stable airway cannot be otherwise established, orotracheal intubation is preferred, using an uncuffed tube in children less than 8 years old. Establishment of a surgical airway can be more difficult than in the adult, because the neck is shorter, the larynx is lower in the neck, and the cricoid and thyroid cartilages overlap, hiding the cricothyroid membrane from palpation. The preferred technique for a surgical airway in children is needle cricothyroidotomy, where a large intravenous catheter needle is used, and then the needle is removed and the plastic sheath advanced. After ventilation and stabilization, that can be converted to a standard tracheotomy.

Closed head injury is the most common cause of death in the pediatric trauma patient, and hemorrhage is the second most common. In the pediatric patient with volume loss, tachycardia occurs first and hypotension does not occur until ~40% of blood volume is lost, at which point circulatory collapse may be impending. Fluid resuscitation is achieved using crystalloid, with a typical initial bolus of 20 mL/kg of body weight, followed by repeated boluses if necessary. The secondary survey and definitive treatment are then performed.

PREHOSPITAL RESUSCITATION

More than half of the deaths in trauma patients occur within several minutes of the accident, which can be classified as immediate death.[3] Therefore, the on-the-scene management and prehospital (in the ambulance) care of the trauma patient have significant implications for eventual survival. There have been significant advances and changes in the prehospital management of trauma patients in the past few decades.

A classic debate was between "scoop and run" versus "scene stabilization." It could be argued that the only definitive treatment is at the hospital, so no delays in transport are needed and the emphasis should be on rapid delivery; on the other hand, transport of unstable patients may exacerbate their physiologic instability, and if patients can be stabilized with simple measures, then that might be beneficial.[7] A variation of this theme can also occur in the emergency center, where the debate is between a prolonged stay with continued attempted resuscitation versus immediate transfer to the operating room or angiography suite, or wherever else definitive care can be rendered.

Some recent evidence indicates that on the prehospital side, controlled hypotension or no resuscitation may be beneficial.[2,7] This makes intuitive sense: if there is a vascular or visceral injury causing hemorrhage and hypotension, then attempts to restore blood pressure and pulse using crystalloid hydration will dilute the available blood and clotting factors, increase bleeding (because of the increasing blood pressure), and exacerbate the cycle of bleeding, the loss of clotting factors, and dilution. On the other hand, a low-blood-flow state decreases further bleeding, preserves the remaining blood, and allows some clotting (platelet plugging) to occur at bleeding sites. In the no-fluid-resuscitation scenario, intravenous lines are placed but fluids are not instilled until the patient is at the hospital or in the operating room, where the bleeding can be explored and controlled. Some have argued that neither full-fluids nor no-fluids are ideal, but that controlled hypotension (systolic blood pressure around 70 or 80 mm Hg) is the ideal prehospital strategy.[2]

Other evidence indicates that in patients with extremity injuries, more aggressive hydration and resuscitation might be indicated. In addition, there is a positive survival impact from on-the-scene intubation and ventilation for patients with respiratory arrest. So, some have argued that although minimizing the on-scene time is important, the philosophy should not be scoop-and-run, but rather scoop-and-treat.[7] In summary, the optimal prehospital care for the injured patient is still a work in progress, but significant strides have made, improving overall survival.

TRAUMA CRITICAL CARE

Once trauma patients have been stabilized using the ATLS protocol and they are on their way to definitive management of their injuries, the critical care management of the patients becomes important. Although early death, within a few hours of injury, is often due to hemorrhage, respiratory failure, or cerebral edema, late death after trauma usually represents gradual physiologic failure, particularly multisystem organ failure. There are three major interruptions that can cause significant physiologic deterioration in injured patients: hypothermia, coagulopathy, and acidosis.[4] These have been called the lethal triad or the triad of death.[6] These three conditions exacerbate each other, making eventual survival less likely. For example, hypothermia significantly worsens coagulation enzyme function and

platelet function, and intact coagulation can be critical in a patient with multiple sites of hemorrhage. In addition, rewarming a hypothermic trauma patient can be difficult, because it is the body core temperature that is important; blankets and convective air rewarming systems only warm the skin, and the temperature transfer through body tissue is very slow. Warmed intravenous fluids are very helpful, as is warmed endotracheal air. There are several other methods and new technologies that show promise, such as pleural or peritoneal lavage, cardiopulmonary bypass, and extracorporeal arteriovenous rewarming.[4]

Acidosis is caused by hypoperfusion and secondary cellular damage, direct tissue injury (i.e., crush or blunt trauma) with lactic acid release, and increased oxygen metabolism after reperfusion. Although acidosis itself can be harmful, it is also an indicator of tissue injury and tissue hypoxia.[6] In the management of trauma patients, acidosis should be treated aggressively, primarily by maximizing volume status and perfusion. Studies have shown that prolonged acidosis results in a higher rate of organ failure and poorer survival, compared with patients in whom the acidosis is corrected early.

SUMMARY

Trauma is best considered a multisystem disease. Despite severe injuries and dramatic presentations, a careful and methodical yet urgent approach to evaluation and management can optimize outcomes. Physicians experienced in management of the upper airway can play an important role in the care of trauma patients.

PEARLS: MANAGEMENT PRINCIPLES FOR THE TRAUMA PATIENT

- The ATLS protocol is a contemporary, systematic, widely taught technique of evaluation and treatment of the injured patient.
- The first step in the ATLS protocol is the primary survey of airway, breathing, and circulation.
- The second step is resuscitation, which can occur simultaneously with the primary survey; the airway is established, through passive, active, or surgical techniques, the patient is ventilated if necessary, and blood pressure and pulse are restored through fluid resuscitation and/or correction of other injuries.
- After resuscitation, a secondary survey for other injuries is performed, and finally definitive treatment of injuries is completed.

- In pediatric trauma, the general principles are the same, but positioning the neck and establishing the airway can be different.
- Advances in prehospital management have involved less aggressive fluid and resuscitation and more rapid transfers.

REFERENCES

1. Ball DR, Jefferson P. Intubating laryngeal mask use in neck injury patients. Anaesthesia 2002;57:407–409
2. Scalea T. What's new in trauma in the past 10 years. Int Anesthesiol Clin 2002;40:1–17
3. Koltai PJ, Kispert PH. Principles of trauma. In: Bailey BJ, ed. *Head and Neck Surgery—Otolaryngology,* 3rd ed. Philadelphia: Lippincott-Raven, 2001:717–730
4. Gentilello LM, Pierson DJ. Trauma critical care. Am J Respir Crit Care Med 2001;163:604–607
5. Stallion A. Initial assessment and management of pediatric trauma patient. Respir Care Clin North Am 2001;7:1–11
6. Wetzel RC, Burns RC. Multiple trauma in children: Critical Care Overview. Crit Care Med 2002;30(11 suppl):S468–S477
7. Fowler R, Pepe PE. Prehospital care of the patient with major trauma. Emerg Med Clin North Am 2002; 20:953–974

DIAGNOSTIC IMAGING IN HEAD AND NECK TRAUMA

Carlos A. Farinas, Orlando Diaz-Daza, and Pedro J. Diaz-Marchan

Diagnostic imaging has become indispensable in the evaluation of a patient with head and neck trauma (HNT). Radiologists are frequently able to make precise and significant contributions to patient management and may guide clinicians concerning the choice and sequence of examinations. These factors allow for the making of rapid decisions that may be critical to patient outcome. This chapter reviews the different imaging modalities used in the assessment of the acutely injured patient with HNT.

CONVENTIONAL PLAIN FILM RADIOGRAPHY

Plain film radiography was for a long time the diagnostic modality of choice for head and neck trauma. Today it has been largely replaced by the computed tomography (CT) scan, as the latter provides more accurate information regarding the bony architecture and its disruption than do plain films. Plain film radiography is still the first modality used for the evaluation of HNT in many institutions due to its greater availability. It allows for a general assessment of the face in a short period of time, with lesser cost and reduced radiation exposure to the patient, and, depending on the clinical situation, can be performed with portable equipment.

Plain film radiography has several disadvantages. It has a limited capacity to reveal soft tissue injury, does not permit the localization of injuries, and is constrained by the presence of tissue hemorrhage or edema and overlying complex bony structures. In addition, the patient's condition (spinal or skull injury) may limit placement of the head in the position needed for adequate facial views.

The standard facial series, which include Towne, Caldwell (occipitofrontal), Waters (occipitomental), and lateral views, is useful as the initial screening examination of patients to provide a global overview of the midfacial skeletal structures; it also helps when comparison views are obtained in patient follow-up.

In the *Towne view* the x-ray beam is tilted 30 degrees downward so that the dorsum sella is projected into the foramen magnum (Fig. **2–1A**). It is useful for the evaluation of the ascending rami of the mandible, the posterior fossa of the skull, and the zygomatic arches.

The *Caldwell view (occipitofrontal)* is obtained posteroanteriorly with the x-ray beam angulated 15 degrees caudad to the canthomeatal line. In this view the petrous pyramids are seen projecting through the orbits (Fig. **2–1B**). It is useful for the evaluation of the superior orbital fissure, the orbital floor and the frontal region.[1,2]

The *Waters' view (occipitomental)* uses a posteroanterior (PA) technique with the x-ray beam angulated 37 degrees caudad to the canthomeatal line (Fig. **2–1C**). In this projection the petrous pyramids are projected inferior to the maxillary alveolar ridges, and there should be clear visualization of the entire maxillary sinus. This projection allows optimal evaluation of the midface and great visualization of the orbital floor and rim, the zygoma, and maxillary bone and sinus.[1,2]

The *lateral projection* is conventionally obtained in the left lateral position with the x-ray beam centered at the lateral canthus (Fig. **2–1D**). This view provides useful information regarding the nasopharynx and other parts of the midfacial skeleton, such as the pterygoid processes of the sphenoid bone and the pterygomaxillary fissure.[1,2]

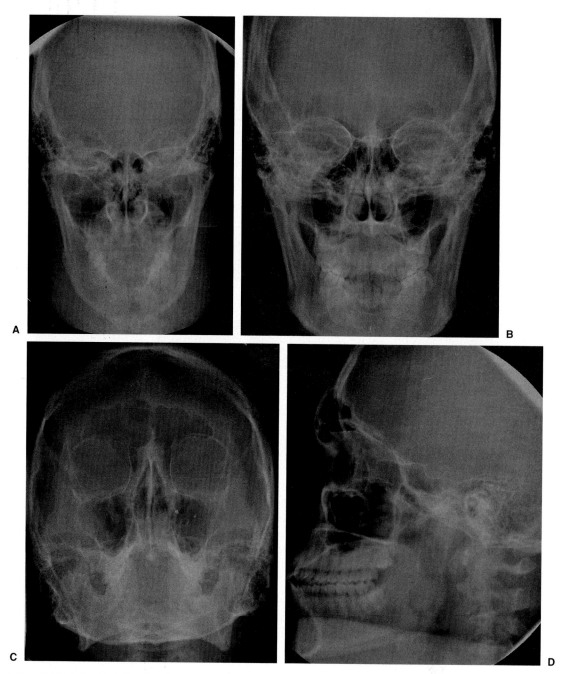

FIGURE 2–1 Facial series: Towne (A), Caldwell (B), Waters (C), and lateral (D).

The *base view (submentovertex)* is useful for the evaluation of the zygomatic arches, the lateral wall of the orbit, and the medial and lateral walls of the maxillary sinus.[1] Proper positioning for this view is difficult to obtain in patients with multiple traumatic lesions, and is contraindicated in patients with cervical spine trauma (Fig. **2–2**).

The *nasal view* has been used for suspected injury of the nasal bones. It consists of an underpenetrated,

cone-down lateral radiograph, which includes the nasal bones and anterior maxillary spine.[1]

With the advent of CT scanning, additional views are almost never necessary.

The *Panorex [panoramic radiograph, orthopantomograms (OPG)]* view is very useful in the evaluation of the mandible, and it is considered the single most helpful radiograph used in the diagnosis of mandibular fractures (Fig. **2–3**).

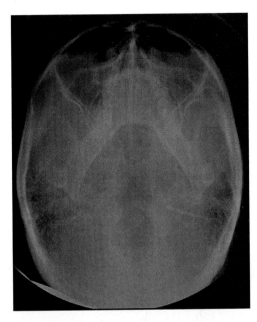

FIGURE 2–2 Submental-vertex view.

COMPUTED TOMOGRAPHY, MAGNETIC RESONANCE IMAGING, COLOR DOPPLER ULTRASOUND, AND ANGIOGRAPHY

The imaging evaluation of patients with head and neck trauma has been transformed since the development of computed tomography (CT) in the 1970s. This revolution was further advanced with the introduction of helical CT in 1989 and multidetector CT in 1998. Helical CT, in general, is now considered the standard imaging modality for facial trauma.[3,4]

HELICAL COMPUTED TOMOGRAPHY

Helical CT was introduced in 1989 after improvements in slip-ring technology and has now become the standard CT imager. Helical or spiral CT allowed data acquisition using a continuously rotating x-ray source and detector array while the patient couch moved through the plane of the rotating beam. This technique resulted in many advantages for the trauma patient. It virtually eliminated data misregistration due to motion artifact because patients could be scanned in a single breath hold. In addition, faster image acquisition allowed the performance of scans of multiple anatomic sites in a short period of time. Reduced scanning time meant that intravenous (IV) contrast could be followed more quickly, resulting in enhanced opacification of vascular and parenchymal structures.[5] Helical CT also allowed greater flexibility in image reconstruction due to the use of interpolation algorithms, which improved reformatted sagittal and coronal views as well as overall resolution.

MULTISLICE COMPUTED TOMOGRAPHY

Introduced in 1998, *multislice CT* is a commonly used term that describes the latest developments in spiral CT concepts, based on the simultaneous acquisition of more than a single slice and the use of multirow detector systems. Multislice CT, therefore, can be seen as the continuation of the exciting innovation that was introduced by spiral/helical CT in the 1990s. This modality has completed the paradigm shift from a slice-based to a volume-based technique. The data acquisition system in a single slice helical scanner allows the registration of one channel of image information of the scanned body part per gantry rotation. In multislice CT scanners multiple rows of detectors have replaced the single detector in the original helical CTs.[6] The currently used 16-detector scanners collect 16 simultaneous channels of information per gantry rotation, so the scan time has been reduced to one-sixteenth of the original single detector scanner. This marked reduction in

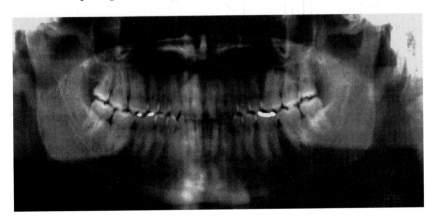

FIGURE 2–3 Normal Panorex view.

time allows the scanning of a larger anatomic volume with a single breath hold and the use of smaller doses of intravenous contrast. Multislice CT also makes it possible to acquire very thin slices, which result in higher resolution and the capability of doing coronal, sagittal, or three-dimensional (3D) reconstructions to evaluate complex facial fractures or complex structures such as the temporal bone.[7] This capability has been the primary reason for the dramatic rise in clinical indications for CT angiography.

In summary, CT can show osseous anatomy to greater advantage than a craniofacial series and has the added benefit of showing the soft tissues of the head and neck in great detail, including the optic globes, nerves, and extraocular muscles. At our institution we perform facial CTs and review the images using soft tissue and bone window settings. Three-dimensional reformations are completed at the workstation and can be seen in different projections according to the type of trauma under evaluation, whether osseous or soft tissue (Fig. **2–4**).

COMPUTED TOMOGRAPHY ANGIOGRAPHY

Head and neck trauma may involve lesions in the great vessels, which may be a cause of high morbidity or mortality. Traumatic vascular lesions include subintimal dissection, active extravasation, pseudoaneurysm, occlusion, and fistulas, and may affect the vertebral arteries as well as the common, external, or internal (intra- or extracranial) carotid arteries. Although catheter-based angiography remains the imaging procedure of choice, recent technologic breakthroughs in multidetector CT scanners have made possible the rapid rise of CT angiography (CTA) as an important screening modality in these clinical situations.

Computed tomography angiography offers several advantages over other imaging modalities, such as conventional or magnetic resonance angiography. It has greater 24-hour availability in many institutions and is a faster procedure, features that are particularly important in the setting of trauma where a rapid diagnosis is critical. In addition, it adds the cross-sectional data available in the axial CT to the luminal information, which permits visualization of vessel walls and anatomic relationships with surrounding structures.[8] It is also a noninvasive study with lower cost than conventional angiography. Finally, the reconstructed 3D images are easier for clinicians to understand, which has contributed greatly to the universal acceptance of this technique.

The value and efficacy of helical CT angiography in the initial evaluation of patients with penetrating neck injuries has been recently documented.[9] The main drawback is that the use of a short bolus of intravenous contrast coupled with a short scanning time has to be accurately timed, or it may result in either poor opacification of the arterial system if the scan is performed too early, or drop-off in luminal enhancement on later images. Both circumstances may interfere with an accurate rendering of 3D images and possibly result in nondiagnostic tests.[8]

Several 3D reformatting techniques are currently used in our hospital to better define vascular structures and surrounding anatomy, including multiplanar reformation (MPR), maximum intensity projection (MIP), and volume rendering (VR) (Fig. **2–5**).

MAGNETIC RESONANCE IMAGING

Magnetic resonance imaging plays a lesser role in HNT. Its main function is detecting cerebral lesions associated with head and neck traumatic injuries and diagnosing traumatic encephaloceles.

MAGNETIC RESONANCE ANGIOGRAPHY

This imaging technique is not used frequently in the setting of trauma due to its sensitivity to movement, which creates pitfalls or artifacts, and the length of time needed to perform the study. It is more expensive than CT angiography, which raises concerns in the current era of cost management. Finally, ~5% of patients are unable to undergo examinations due to claustrophobia in the closed magnetic resonance (MR) units.

In magnetic resonance angiography (MRA), there are three principal techniques:

Two-dimensional (2D) and 3D time-of-flight (TOF) sequences (Fig. **2–6A**) have remained the principal imaging methods used in the evaluation of intra- and extracranial circulation. Two-dimensional TOF has shown greater sensitivity to slower flow, whereas 3D TOF demonstrates an ample range of flow velocities and superior accuracy in outlining the morphology of the internal and external lumina.[10,11]

Contrast-enhanced MRA (Fig. **2–6B**) has been the focus of recent interest and current development. This technique has the advantage of a short acquisition time and provides better assessment of stenoses than nonenhanced MRA.

Phase-contrast MRA is so named because of the contrast obtained between the magnetic properties of moving blood and the stationary vessel

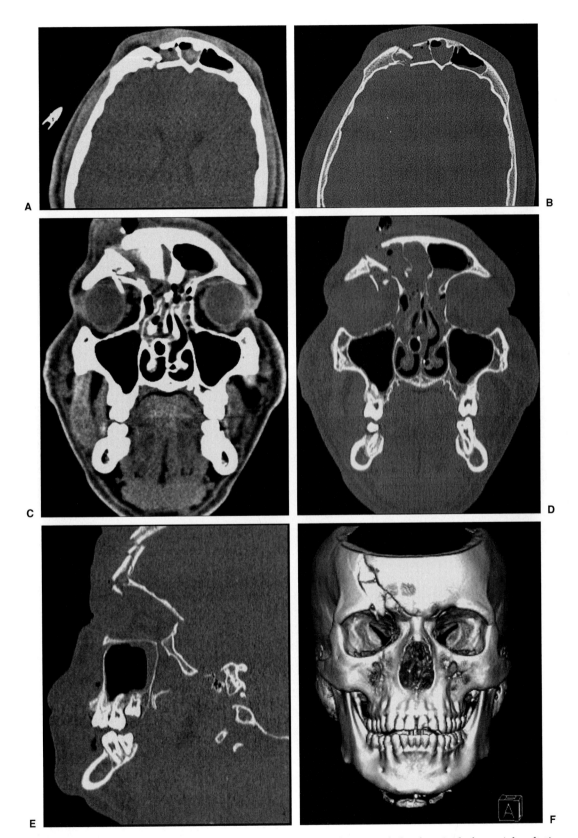

FIGURE 2–4 Routine computed tomography (CT) evaluation of the face includes axial soft tissue (A) and bone window (B) images. These are used to obtain coronal views (C,D), sagittal view (E), as well as 3D reconstructions (F). These images demonstrate a focally depressed comminuted right frontal fracture with bone fragments displaced inferiorly into the orbit.

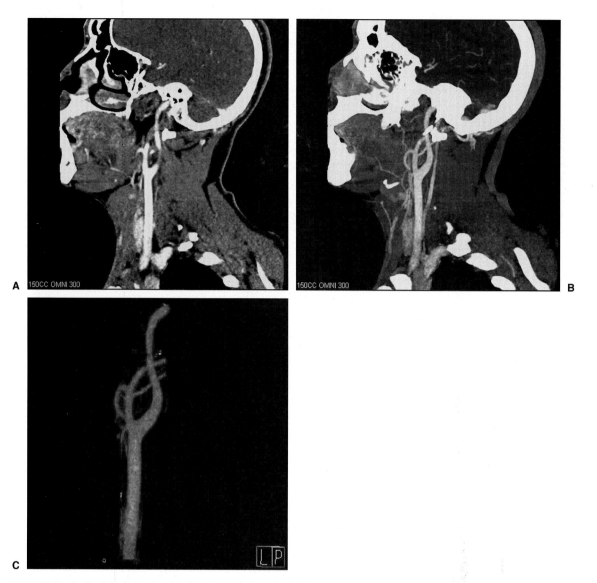

FIGURE 2–5 Noninvasive evaluation of the carotid arteries is possible on computed tomography angiography (CTA) using multiplanar reformation (MPR) (A), maximum intensity projection (MIP) (B), or volume rendering (VR) techniques (C).

wall. It has the advantage of providing information about velocity and direction of flow.

COLOR DOPPLER ULTRASOUND

Color Doppler ultrasound (US) has been utilized as a noninvasive test for the diagnosis of traumatic vascular injuries.[12,13] This technique is able to provide sufficient information about vascular wall, flow, lumen, and possible thrombi in patients with carotid artery dissection.[14] Its main drawback is that it is operator dependent and may be a lengthy procedure, even with experienced personnel, which limits its value in unstable patients. Another drawback is that the presence of subcutaneous emphy-

sema or large hematomas in the scanned area may diminish the ability to detect injuries.[9]

DIGITAL SUBTRACTION ANGIOGRAPHY

Digital subtraction angiography (DSA) still remains the "gold standard" for assessment of the extra- and intracranial vascular system.[10] It utilizes digital images obtained before and after the injection of contrast and subsequent electronic removal of noncontrast images of osseous structures. This technique allows for a shorter examination time, decreased contrast dose, and improved contrast resolution when compared with conventional angiography. Although it has a low reported incidence of

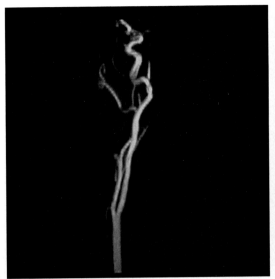
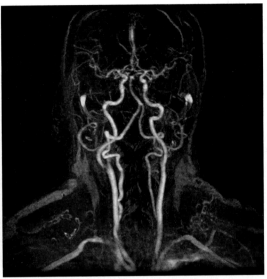

FIGURE 2–6 Magnetic resonance angiography (MRA) images. A: Image was generated using time-of-flight (TOF) methodology and shows a lateral view of the cervical carotid bifurcation. B: Image was generated using MRA with contrast, and shows the cervical region from the thoracic inlet to the circle of Willis.

complications of 0.16% to 2.0%,[15] it still is an invasive procedure with the inherent risks of vessel wall injury, bleeding, and thrombosis, among others. These complications may be disastrous and lead to permanent damage when the central nervous system is involved. Finally, angiography is only able to provide information about the vessel lumen. Whereas angiography was performed in the past on all cases for diagnostic purposes, the recent developments in vascular imaging with CT and MR have pushed these noninvasive modalities to the forefront, especially for screening purposes. DSA is still used when noninvasive imaging fails to provide diagnostic information or when endovascular treatment is needed or planned.

Pearls: Diagnostic Imaging

- Plain x-rays were traditionally used in the evaluation of facial trauma, and still play a role in screening and evaluation of some injuries.
- CT scanning has become the gold standard for evaluation of head and neck trauma, as it allows imaging of bone and soft tissue. Recent advances in CT technology, such as the helical scan, have improved the speed and efficacy of imaging in multiple planes.
- CT angiography, magnetic resonance angiography, and color Doppler ultrasound are all useful techniques for evaluation of vascular injury. The gold standard for vascular evaluation, however, is digital subtraction angiography.

References

1. Pathria M, Blaser S. Diagnostic imaging of craniofacial fractures. Radiol Clin North Am 1989;27:839–853

2. Harris JH, Castillo M, Smith M. Face, including intraorbital soft tissues and mandible. In: Harris JH, Harris WH, eds. *The Radiology of Emergency Medicine,* 4th ed. Philadelphia: Lippincott Williams & Wilkins, 2000:49–135

3. Thai KN, Hummel RP III, Kitzmiller WJ, Luchette FA. The role of computed tomography scanning in the management of facial trauma. J Trauma 1997;43:214–217

4. Turestchek K, Wunderbaldinger P, Zontisch T. Trauma of facial skeleton and calvaria Radiologe 1998;38:659–666

5. Novelline R, Rhea J, Rao P, Stuk J. Helical CT in emergency radiology. Radiology 1999;213:321–339

6. Rydberg J, Liang Y, Teague S. Fundamentals of multichannel CT. Radiol Clin North Am 2003;41:465–474

7. Philipp M, Funovics M, Mann F, et al. Four-channel multidetector CT in facial fractures: do we need 2 × 0.5 mm collimation? AJR Am J Roentgenol 2003;180:1707–1713

8. Chow L, Rubin G. CT angiography of the arterial system. Radiol Clin North Am 2002;40:729–749

9. Múnera F, Soto JA, Palacio DM, et al. Penetrating neck injuries: helical CT angiography for initial evaluation. Radiology 2002;224:366–372

10. Phillips C, Bubash L. CT angiography and MR angiography in the evaluation of extracranial carotid vascular disease. Radiol Clin North Am 2002;40:783–798

11. Patel MR, Kuntz KM, Klufas RA, et al. Preoperative assessment of the carotid bifurcation: can magnetic resonance angiography and duplex ultrasonography replace contrast arteriography? Stroke 1995;26: 1753–1758

12. Montalvo B, Leblang S, Nuñez DB, et al. Color Doppler sonography in penetrating injuries of the neck. AJNR Am J Neuroradiol 1996;17:943–951

13. Corr P, Abdool Carrim AT, Robbs J. Colour-flow ultrasound in the detection of penetrating vascular injuries of the neck. S Afr Med J 1999;89: 644–646

14. Pannone A, Bertoletti GB, Nessi F, et al. Carotid artery dissection: correlation of different diagnosis techniques. Minerva Cardioangiol 2000;48:19–27

15. Douglas P. Emergent radiological evaluation of the gunshot wound. Radiol Clin North Am 1992;30: 307–323

Chapter 3

BIOMECHANICS OF FRACTURE HEALING IN THE CRANIOFACIAL SKELETON

Eric T. Becken, Peter A. Hilger, and Anthony E. Brissett

The craniofacial skeleton serves three distinct yet equally important purposes. First, its hemispherical shape and multilayered bone provides protection for the vital structures of the head and upper neck including the central nervous system, ocular system, and upper aerodigestive tract. Second, the craniofacial skeleton provides a foundation for aesthetic features of the human face. Third, it provides a framework, lever, and fulcrum point for mastication. Given these vital roles, trauma or other disruption of the craniofacial skeleton has important and life-threatening consequences. This chapter assists the head and neck trauma surgeon by describing the mechanical and biochemical concepts that contribute to or condemn the healing of fractures within the craniofacial skeleton.

STRUCTURE AND COMPOSITION

Bone is a highly specialized form of connective tissue. In addition to its protective and structural functions, it also acts as a repository for inorganic ions. At its most simplistic level, bone is composed of an organic matrix that is strengthened by deposits of inorganic calcium salts. The inorganic portion of bone constitutes 65 to 70% of its dry weight, whereas the remainder consists of organic materials. Type I collagen constitutes 90% of the organic matrix, with the remaining 10% being composed of proteoglycans, glycoproteins, and other noncollagenous proteins. Impregnating and surrounding the collagen is a variety of calcium phosphates, the most common being hydroxyapatite. This combination of organic matrix and mineral components interact with cellular elements to form a solid and adaptable structural element in the human body.

Bone contains four different cell types, all of which have distinct functions. Osteoblasts, osteoclasts, and bone lining cells are present on the surface of the bone, whereas osteocytes occupy the interior of the bone (Fig. 3–1). Osteoblasts secrete type I collagen and other noncollagenous proteins. As a result, they are responsible for the production of bone matrix and the regulation of mineralization that occurs during fracture repair. Osteoclasts, a derivative of mononuclear cells, are large multinucleated cells active in areas of bone absorption. Bone lining cells are flat elongated cells that cover all surfaces of bone, including the vascular channels and control the movement of ions between the body and the bone. Osteocytes are the cells within the body of the bone. They are derived from osteoblasts and occupy the lacunae within the bone matrix. Osteocytes are responsible for the maintenance of bone matrix by establishing an equilibrium between synthesis and resorption.

The gross structure of bone can be divided into either cortical or cancellous bone. This division does not reflect the cellular origin or composition, but simply reflects architectural differences. Cortical bone, or compact bone, is found on the outer surface of bone, adjacent to the periosteum. Cancellous bone, located in the medial aspect of the bone, consists of a network of trabeculae. The arrangement, density, and size of the trabeculae vary with the age, site, and loading conditions of the bone. The transition zone between theses two types of bone remains in a state of flux. In one area, osteoblasts may fill the trabeculae of the cancellous bone to form cortical bone, whereas other areas may have osteoclasts creating cavities in cortical bone that are subsequently filled with cancellous bone.

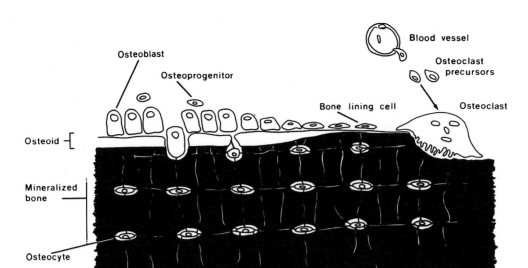

FIGURE 3–1 The origin and location of the cellular elements of bone. (From Marks SC, Popoff SN. Bone cell biology: the regulation of development, structure, and function in the skeleton. Am J Anat 1988;183:1–44, with permission of Wiley-Liss, Inc., a subsidiary of John Wiley & Sons, Inc.)

At the microscopic level, bone is described as either woven or lamellar bone. These terms are derived from the orientation and arrangement of the collagen bundles. Woven bone is composed of bundles of collagen fibers that are woven into neighboring connective tissue. It forms rapidly in humans, 3 to 5 μm per day, and is well suited for bone repair. This rapid rate of growth occurs at the expense of biomechanical strength. To remedy this problem, woven bone often undergoes remodeling to better suit the biomechanical needs of the area under repair. Woven bone is ubiquitous in the embryonic skeleton, whereas in the adults it is only found at the insertion of tendons and ligaments as ossified collagen bundles.

Lamellar bone, which is a major portion of both cortical and cancellous bone in adults, is more highly organized and specialized than woven bone. The formation of lamellar bone proceeds at a rate of only 1 to 2 μm per day. This slower rate of bone formation results from the deposition of bone in a layered fashion onto a preformed solid scaffold and continues in a parallel manner. Any irregularities result in an area of woven bone deposition. The interspersed areas of woven bone are later remodeled to lamellar bone. The orientation and configuration of the collagen bundles within lamellar bone make it appropriate for the mechanical stresses of its corresponding site.

Remodeling of bone is a closely orchestrated process that occurs between osteoblasts and osteoclasts and can be described as a slow renovation of an existing structure while continuing to fulfill its structural and protective duties. This process takes place on both the outer surface as well as the interior aspects of cortical bone. Osteoclasts create channels followed by osteoblasts laying down new bone concentrically on the walls of the channels. This continues until the lumen is narrowed to the diameter of the central capillary. This newly formed structure is named an osteon or haversian system.

The blood supply inside of the bone is from the artery and vein that travel through the haversian systems and are interconnected by vascular channels referred to as Volkmann's canals (Fig. 3–2). Multiple canaliculi connect the haversian system to lacunae where the osteocytes reside. The maximum diameter of an osteon or haversian system is limited by vascular perfusion of 100 and 200 μm in cortical and cancellous bone, respectively. The blood supply to cortical bone is dependent on long low-pressure connections, which are more susceptible to disruption. The vascular supply of cancellous bone is without significant branching and thus has a more robust blood supply, which allows revascularization to proceed more rapidly following an injury. The blood supply of the craniofacial skeleton resembles cancellous bone due to a large surface area to bone volume. The one exception is the mandible, which has a mixture of cancellous and cortical types of blood supply and is subsequently more vulnerable to complications resulting from poor vascular supply.

EMBRYOLOGY AND DEVELOPMENT

The craniofacial skeleton is primarily derived from neural crest cells. The mesenchyme begins in neural crest cells that originate in the neuroectoderm of the forebrain, midbrain, and hindbrain. From these

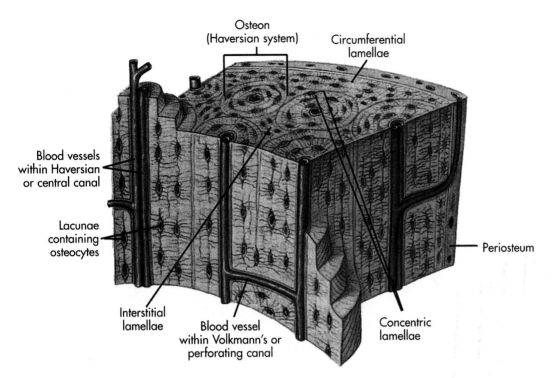

FIGURE 3–2 A schematic of compact bone showing the vascular supply. The primary vessels course through the haversian system with the connecting vessels running within Volkmann's canals. (Reprinted from Thibodeau GA, Patton KT. *Anthony's Textbook of Anatomy and Physiology.* New York: Elsevier: 1996:215, with permission of Elsevier.)

structures, the neural crest cells migrate ventrally into the pharyngeal arches and rostrally around the forebrain and optic cup. By the fourth or fifth week of development the pharyngeal arches are formed and give the characteristic external appearance of the embryo. From this mesenchyme, two distinct mechanisms of bone formation are seen: membranous and endochondral bone formation. The only exception is the skull base and a portion of the occipital region, which arise from paraxial mesoderm.

The majority of the craniofacial skeleton is derived from membranous bone formation, including the frontal, parietal, and nasal bones, as well as the zygoma, maxilla, and mandible. Endochondral bone formation is responsible for the occipital bone, cranial base, and nasal septum.

During membranous bone formation, ossification occurs by direct mineral deposition into the mesenchymal matrix followed by the transformation of mesenchymal cells into osteoblasts.[1] Conversely, endochondral bone formation begins with a cartilaginous template that becomes mineralized and then ultimately replaced by bone. During this process, osteoclasts invade and remove the cartilaginous template and are then replaced by osteoblasts, which then form bone. At maturity, the craniofacial skeleton consists of minimal original bone due to the extensive remodeling processes involved in its formation.

FRACTURE HEALING

A fracture results when the mechanical forces acting on a bone overcome its ability for deformation. Varying patterns of mechanical forces—compression, bending, torque, and avulsion—result in specific patterns such as transverse, oblique, impacted, or comminuted fractures. The loss of structural support, disruption of the soft tissue envelope, and neurovascular structures contribute to complications and increased morbidity. In addition, fracture repair may be compromised due to an interruption of the intracortical blood supply at the fragment ends.

Fracture healing is a biomechanical and biochemical process that results in the restoration of form and function of the original structure. There are three necessities for healing: an adequate supply of functional cells for regeneration, an appropriate blood supply, and a stable environment to minimize interfragmentary movement. An important difference between fracture healing and soft tissue healing is the resulting tissue. As opposed to scar formation in soft tissue repair, bone has the capacity to produce a structure that resembles its appearance prior to the injury. Bone is clinically healed when it resumes function; however, complete biologic healing and remodeling may require much more time.

Although fracture healing should be understood to be a continuum between primary and secondary healing, these two patterns of healing exist at either end of the spectrum (Table 3–1). Within any given fracture, there is a range of conditions that extend from no interfragmentary motion to high interfragmentary motion. In addition, different tissues possess varying tolerances to deformation. Connective tissue tolerates conditions with high deformation, whereas bone tolerates very little deformation. As a result, areas with minimal or no interfragmentary motion can heal primarily, whereas high interfragmentary motion areas heal secondarily. This means that various fractures, or even the same fracture in a different area, will undergo different modes of healing.

PRIMARY BONE HEALING

Perfect alignment of the entire fracture is not possible to achieve. In fact, direct contact between fragment ends is restricted to only small portions of the fracture. The remainder consists of a gap of varying width. If a zone is completely immobilized, whether from the beginning of healing or secondarily from bony bridging at other sites, direct intracortical remodeling across the fracture plane may take place. Fracture healing without the intermediate steps of tissue differentiation is called direct or primary bone healing, and is shown in Fig. 3–3A. In small, immobilized gaps lamellar bone fills and directly bridges the gap (Fig. 3–3B). This is followed by secondary remodeling in the axis of the bone, which gradually leads to the reconstruction of the original structural and functional integrity of the bone. Pure primary healing of a fracture is relatively rare. Further away from the contact areas of the fracture there is a higher chance of interfragmentary motion to various degrees. Additionally, the gap is often wider. Larger immobilized gaps initially result

TABLE 3–1 THE BASIC STEPS IN EITHER PRIMARY OR SECONDARY FRACTURE REPAIR

Primary healing

Direct bone formation

Secondary healing

Hematoma formation

Soft callus

Hard callus

Remodeling

in woven bone formation followed by the creation of lamellar bone secondarily (Fig. 3–3C).

SECONDARY BONE HEALING

When interfragmentary motion exceeds the limits of primary bone healing a process referred to as secondary healing is required to bridge the fracture zone. The formation of cartilage, followed by its transformation to endochondral bone, is the primary mechanism for this type of repair. A cascade of tissue differentiation results in a progressive increase in stability and function. This cascade begins with hematoma formation, followed by soft callus formation and hard callus formation, and concludes with the remodeling phase (Fig. 3–3D).

Immediately ensuing after trauma, the attached muscle and surrounding soft tissue create a hematoma. Activated platelets and osteocytes release inflammatory mediators and cytokines such as platelet-derived growth factor (PDGF), and transforming growth factor-β (TGF-β), which triggers the influx of inflammatory cells into the fracture zone. In addition, osteocytes also release bone morphogenetic proteins, insulin-like growth factors, and fibroblast growth factors. This cytokine cascade recruits the cells of repair such as fibroblasts, endothelial cells, and osteoblasts, into the fracture zone to form the soft callus (Table 3–2).

The soft callus phase, also known as the proliferative phase, begins with angiogenesis. During this phase, the soft callus becomes vascularized by the formation of arterioles and venules. Following neovascularization, cartilage is formed within and adjacent to the callus, creating a relatively avascular zone. Small lacunae begin to form around these cells and as their nuclei hypertrophy they begin to resemble chondrocytes. This continues until the fracture zone is filled with cartilage.

Hard callus formation is the third phase that occurs during the process of secondary bone healing. During this stage, osteoblasts rapidly form woven bone through a cartilaginous intermediary. However, in the subperiosteal region, woven bone is formed directly from mesenchymal tissue. The former represents endochondral bone formation, whereas the latter is referred to as intramembranous formation.

The final phase of fracture repair is remodeling. Remodeling is required to remove mechanically disadvantaged woven bone and replace it with highly ordered and superior lamellar bone. This process of remodeling occurs through the concerted actions of osteoclasts and osteoblasts. Once remodeling is completed, a fracture is biologically healed

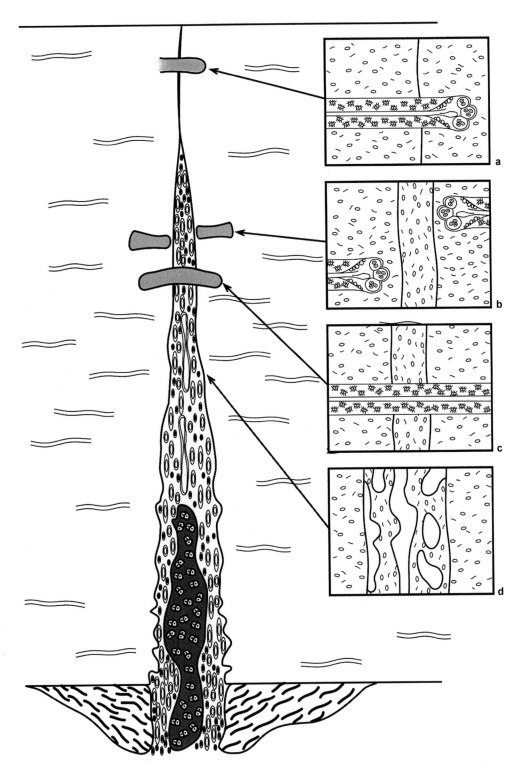

FIGURE 3–3   Patterns of fracture healing. a: Direct intracortical remodeling across the fracture plane. b: Lamellar bone formation. c: Secondary remodeling in the axis of the bone. d: Wide gaps can be healed by the formation of woven bone. (From Friedman CD. Craniofacial bone healing and repair: basic principles. In: Papel ID, ed. *Facial Plastic and Reconstructive Surgery.* New York: Thieme Medical Publishers; 2002:697–705.)

and the process of bone repair is complete. Under normal circumstances, healing is complete within 4 to 6 weeks in the midface and 10 to 12 weeks in the mandible (Fig. 3–4).

TABLE 3–2 IMPORTANT GROWTH FACTORS THAT STIMULATE AND MODULATE HEALING IN FRACTURE REPAIR

Growth Factor	Source	Responding Cells	Unique Properties
Transforming growth factor -β (TGF-β1 most common isoform in bone)	Most cells in the body	Osteoblasts, osteoclasts, neutrophils, monocytes, and fibroblasts	Potent chemoattractant that attracts multiple cell types to sites of repair and inflammation
			Regulation of cell growth
			Stimulates matrix production
			Inhibits osteoclast activity
			Activity mediated through a serine-threonine kinase receptor
Bone morphogenetic proteins (BMP-2 to -9)	Osteocytes, chondrocytes, kidneys, central and peripheral nervous system, the heart and lungs	Osteoprogenitor cells, chrondroblasts	Subdivision of the TGF-β superfamily
			Stimulates conversion of osteoprogenitor cells and undifferentiated mesenchymal cells to osteoblasts
			Activity mediated through a serine-threonine kinase receptor
Fibroblast growth factors (FGF-1 and FGF-2)	Osteocytes, chondrocytes, endothelial cells, adrenal medulla, pituitary	Most cells of mesoderm or neuroectoderm origin	Function as an autocrine and paracrine cellular regulator
			Stimulate and inhibit osteoblast replication and differentiation
			Decrease collagen synthesis
			Stimulates neovascularization and cell migration
Platelet-derived growth factors (PDGF-AA, -BB, and -AB)	Platelets, osteoblasts, monocytes, macrophages, endothelial cells	Most cells of mesoderm origin	Systemic and local regulator of cellular growth
			Stimulates osteoblast replication and DNA synthesis
			Increases collagen degradation and collagenase expression
			Activates a tyrosine-kinase receptor
Insulin-like growth factor-I and –II (IGF-I and -II)	Osteocytes, osteoblasts, and many other cell types	Osteoblasts and osteoclasts	Autocrine/paracrine regulator of bone formation
			Present during all stages of matrix formation and remodeling, with IGF-II predominating

COMPLICATIONS IN FRACTURE HEALING

Complications in fracture healing include delayed union or nonunion, infection, implant failure, and refracture. Some are related to surgical intervention and fixation, whereas others are related to the inherent qualities of fracture healing.

The stability and functional ability of a fracture line is in a constant state of flux. As healing occurs, bone gradually takes the strain and stress off of an

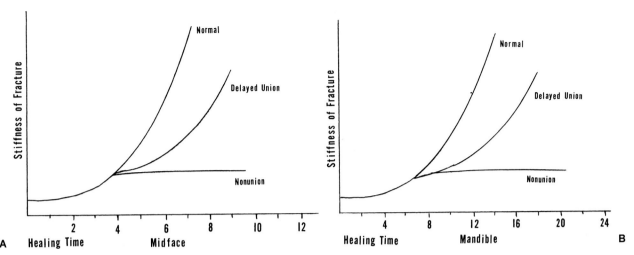

FIGURE 3–4 The time course for fracture healing in the midface (A) and mandible (B). Initially, a fracture has low stiffness and strength. As healing progresses, the functional and structural properties move toward normal bone. If loading of the fracture does not exceed the requirements for mineralization, healing proceeds normally and occurs at approximately 4 to 6 weeks in the midface and 10 to 12 weeks in the mandible. Excessive loading may disturb mineralization and lead to a delayed union or nonunion if healing mechanisms fail. (Reprinted with permission from Prein J, Rahn BA. Scientific and technical background. In: Prein J, ed. *Manual of Internal Fixation of the Cranio-Facial Skeleton.* Berlin: Springer-Verlag; 1998:1–49.)

implant and allows for greater stresses. If healing does not occur, continued stress and strain on an implant ultimately result in failure of the implant. Remodeling and full load bearing in the mandible can take up to 6 months, although other non–load-bearing areas of the craniofacial skeleton require significantly less time. However, with the advent of rigid internal fixation, limited use and load bearing can begin immediately following fracture fixation.

A functional bony union that does not occur within the normally anticipated time frames is referred to as a delayed union. A nonunion or fibrous union is the absence of healing, and requires intervention. An important concept is that the fibrous tissue in a nonunion represents the earliest stages of tissue differentiation in fracture healing. However, excessive interfragmentary movements prevent mineralization.

Infection has been reported to occur in ∼3.2 to 12.7% of all mandible fractures treated with open reduction and internal fixation (ORIF).[2] Extensive trauma or soft tissue loss predisposes an injury to infection due to the absence of protective covering and blood supply. Often these infections begin in the soft tissue and secondarily extend to the bone.

Implant failure or screw loosening is a potential source of complications. This can be caused by the inappropriate choice of plates or screws or mechanical failure. There are many technical issues involving the choice, placement, and fixation of implants that may impact on fracture healing in the craniofa-

cial skeleton, but they are outside the scope of this chapter.

FRACTURE FIXATION

The treatment of midface and mandibular fractures has progressed from closed treatment, using a Barton's dressing, to mandibular-maxillary fixation (MMF), to open reduction with wire fixation. Now the standard of care is ORIF using titanium plates and screws. Although some nondisplaced, closed fractures may continue to be treated conservatively with MMF or even diet modifications, there are multiple indications for operative intervention. This list includes multiple fractures, comminuted fractures, pan-facial fractures, fractures with bony defects, a fracture of an atrophic mandible, infected fractures, and bony nonunion.

The main goal of ORIF is the immediate return of form and function with the minimization of late-onset complications. This is accomplished by reducing and stabilizing the fracture in a position that is conducive to either primary or secondary bone healing. Rigid internal fixation provides the optimal environment for appropriate bony union. Many manufacturers produce titanium plates and screws of differing strengths and dimensions depending on the specific fracture and fracture site. Choices include small miniplates for treatment of midface fractures, to large locking plates for the treatment of mandible fractures that are either comminuted or have significant bony defects. Additional options include compression plates for mandibular fractures. These are specially designed to increase the friction at the contact zone and decrease interfragmentary movement, thereby enhancing healing and maintaining function. Additional plating options include monocortical and bicortical screw fixation. In vitro studies have shown that bicortical screws with a compression plating system provide the most stable repair.[3] Other in vitro studies demonstrate that both bicortical compression and monocortical plating systems meet or exceed currently identified postoperative functional requirements for mandible fractures.[4] In fact, many facial plastic and reconstructive surgeons follow the methods outlined by Champy et al,[5] employing monocortical miniplates along the lines of osteosynthesis with excellent functional and structural results.

AUGMENTING FRACTURE REPAIR

In general, fractures of the craniofacial skeleton achieve bony union quickly and without undue complications. However, certain patients do poorly. Malnutrition, poor vascular supply, diabetes mellitus, and other metabolic conditions can condemn the fracture repair. For these patients there are some unique and emerging treatment strategies that may augment healing of the fracture.

One strategy is the use of physical methods. Mechanical loading accelerates fracture healing.[6] This is accomplished by early mobilization and functional use of the mandible following ORIF. Another physical method is ultrasound therapy. A meta-analysis concluded that 20-minute daily sessions of low-intensity, pulsed ultrasound decreased the mean time to heal.[7] These studies primarily evaluated nonsurgically treated fractures of the axial skeleton, and further investigation is needed to demonstrate its utility in the craniofacial skeleton. A third strategy is the use of electromagnetic fields. In vitro experiments have shown that osteoblasts exposed to electromagnetic fields increase their secretion of growth factors, including bone morphogenetic proteins, TGF-β, and insulin-like growth factors. Although the underlying effect of electromagnetic fields on the biochemistry of the cell is not well understood, this technique has been used in skeletal orthopedics on delayed or nonunion fractures for many years.[6]

The use of biologic methods to assist with the healing of large defects or nonunions represents an additional treatment strategy to support and enhance fracture repair. The goal of this approach is to provide the key components that can assist in creating bone. This includes the use of osteoconductive or osteoinductive bone substitutes, and growth factors. Osteoconductive materials support the growth of bone over its surface, whereas osteoinductive materials undergo direct chemical bonding to the surface of the bone without an intervening layer of fibrous tissue. The ideal biomaterial for a bone substitute must be biocompatible without causing hypersensitivity reactions, easily contoured, and porous to allow the ingrowth of blood vessels.

The most common biomaterial used in the craniofacial skeleton are the calcium phosphate–based bone substitutes, including tricalcium phosphates, various forms of hydroxyapatite (HA), and newer agents such as Norian SRS (Norian Corp., Cupertino, CA) and Embarc (Walter Lorenz Surgical, Jacksonville, FL).

Tricalcium phosphate is one of the earliest calcium phosphates to be used as a bone substitute. Various forms of HA have been used clinically. It is biocompatible, resists absorption, and is both osteoconductive and osteoinductive. It is available in ceramic and nonceramic forms as well as dense and porous forms. The most clinically useful form in the head and neck region is the nonceramic HA, which is also known as HA cement (HAC). It is produced as a paste that is readily sculpted in situ. Although it is relatively strong, it is not recommended for use in stress-bearing areas such as the mandible, but is appropriate for the repair of defects in the remainder of the craniofacial skeleton in both the adult and pediatric patient populations. Newer calcium phosphate–based bone substitutes include Norian SRS and Embarc. Both are implanted as a paste, set rapidly, and are remodeled into new bone.

In addition to synthetically created or modified bone substitutes, there are also autogenous bone grafts, demineralized bone, and bone morphogenetic proteins (BMPs) to assist in the process of bone healing and fracture repair. Autogenous bone grafts, especially calvarial bone grafts, are ideal in the craniofacial skeleton. They are often in the operative field and are resistant to resorption. Alternative donor sites for autogenous sites are less favorable, given the need for additional surgical sites and the attendant morbidity and rapid absorption for iliac crest grafts and rib grafts, respectively. Demineralized bone is a time-tested alternative to autogenous bone grafts. Unfortunately, high rates of resorption limit its clinical applications.

Bone morphogenetic proteins are a subgroup of the TGF-β family and play a critical role in cellular growth and differentiation. In addition to bone, they can be found in many tissues including the kidneys, central and peripheral nervous system, the heart, and lungs. There are eight classes of BMPs that are known to function as osteogenic regulators. In general, BMPs are vital to the conversion of osteo-progenitor cells to osteoblasts, and subsequently stimulate bone formation. BMP-3, which is also known as osteogenin, has been shown to have the highest osteoinductive activity. It has been paired with tricalcium phosphate and used in animal models, which had increased new bone growth as compared with controls.[8] Other BMPs, BMP-2, -4, and -7, have also shown promise as osteoinductive growth factors and are thought to act synergistically in the repair of a fracture. Further study is needed to determine the optimal mixture and carrier system for use in the craniofacial skeleton.

PEARLS: BIOMECHANICS OF FRACTURE HEALING

- Basic principles of bone biology and fracture healing are key components of a facial plastic and reconstructive surgeon's knowledge base.
- Bone is a complex and highly ordered form of connective tissue consisting mainly of type I collagen and hydroxyapatite.
- A fracture results when the mechanical forces acting on a bone overcome its ability for deformation.
- There are two distinct mechanisms of bone formation, membranous and endochondral, with membranous comprising the majority of the craniofacial skeleton.
- Primary fracture healing occurs in fragments that are in close contact and immobilized. The secondary bone-healing cascade occurs in areas that are not suitable for primary healing.

- Additional fracture repair strategies can be achieved by both physical and biologic methods including ultrasound, electromagnetic stimulation, bone substitutes, and bone morphogenetic proteins.

REFERENCES

1. Karaplis AC. Embryonic development of bone and the molecular regulation of intramembranous and endochondral bone formation. In: Bilezikian JP, Raisz LG, Rodan GA, eds. *Principles of Bone Biology.* San Diego: Academic Press; 2002:33–58

2. Valentino J, Levy FE, Marentette LJ. Intraoral monocortical miniplating of mandible fractures. Arch Otolaryngol Head Neck Surg 1994;120:605–612

3. Shetty V, McBrearty D, Fourney M, Caputo AA. Fracture line stability as a function of the internal fixation system: an in vitro comparison using a mandibular angle fracture model. J Oral Maxillofac Surg 1995;53:791–801

4. Haug RH, Fattahi TT, Goltz M. A biomechanical evaluation of mandibular angle fracture plating techniques. J Oral Maxillofac Surg 2001;59:1199–1210

5. Champy M, Lodde JP, Schmitt R, Jager JH, Muster D. Mandibular osteosynthesis by miniature screwed plates via a buccal approach. J Maxillofac Surg 1978;6:14–21

6. Hannouche D, Petite H, Sedel L. Current trends in the enhancement of fracture healing. J Bone Joint Surg Br 2001;83:157–164

7. Busse JW, Bhandari M, Kulkarni AV, Tunks E. The effect of low-intensity pulsed ultrasound therapy on time to fracture healing: a meta-analysis. Can Med Assoc J 2002;166:437–441

8. Breitberg AS, Staffenberg DA, Thome EHM, et al. Tricalcium phosphate and osteogenin: a bioactive onlay bone graft substitute. Plast Reconstr Surg 1995;96:699–708

Chapter 4

FRONTAL SINUS TRAUMA

Danny J. Enepekides and Paul J. Donald

Of all the bones constituting the facial skeleton, the frontal is the strongest. Therefore, it is not surprising that the majority of frontal sinus injuries are accompanied by other maxillofacial fractures. Frontal sinus fracture requires considerable force and, as such, is indicative of serious injury. Transmission of energy to the anterior cranial fossa is common, resulting in associated intracranial injuries. These injuries are most often the result of blunt trauma. Despite improved automobile safety standards and the implementation of enforced seatbelt laws, motor vehicle accidents (MVAs) remain the most frequent etiology. Penetrating trauma, usually the result of violent crime, represents an equally important but far less frequent cause.

Successful management of frontal sinus trauma requires a sound understanding of paranasal sinus anatomy and pathophysiology. The inappropriate management of these injuries rarely leads to acute sequelae. Rather it often leads to mucocele formation and serious infectious complications years later. Therefore, it behooves the trauma surgeon to carefully evaluate, accurately classify, and meticulously treat these injuries.

ANATOMY

When present, the frontal sinus occupies the central brow. The sinus begins to develop in the fourth month of gestation and continues to grow into adolescence. Its growth is usually complete by the age of 18 years in men and 14 years in women.[1] Complete absence of the sinus has been found in approximately 15% of Caucasians. Curiously, it is absent in ~35% of individuals of other ethnicity.[2] Unilateral aplasia of the sinus is very rare, seen in only 3 to 4% of the population.[3]

Embryologically, the frontal sinus develops either as an expansion of frontoethmoidal air cells into the dense frontal bone or by superior extension of the frontal recess.[4] The frontal recess represents the most anterosuperior portion of the infundibulum of the middle meatus. There is significant variability in the size of the frontal sinus. When present, the average sinus measures 28 mm in height, 27 mm in width, and 17 mm in depth.[2] This variability in size may influence the likelihood of fracture. Although the arched configuration of the sinus's anterior wall efficiently distributes forces of impact across the brow, fracture is more likely in the presence of a well-aerated sinus as compared with a contracted or atretic one.

The frontal sinus, illustrated in Fig. 4–1, can be conceptualized as a pyramid. Its anterior wall is thickest. The arched configuration of the frontal bone gives the anterior wall considerable strength. The posterior table or wall is the thinnest. Medially, its intracranial relationships include the sagittal sinus superiorly and the frontal crest and emissary vein to the sagittal sinus inferiorly. Laterally, the posterior wall extends to varying degrees over frontal dura. The transosseous veins of Breschet traverse the posterior wall and drain directly to the subdural space. These veins serve as a direct path of spread for infection from the sinus interior to the subdural space. The floor of the sinus forms a variable amount of the medial orbital roofs. Laterally, the anteroposterior dimensions of the sinus may extend all the way back to the lesser wing of the sphenoid. In the midline the floor of the sinus forms the anterosuperior portion of the nasal roof anterior to the cribriform plate and crista galli.

The frontal sinus is typically divided into two unequal halves by an intersinus septum. Supernumerary septa may be present but are usually

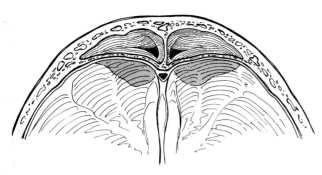

FIGURE 4–1 Axial anatomy of the frontal sinus. (From Donald PJ, Gluckman JL, Rice DH. *The Sinuses.* New York: Raven Press, 1995:44, with permission.)

incomplete. Paired nasofrontal ducts drain the sinus interior. In 25% of cases the sinus drains through true ostia into the anterosuperior portion of the middle meatus. However, the majority drain into the anterosuperior portion of the infundibulum through convoluted frontoethmoid air cells that form the frontal recess.[3]

The internal carotid arterial system supplies the frontal sinus via the supraorbital branch of the ophthalmic artery. The anterior ethmoid artery may also make a minor contribution. The sinus is drained via the angular, anterior facial, and superior ophthalmic veins. In addition the veins of Breschet drain the sinus interior. Mosher and Judd[5] first described these transosseous venous channels in 1933. These channels penetrate the thin posterior wall of the sinus, typically accompanied by imbrications of sinus mucosa, and terminate in the subarachnoid space.

The first division of the trigeminal nerve via the supraorbital and supratrochlear nerves supplies sensory innervation to the forehead. The supraorbital nerve passes through the supraorbital notch or foramen and supplies sensation to the majority of scalp. The supratrochlear nerve exits the orbit between the trochlea and the supraorbital notch, passing medial to the supraorbital neurovascular bundle. It supplies the midline skin of the lower forehead.

MUCOSAL RESPONSE TO TRAUMA

The successful management of frontal sinus trauma must address the extent of both bony and mucosal injury. This is due to the frontal sinus mucosa's unique response to trauma. The frontal mucosa tends to from cysts in response to trauma. Although the majority of mucoceles form in the setting of nasofrontal duct obstruction, mucosal injury in and of itself may lead to cyst formation. This was clearly demonstrated by the work of Lotta and Schall,[6] Schenck,[7] and Donald.[8] The resultant inflammatory reaction at the cyst's periphery leads to osteoclast activation and bone resorption. Erosion proceeds in the paths of least resistance into the anterior cranial fossa, medial orbit, or nasal vault. Over time, this results in clinically apparent mucocele and puts the patient at risk of serious infectious complications.

Another important characteristic of frontal mucosa is its tenacity. The variability of the sinus's interior, with its nooks and crannies, may make complete removal of the mucosa difficult. In addition, as shown by Donald,[8] imbricated tongues of mucosa accompany the veins of Breschet.[8] Incomplete removal of this mucosa may lead to mucocele formation and is an important aspect of the sinus obliteration procedure.

PRESENTATION AND EVALUATION

Fracture of the frontal sinus requires between 800 and 1600 pounds of force.[9] This variability is related in part to the degree of sinus pneumatization. The majority of frontal sinus injuries are accompanied by other maxillofacial fractures. This was highlighted in a large series from the University of California at Davis in which 69% of patients with frontal sinus fractures had at least one other maxillofacial injury.[10]

The majority of patients with frontal sinus fractures are victims of polytrauma and may have life-threatening injuries. Many present with associated head injury and altered levels of consciousness. Some may be comatose. Careful and complete evaluation of the brain and cervical spine are essential in all patients, especially the unconscious.

Certain clinical findings should raise suspicion for frontal sinus injury. Swelling of the forehead is omnipresent unless patients are evaluated immediately posttrauma or several days later. Palpable step-offs at the brow or over the sinus proper may be present. Coexisting subgaleal hematoma often obscures this finding. Lacerations over the sinus should also raise concern about an underlying fracture. Often, the anterior table can be directly examined and palpated through the laceration. When compound, the injury is usually obvious. In the most severe case, the through-and-through injury where an open fracture transgresses both the anterior and posterior walls of the sinus, bone, cerebrospinal fluid (CSF), or brain matter may be seen within the wound. CSF rhinorrhea may be seen in cases of posterior wall injury. Epistaxis is more often than not indicative of other associated midface injuries. Patients may also complain of anosmia. This may simply be the result of mucosal edema and nasal obstruction. However, it may also be indicative of anterior skull base injury with fracture of the cribriform plate. In the unconscious polytraumatized patient, frontal sinus fracture may be an incidental radiographic finding during the trauma evaluation.

Whenever possible, careful evaluation of forehead sensation and movement should be performed and documented. Injuries to the front wall of the sinus may involve the supraorbital foramen or notch, resulting in hypesthesias of the forehead. In the presence of a laceration it is useful to note whether the entire forehead is numb or just that above the laceration. The latter suggests injury to the nerves at the level of the laceration, whereas the former implies a more distal injury of the nerve within the foramen or notch. Similarly, paresis or paralysis of the forehead should be documented. Documentation of these findings is important given that these neuropathies may be the result of the initial trauma or the subsequent surgical repair.

Despite clinical impressions, the definitive diagnosis of frontal sinus fracture requires diagnostic imaging. In the past, plain films of the facial skeleton were relied on to demonstrate these injuries. In particular, the Caldwell view could reveal fracture lines and opacification of the sinus. These studies have now become obsolete. The current gold standard for the radiographic evaluation of all craniofacial trauma is high-resolution computed tomography (CT). Both axial and coronal fine-cut, 1- to 2-mm images are necessary for complete evaluation of the frontal sinus. However, true coronal images are not possible when cervical spine precautions are necessary. In such situations, coronal reconstructions may be used. Most fractures of the frontal sinus are easily seen on CT. However, linear nondisplaced fractures of the posterior wall may difficult to appreciate. Therefore, CT findings notwithstanding, it is critical to confirm the integrity of the sinus interior and its posterior wall in all cases of anterior wall fracture requiring surgical repair. Currently, magnetic resonance imaging (MRI) plays a very limited role in the evaluation of frontal trauma. It may complement CT when intracranial injury is suspected.

FRACTURE CLASSIFICATION AND TREATMENT

The classification scheme for frontal sinus fracture is an anatomic one based on the extent of injury as determined by clinical, radiographic, and intra-operative findings. The four subtypes, which are not mutually exclusive, are anterior wall, posterior wall, nasofrontal duct, and through-and-through injuries. Each injury may be further subclassified as nondisplaced, displaced, comminuted, or compound.

ANTERIOR WALL FRACTURE

Anterior wall fractures represent approximately one third of all frontal injuries.[11] These fractures may be nonpalpable in the presence of subgaleal hematoma and forehead edema but are easily seen on CT scan (Fig. 4–2). Isolated nondisplaced anterior wall fractures do not require intervention. Left alone, these injuries do not result in cosmetic deformity. Furthermore, entrapment of sinus mucosa within a nondisplaced fracture of the anterior wall is uncommon. Consequently, mucocele formation is unlikely. Conversely, all displaced injuries of the anterior wall must be surgically addressed. In such cases, cosmetic deformity, risk of mucocele formation, and the need to examine the sinus interior all mandate surgical treatment.

The surgical approach to the frontal sinus must be individualized. The patient's hairline, sex, and injury will determine which approach is most appropriate. The most frequently used incisions include the infrabrow, midforehead, and bicoronal (Fig. 4–3). In the presence of a compound fracture, the sinus may be approached through the laceration. In almost all cases, the laceration must be extended to properly expose the fracture and allow repair. Caution is

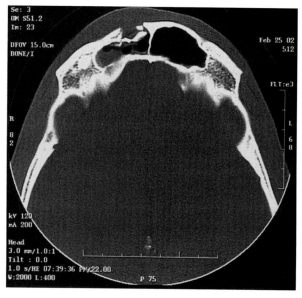

FIGURE 4–2 Axial computed tomography (CT) scan of a displaced anterior wall fracture.

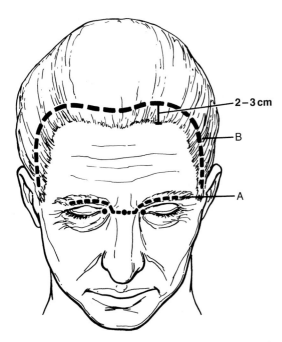

FIGURE 4–3 The infrabrow (A) and bicoronal scalp (B) incisions for exposure of the frontal sinus. The midforehead incision may be placed in any of the brow's mimetic lines. (From Donald PJ, Gluckman JL, Rice DH. *The Sinuses.* New York: Raven Press, 1995:380, with permission.)

warranted when such an approach is used. In most cases, this approach affords the surgeon adequate exposure to repair the anterior wall. However, when unexpected nasofrontal duct or posterior wall injuries are encountered, this exposure is limiting, and sinus obliteration is difficult. Frequently, meticulous closure of the laceration in conjunction with a bicoronal approach results in both improved exposure and cosmesis. The bicoronal scalp incision is the most commonly used. When performed properly, it allows unparalleled exposure of the frontal bone and results in an aesthetically pleasing scar that may be hidden in the hairline. The incision is made ~ 2 cm behind the hairline. The scalpel blade should be beveled in the plane of the hair follicles to avoid hair loss along the incision and a noticeable scar. If necessary, the incision may be carried down into a preauricular skin crease allowing exposure of the zygomatic arch. The scalp flap is then elevated in a subgaleal plane to the level of the brow. It is very important to prevent injury to the supraorbital neurovascular pedicle at this point. Laterally, the scalp flap may be raised deep to the superficial layer of the deep temporal fascia to minimize risk to the frontal division of the facial nerve. The pericranium is left intact over the calvarium. Alternatively, the infrabrow incision, also known as the butterfly incision, may be used. This incision is made at the

inferior margin of the eyebrows and connected in the midline across the glabella. This approach leaves a less acceptable scar and provides limited exposure. It also puts both the supraorbital and supratrochlear nerves at risk of injury. Finally, a midbrow incision may be used. This should only be considered in balding males with deep forehead rhytids. The midforehead approach shares all the limitations of the translaceration approach and should be used only in a select group of patients with minimally displaced anterior wall fractures.

As illustrated in Fig. 4–4, once exposed the depressed bone fragments should be gently elevated with a bone hook. Frequently, bone fragments may have prolapsed into the sinus interior. The sinus interior should then be carefully examined. This is simply done when a large anterior wall fracture is present. However, such examination through a smaller fracture may prove difficult. These circumstances lend themselves to endoscopic techniques using 0- and 30-degree endoscopes. Particular attention is paid to the posterior wall and nasofrontal ducts. Small amounts of methylene blue may be instilled into the sinus. Egress of the blue dye into the middle meatus confirms duct patency. If the injury is limited to the anterior wall, all damaged mucosa must be removed from the fragments, the bone burred down with a drill, and the fracture reduced and plated. If a fragment is of considerable size, simply removing a rim of mucosa at its periphery with a drill may be sufficient. When comminuted, all fragments should be pieced back together. Injudicious use of irrigation and suction may result in fragment loss. Such injuries are challenging. Severe comminution of the anterior wall is rarely isolated. Small fragments may be difficult to plate together and it may be preferable to use 26- or 28-gauge wire. Missing bone results in gaps in the anterior wall of the sinus. Such gaps may result in unsightly forehead depressions as posttraumatic and surgical edema subsides. When larger than 1 cm they should be repaired. This may be done using calvarial bone grafts. Grafts from the outer table of the skull are easily harvested when using a bicoronal scalp incision. Alternatively, titanium mesh may be used.[12] When severely comminuted, sinus obliteration should be considered, as many of the sinuses will be nonfunctional and problematic.

Isolated compound fractures of the anterior wall of the frontal sinus are very rare. Controversy exists regarding the management of these rare injuries, especially when large segments of bone are missing. There are two schools of thought. Calvarial grafts may replace missing bone. In most

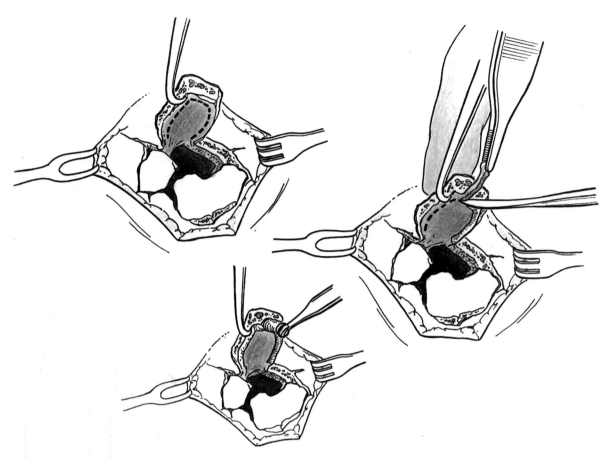

FIGURE 4–4 Depressed fragments of bone are gently elevated with a bone hook and all traumatized mucosa is removed. (From Donald PJ, Gluckman JL, Rice DH. *The Sinuses.* New York: Raven Press, 1995:381, with permission.)

instances the sinus should be obliterated following removal of all sinus mucosa and plugging of the nasofrontal ducts. Fat may be used. However, when significant portions of the anterior wall have been devascularized, there may be insufficient vascular supply to sustain a fat graft and partial resorption of the fat may result, leading to mucosal ingrowth and mucocele formation. Therefore, whenever possible, a vascularized pericranial flap should be used to obliterate the sinus interior. (The obliteration procedure is discussed in detail below.) Alternatively, these complicated fractures can be managed by Riedel ablation. This involves removal of the remaining anterior sinus wall, removal of all sinus mucosa, drilling down the bone of the sinus interior, and obliteration of the nasofrontal ducts. The bicoronal scalp flap is then allowed to collapse onto the posterior sinus wall. As shown in Fig. **4–5**, this procedure results in significant cosmetic deformity requiring future secondary reconstruction. It should be reserved for those cases involving delayed treatment and significant contamination of the wound.

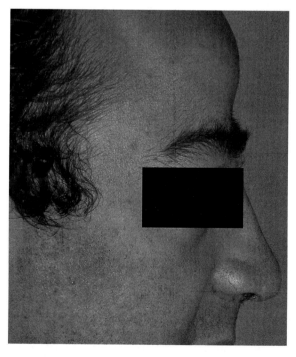

FIGURE 4–5 The Riedel deformity.

POSTERIOR WALL FRACTURE

Fractures of the posterior wall of the frontal sinus have a significant potential for serious late infectious complications. For this reason, management of non-displaced posterior wall fractures remains quite controversial. Unlike nondisplaced anterior wall fractures, fractures of the posterior wall frequently result in mucosal trauma and entrapment. Therefore, even in the presence of a patent nasofrontal duct, mucoceles may form. In addition, the frontal dura is tightly adherent to the posterior wall of the sinus. Even small nondisplaced fractures may cause dural tears and CSF leak. Missing such an injury could prove disastrous, and become evident only when the patient develops meningitis. For these reasons, we feel that nondisplaced posterior wall fractures should be treated surgically, usually by sinus obliteration. Alternatively, these injuries may be observed. Observation of such fractures requires a reliable patient who will attend follow-up appointments regularly. Interval CT scans are necessary to prevent delayed diagnosis of mucocele. This treatment is not truly nonsurgical. Examination of the sinus's posterior wall is still necessary to rule out significant mucosal tears and CSF leak. This can be done endoscopically through a small frontal trephine. If the posterior wall appears completely intact, the patient is observed. The argument for such an approach is that many patients have retained a functioning frontal sinus and thus sinus obliteration can be avoided. For those who develop mucoceles, sinus obliteration is necessary, the same operation that would have been done at the outset. Unfortunately, given the demographics of this patient population, careful follow-up may prove difficult, and some patients may return only when they have developed serious complications.

There is no controversy surrounding displaced posterior wall fractures. All such injuries must be explored and treated surgically. Often, these injuries are associated with anterior wall fractures (Fig. 4–6). The surgical approach to the posterior wall of the sinus is via an osteoplastic flap of its anterior wall. The sinus is approached through a standard bicoronal scalp incision. The flap is elevated to the level of the supraorbital rims, leaving the pericranium down. An accurate template of the frontal sinus is essential. Traditionally, a 6-foot penny Caldwell radiograph is used. A cutout of the sinus and the supraorbital rims is prepared from this 1:1 image and sterilized. Inclusion of the supraorbital rims allows accurate placement of the template on the skull. Alternatively, an endoscope may be inserted into the sinus via a trephine and the sinus transilluminated. This allows excellent visualization of the sinus confines, especially when well pneumatized. Image guidance may also allow very accurate localization of the sinus but requires sophisticated equipment and familiarity with its use. The outline of the sinus is then marked onto the skull with methylene blue. The pericranium is incised along the outline. On occasion a pericranial flap is needed for reconstruction. In such cases it is advisable to carefully lift the pericranium off of the calvarium as a separate flap rather than incising it along the outlines of the sinus. However, there is a theoretical risk of bone flap resorption when the osteoplastic flap is devoid of an intact periosteal cover. As illustrated in Fig. 4–7, the osteotomy is then made using a saw or cutting drill bit. It is essential to angulate the cutting instrument toward the sinus interior to avoid inadvertent injury to the dura and brain. A second osteotomy is made through the dense bone of the brow and nasion above the level of the sinus floor. Finally, an osteotome is used to cut the intersinus septum. The osteotome should be directed toward the superior aspect of the nasion to avoid injury to the nasofrontal ducts and sinus floor. Gentle downward pressure is used to fracture the osteoplastic flap. If devoid of pericranium, the bone flap should be kept wrapped in a moist sponge.

Once the osteoplastic flap has been successfully elevated, the sinus interior is carefully examined. The mucosa of the posterior wall is very gently elevated off the bone to expose the fracture. In the case of nondisplaced fractures without CSF leak, all of the sinus mucosa must be removed. This requires drilling off ~1 to 2 mm of bone to remove the

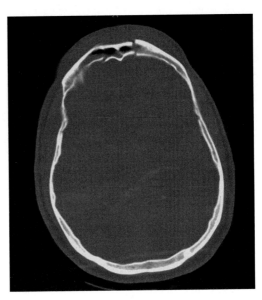

FIGURE 4–6 Axial CT scan of an anterior wall–posterior wall displaced frontal sinus fracture.

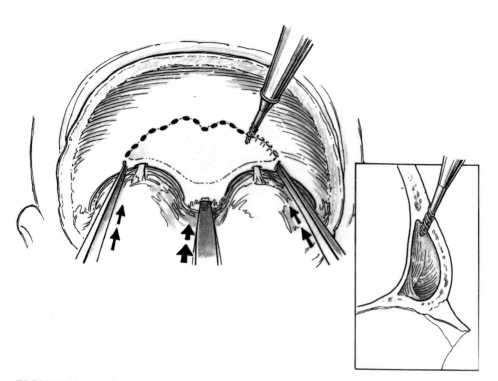

FIGURE 4–7 The osteoplastic flap procedure. The outline of the sinus is transferred to the brow and the sinus is entered with a drill. It is important to angulate the drill into the sinus interior (inset) to avoid accidental intracranial injury. (From Donald PJ, Gluckman JL, Rice DH. *The Sinuses.* New York: Raven Press, 1995:385, with permission.)

aforementioned imbrications of mucosa in the foramina of Breschet. The remaining sinus mucosa, including that on the interior surface of the osteoplastic flap, should be removed judiciously and the bone should be polished with the drill. The nasofrontal ducts are plugged with free temporalis muscle grafts. Failure to obliterate the nasofrontal

ducts may result in ascending infection or mucosal ingrowth and mucocele formation. The sinus interior is then packed with abdominal fat harvested from the left lower quadrant (Fig. **4–8**). The osteoplastic flap is then plated back into position.

Should a CSF leak be diagnosed, the bone of the posterior sinus wall must be carefully elevated to

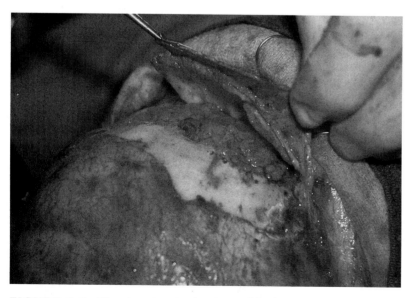

FIGURE 4–8 The sinus interior has been obliterated with abdominal fat and the osteoplastic flap is being replaced. Note that the pericranium remains intact over the bone flap.

expose the dural tear. Small linear dural tears may be closed with simple interrupted dural sutures. Once a watertight closure has been achieved the repair should be augmented with fascia. Urgent neurosurgical consultation is indicated for more complex dural tears, frontal lobe injuries, or laceration of the superior sagittal sinus. Complex dural injuries require duraplasty with fascia lata, temporalis fascia, or lyophilized dura. The repair should ideally be augmented with a second layer of fascia and fibrin glue.

Sinus obliteration is ill-advised when considerable portions of the posterior wall are missing or devascularized. Donald and Ettin[13] demonstrated that fat graft absorption is likely when significant amounts of the posterior wall are missing. Both dura and devascularized bone offer little blood supply to the fat graft. Subsequent loss of the graft leads to ingrowth of epithelium and mucocele formation. Therefore, when there are small dehiscences of the posterior wall, consideration should be given to sinus obliteration with a vascularized pericranial flap. When more than 25% of the posterior wall is missing, the sinus should be cranialized. The procedure is outlined in Fig. 4–9. This requires complete removal of the posterior wall and sinus mucosa and obliteration of the nasofrontal ducts. The frontal lobes of the brain are then allowed to expand into the dead space previously occupied by the frontal sinus. The nasofrontal ducts, although obliterated, may be further separated from the brain by slipping a pericranial flap over the sinus floor underneath the frontal dura. The osteoplastic flap is then replaced.

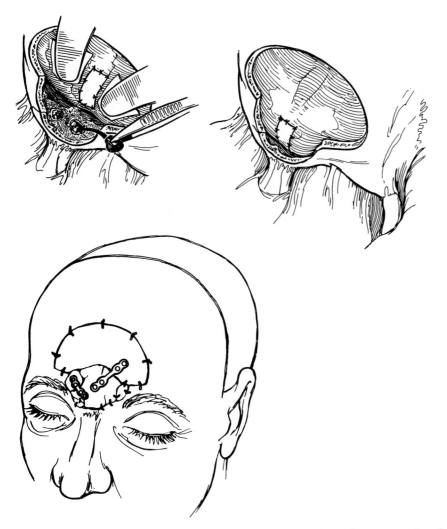

FIGURE 4–9 The cranialization procedure. The osteoplastic flap is created and the posterior wall of the sinus is taken down completely. In this illustration a small duraplasty has been performed. The sinus mucosa is completely removed. The nasofrontal ducts are then obliterated with muscle plugs. The osteoplastic flap is then replaced. (From Donald PJ, Gluckman JL, Rice DH. *The Sinuses.* New York: Raven Press, 1995:393, with permission.)

Nasofrontal Duct Injury

Nasofrontal duct injuries are rarely isolated. Most accompany other fractures of the sinus and as such are appreciated at the time of surgical exploration. Diagnosis of an isolated injury to the duct requires a high index of suspicion. Many such injuries become evident only when they manifest as mucoceles or infectious complications thereof, many months after the insult. The diagnosis is suggested by opacification of a traumatized sinus that persists for 10 or more days. Fractures through the ducts may be seen on coronal and, less commonly, axial CT scans. However, these injuries may be minimally displaced or limited to the mucosa and, as such, poorly seen on CT. When suspected, the diagnosis should be confirmed by inspection of the sinus interior. This is easily accomplished by placing a 30-degree endoscope into the sinus via a trephine. Instilling methylene blue into the sinus interior and watching its egress into the middle meatus can then confirm patency of the ducts.

When injuries to the nasofrontal duct accompany other sinus fractures, the management is very straightforward. The sinus is either obliterated or cranialized depending on the extent and type of associated fracture. Regardless of treatment, the ducts must be denuded of all mucosa and plugged. The real controversy surrounds the management of minor injuries to the duct. For many rhinologists, sinus obliteration for unilateral minor injuries of the duct is too aggressive; once patency of the duct has been confirmed, careful and regular patient follow-up may be an acceptable alternative. These rhinologists' argument is that, should a reliable patient develop a mucocele, sinus obliteration or marsupialization of the mucocele may be performed prior to any infectious complication. Alternatively, in experienced hands, endoscopic frontal sinusotomy may be considered. This technically demanding procedure requires experience in sinus endoscopy, specialized instrumentation, and an in-depth appreciation for paranasal sinus and anterior skull base anatomy.[14-16] It has largely replaced the classic open sinusotomy procedures described by Lynch, Sewall, Boyden, and Lothrop that were previously considered the gold standard. Once again, patient reliability is an essential selection criterion given the risk of eventual duct restenosis and mucocele formation.

Given the frequent unreliability of the trauma patient, these injuries should be approached with healthy respect. Avoiding potentially serious late infectious sequelae of frontal sinus injury and patient safety should be paramount in the decision-making process. Therefore, sinus obliteration for most nasofrontal duct injuries is very appropriate.

Alternative, more conservative, approaches should be reserved for a select few cases of minimal injury in motivated patients.

Through-and-Through Fracture

The through-and-through fracture is the most devastating of all frontal injuries and involves displaced fractures of both sinus walls (Fig. 4–10). These injuries require tremendous force and are most often open. Typically, there is associated intracranial injury manifesting as either CSF leak or brain matter within the wound. Almost half of these cases result in death at the scene of the accident or shortly thereafter. Management of these injuries is complex and requires a team approach.[17] Immediate neurosurgical consultation is essential. Devitalized brain must be debrided. Hemorrhage from torn cortical veins or from the sagittal sinus must be controlled. Sagittal sinus injury is very serious. Ligation of the proximal third of the sinus may be done at some risk of venous congestion and cerebral infarction. The risk is increased in the face of elevated intracranial pressures. Ligation of the sinus posterior to the coronal suture line usually results in death.[18] Complex dural injuries are frequently encountered and primary dural closure is rarely possible. Once all devitalized dura has been removed, a duraplasty using temporalis fascia, fascia lata, or lyophilized dura must be performed. A watertight closure is necessary to help prevent postoperative CSF leak and minimize the risk of meningitis. Lumbar or intraventricular drains may be used to decrease intracranial pressure and help reduce the risk of postoperative CSF leak.

Given the complexity of these injuries, excellent exposure is essential. Whenever possible, lacerations should be conservatively debrided and meticulously closed. A bicoronal scalp incision provides needed exposure and allows simultaneous elevation of a pericranial flap. In many cases, treatment of the intracranial injuries require a frontal craniotomy. Frontal sinus cranialization is most often necessary. The frontal lobes are allowed to prolapse into the sinus interior. The additional intracranial space is usually welcome in such cases as there is often associated cerebral edema. It is crucial to minimize intracranial dead space. As the authors have highlighted elsewhere, failure to do so in anterior skull base surgery predisposes to infectious complications.[19] Therefore, fat grafts should be used to obliterate all dead space. Unfortunately, free fat grafts often absorb when placed against dura, especially when large duraplasties have been performed. The longest possible pericranial flap should be raised. It is passed through the craniotomy and

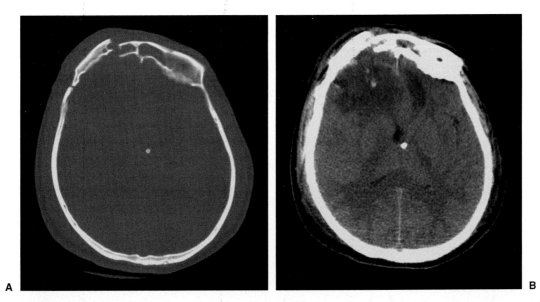

A   B

FIGURE 4–10 A: Axial CT scan of a through-and-through frontal sinus injury. B: Note the associated extensive frontal lobe cerebral injury and edema.

tucked underneath the frontal lobe dura (Fig. **4–11**). The fat graft is then placed on top of the pericranial flap. The remaining flap may be used to augment the duraplasty or may be folded over the top of the fat graft, further improving its blood supply. The pericranium is held in place with either fibrin glue or sutures.

Reconstruction of the frontal sinus's anterior wall may be challenging but is crucial to protect the prolapsed brain from further injury. To this end, all of the bone fragments of both the anterior and posterior walls should be preserved. Often, there may be significant defects in the anterior wall and the wound may be heavily contaminated.

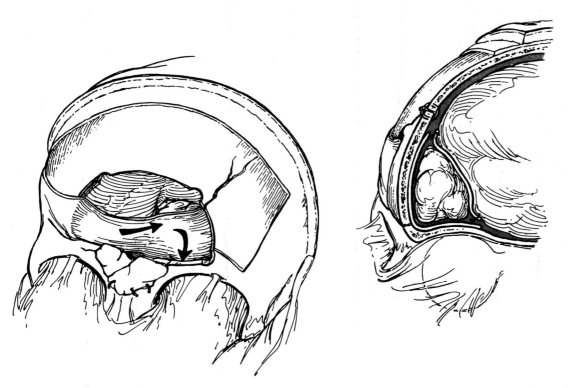

FIGURE 4–11 The pericranial flap is elevated and pedicled, in this case, on the right supraorbital vessels. The flap is then tucked in underneath the osteoplastic flap and used to wrap the fat graft and help obliterate the nasofrontal ducts. (From Donald PJ, Gluckman JL, Rice DH. *The Sinuses.* New York: Raven Press, 1995:397, with permission.)

Fortunately, the work of Nadell and Kline[20] has established the safety of using iodine-povidone–cleansed bone fragments for anterior wall reconstruction. In addition, calvarial outer table grafts may be harvested to fill any persistent dehiscences. Alternatively, titanium mesh may be used to recontour the forehead. In the most severe cases, when there has been extensive soft tissue loss, local flaps, such as rotational scalp flaps, or microvascular free tissue transfer may be needed to cover the reconstruction and protect the brain.

ENDOSCOPIC TREATMENT OF FRONTAL SINUS TRAUMA

Advances in endoscopic and minimally invasive surgery have all been driven by a desire to minimize surgical morbidity. The application of these techniques to the management of facial trauma has been a natural progression based on experience gained from endoscopic sinus and facial rejuvenation surgery. With respect to frontal sinus trauma, the use of such techniques remains controversial. Several authors have described techniques applied to small numbers of patients with encouraging results.[11,21–24] Preservation of a functional frontal sinus with adequate fracture reduction and cosmesis has been the goal. To date, the majority of reports limit selection criteria to minimally displaced anterior table fractures. Given that frontal trauma is most often a high-velocity injury, such limited fractures are not commonplace.

To describe these approaches as purely endoscopic is misleading. In fact, they are endoscopically assisted procedures that require several small incisions to gain access to and manipulate the fragments of the fractured anterior frontal wall. Typically, three separate 5-mm incisions, one central and two lateral, are made in or just behind the hairline. Elevating the soft tissues of the brow in either a subperiosteal or supraperiosteal plane then creates the optical cavity. If elevation is performed supraperiosteally, care should be taken as the supraorbital rims are approached to avoid injury to the supraorbital and supratrochlear neurovascular bundles. Visualization is best with a 30-degree endoscope to compensate for the convexity of the frontal bone. Once the fracture has been exposed, small stab incisions may be made within the mimetic lines of the forehead to allow introduction of drill guides and bone hooks for manipulation and fixation of the fracture. Manipulation of bone fragments may be difficult. Threaded Steinmann pins or 1.5-mm screws can be placed percutaneously and used to guide the fragment into

position. Once adequately reduced, 1.5-mm miniplates contoured to the brow can be inserted through one of the forehead incisions and percutaneously screwed in place effectively reducing the fracture. An alternate approach to minimally displaced anterior wall fractures is simply to allow the fracture to heal and then recontour the brow endoscopically. This can be achieved using polyglactin mesh or porous polyethylene implants.

These techniques can be applied only to a select subset of patients. The success of such endoscopic approaches relies as much on selection criteria as on surgical expertise. To date the majority of reports limit selection to minimally displaced anterior wall fractures with preservation of frontal outflow.[21–24] In addition, only the most reliable patients should be offered such treatment because follow-up is essential given the risk of chronic frontal sinusitis and mucocele. It is this risk that makes endoscopic management controversial. Although a departure from classic teaching, many of the principles must be adhered to regardless of approach. Therefore, endoscopic reduction of the anterior wall is contraindicated in cases of significant comminution and mucosal injury.

Until recently, injury to the nasofrontal ducts was also an absolute contraindication to simple reduction of the anterior table and preservation of the sinus. The established effectiveness of endoscopic nasofrontal sinusotomy as a treatment for chronic frontal sinusitis[16] has been applied to frontal sinus trauma. It is recognized that many cases of traumatic nasofrontal duct obstruction are due to mucosal edema. Smith et al[25] have reported a novel approach to the anterior wall fracture with nasofrontal duct obstruction. In a small series of seven patients with such injuries, open reduction and internal fixation (ORIF) of the anterior wall fracture was performed without sinus obliteration. The patients were then treated medically for their nasofrontal duct obstruction with 4 weeks of broad-spectrum antibiotics. Serial CT scans at 8 weeks, 16 weeks, 6 months, and 1 year were used to confirm patency of the frontal sinus outflow tract. In five patients spontaneous ventilation of the sinus occurred and no further treatment was necessary. Two patients developed frontal sinusitis and required endoscopic frontal sinusotomy with restoration of sinus outflow. Both patients had associated naso-orbital-ethmoid fractures.

It remains to be seen whether or not these new techniques represent a true paradigm shift in the treatment of limited frontal sinus fracture. As experience increases and the long-term results are analyzed, a clearer picture should develop. However, we feel that serious injuries, especially those of the posterior wall, must be treated with traditional open approaches to avoid potentially devastating complications.

COMPLICATIONS OF FRONTAL SINUS FRACTURE

The complications of frontal sinus trauma are almost always the result of inadequate initial care. They range from minor cosmetic deformities of the brow to life-threatening intracranial infections. More often than not, they manifest as late complications. In a patient population typically noncompliant with regular follow-up, this becomes a very serious issue.

Cosmetic deformities are most often due to defects in the anterior wall of the sinus. Even those as small as a centimeter may become noticeable as forehead edema subsides. This can be avoided by carefully replacing all bone fragments during fracture repair. When defects are present, it behooves the surgeon to replace missing bone with bone grafts or titanium mesh. Similarly, iatrogenic injury to the frontal division of the facial nerve may also significantly impact the aesthetics of the brow. This injury results in unilateral brow ptosis and paralysis of the ipsilateral forehead. This complication can be avoided by carefully elevating the bicoronal scalp flap as described.

Mucoceles may result from nasofrontal duct obstruction, trauma to the sinus mucosa, or both. These benign cysts expand and erode bone along paths of least resistance. Typically, this results in erosion of the medial orbital roof and frontal sinus floor, causing downward and outward displacement of the globe. In addition, erosion of the frontal sinus's posterior wall may result in intracranial extension. Mucoceles are clinically significant because of their propensity to become infected, leading to mucopyocele formation and the secondary infectious complications that may ensue, which may be divided into extracranial complications and intracranial complications. The extracranial complications include orbital cellulitis, subperiosteal abscess, orbital abscess, and frontal osteomyelitis, also referred to as Pott's puffy tumor. The intracranial infectious complications include meningitis, subdural and epidural abscess, brain abscess, and cavernous or sagittal sinus thrombophlebitis. In addition to culture-directed antimicrobial therapy, the offending sinus must always be addressed surgically. The management of these infectious sequelae is complex and beyond the scope of this chapter.

SUMMARY

The successful management of frontal sinus trauma requires careful preoperative and, often, intraoperative assessment of fracture type and location. An organized and logical approach to these injuries based on fracture type allows the surgeon to make necessary decisions to effectively treat these injuries. The surgeon requires a healthy respect for trauma to the frontal sinus and an awareness of the potentially life-threatening complications that may result from improper initial management. Although it is rewarding to restore health, function, and cosmesis to these patients, it is imperative to understand that the majority of complications due to frontal sinus trauma manifest months after the injury. Unfortunately, many such patients are unreliable and postoperative follow-up is difficult. For this reason, it is incumbent upon the surgeon to make sound treatment decisions and reserve less traditional approaches, such as endoscopic treatment, only for the most reliable patients.

PEARLS: FRONTAL SINUS TRAUMA

- Frontal bone and frontal sinus anatomy can be variable.
- Damage to the frontal sinus mucosa alone can cause mucocele formation.
- Nasofrontal duct obstruction causes mucocele formation.
- The frontal sinus mucosa is tenaciously adherent to the bone and imbricates into the bony foramina of Breschet, necessitating meticulous removal of sinus mucosa as part of obliteration.
- CT scan, with axial and coronal views, is the appropriate imaging technique for evaluation.
- Treatment of frontal sinus trauma differs according to the classification of the fracture: anterior table versus posterior, displaced versus nondisplaced, comminuted versus noncomminuted.
- Techniques to treat frontal sinus injuries include ORIF alone, sinus obliteration, sinus cranialization, sinus ablation, and endoscopic frontal sinusotomy.
- In patients who are unlikely to be compliant with regular follow-up, definitive treatment at initial surgery is mandatory.

REFERENCES

1. Yuge A, Takio M, Masami T. Growth of frontal sinus with age—an x-ray tomographic study. In:

Myers E, ed. *New Dimensions in Otolaryngology–Head and Neck Surgery*, vol 2. New York: Excerpta Medica, 1985:326–327

2. Lang J. *Clinical Anatomy of the Nose, Nasal Cavity and Paranasal Sinuses*. New York: G. Thieme Verlag, 1989: 62–69

3. Novak R, Mehls G. Die aplasien der sinus maxillares und frontales unter besenderer Berucksichtigung der pneumatisation bei spalttragern. Anat Anz 1977;142: 441–450

4. Van Alyea OE. Maxillary and frontal sinuses. In: English, GM ed. *Otolaryngology*. Hagerstown, MD: Harper and Row, 1977

5. Mosher HP, Judd DK. An analysis of seven cases of osteomyelitis of the frontal bone complicating frontal sinusitis. Laryngoscope 1933;43:153

6. Lotta JS, Schall RF. The histology of the epithelium of the paranasal sinuses under various conditions. Ann Otol Rhinol Laryngol 1934;43:945–971

7. Schenck NL. Frontal sinus disease: III. Experimental and clinical factors in failure of the frontal osteoplastic operation. Laryngoscope 1975;85:76–92

8. Donald PJ. The tenacity of the frontal sinus mucosa. Otolaryngol Head Neck Surg 1979;87:557–566

9. Nahum AM. The biomechanics of maxillofacial trauma. Clin Plast Surg 1975;2:59–64

10. Wallis A, Donald PJ. Frontal sinus fractures: a review of 72 cases. Laryngoscope 1988;98:593–598

11. Lappert PW, Lee JW. Treatment of an isolated outer table frontal sinus fracture using endoscopic reduction and fixation. Plast Reconstr Surg 1998;102: 1642–1645

12. Lakhani RS, Shubuya TY, Mathog RH, Marks SC, Burgio DL, Yoo GH. Titanium mesh repair of the severely comminuted frontal sinus fracture. Arch Otolaryngol Head Neck Surg 2001;127:665–669

13. Donald PJ, Ettin M. The safety of frontal sinus obliteration when sinus walls are missing. Laryngoscope 1986;96:190–193

14. Smith TL, Han JK, Loehrl TA, Rhee JS. Endoscopic management of the frontal recess in frontal sinus fractures: a shift in the paradigm? Laryngoscope 2002; 112:784–790

15. Kuhn FA, Javer AR. Primary endoscopic management of the frontal sinus. Otolaryngol Clin North Am 2001;34:59–76

16. Weber R, Draf W, Kratzsch, Hosemann W, Schaefer SD. Modern concepts of frontal sinus surgery. Laryngoscope 2001;111:137–146

17. Donald PJ, Bernstein L. Compound frontal sinus injuries with intracranial penetration. Laryngoscope 1978;88:225–232

18. Donald PJ, Gluckman JL, Rice DH. *The Sinuses*. New York: Raven Press, 1995

19. Enepekides DJ, Donald PJ. Long-term outcomes of anterior skull base surgery. Curr Opin Otolaryngol Head Neck Surg 2000;8:130–136

20. Nadell J, Kline DG. Primary reconstruction of depressed skull fractures including those involving the sinus, orbit, and cribriform plate. J Neurosurg 1974; 41:200–207

21. Shumrick KA, Ryzenman JM. Endoscopic management of facial fractures. Facial Plast Surg Clin North Am 2001;9:469–474

22. Forrest CR. Application of endoscope-assisted minimal-access techniques in orbitozygomatic complex, orbital floor, and frontal sinus fractures. J Craniomaxillofac Trauma 1999;5:7–12

23. Graham HD III, Spring P. Endoscopic repair of frontal sinus fracture: case report. J Craniomaxillofac Trauma 1996;2:52–55

24. Chen DJ, Chen CT, Chen YR, Feng GM. Endoscopically assisted repair of frontal sinus fracture. J Trauma 2003;55:378–382

25. Smith TL, Han JK, Loehrl TA, Rhee JS. Endoscopic management of the frontal recess in frontal sinus fractures: a shift in the paradigm? Laryngoscope 2002; 112:784–790

Chapter 5

NASAL AND NASO-ORBITAL-ETHMOID FRACTURES

John C. Oeltjen and Larry Hollier

Nasal fractures rank third in incidence to that of clavicle and wrist fractures.[1] For the physician treating maxillofacial traumas, injuries of the nose and the region lateral to the nose and medial to the eye, the naso-orbital-ethmoid (NOE) region, are common in occurrence, but returning patients to their premorbid state both functionally and aesthetically is a therapeutic challenge.

Although nasal fractures are common, the treatment of the acutely fractured nose has essentially not changed over the past five thousand years.[2] The Edwin Smith papyrus from ancient Egypt details the technique of repositioning the deviated nasal bones with fingers or an elevator followed with insertion of intranasal stabilization splints and placement of a firm dressing over the nose. Packing consisted of linen saturated with grease and honey, external splints of stiff rolls of linen laid on either side of the nose.[3]

The frequency of sports-related nasal injuries in ancient Greece prompted Hippocrates to study the structural violations of the injury, specifically the bony and cartilaginous components. In addition, he provided a structured approach to the care of individual types of fractures from simple application of poultice and bandaging to reshaping and reconstruction of the fractured and deviated nose. The Hippocratic methods constitute the scaffolding on which today's approaches to nasal fractures are designed.[4]

Nasal and NOE fractures result from blunt trauma, particularly motor vehicle accidents (MVAs), sports-related injuries, and altercations.[5] Childhood injuries tend to result more from sports injuries and play accidents, whereas adults sustain a majority of the facial injuries in altercations and sports-related injuries.[6] Although the use of restraining devices and airbags has significantly reduced the number of facial fractures in MVAs,[7] the use of airbags does not appear to change the pattern of facial fractures when they occur.[8] Lastly, many nasal and septal fractures are unrecognized and therefore untreated at the initial injury but later account for a high percentage of the septoplasty procedures performed for nasal obstruction and deviation.[9]

ANATOMY

Crucial to the treatment of nasal and NOE fractures is a detailed understanding of the anatomy of the region. This includes not only the underlying bony and cartilaginous structures but also the medial canthus.

The bony support structure in the compact midface region consists of the nasal bones, the frontal process of the maxilla, the internal angular process of the frontal bone, the lacrimal bone, the ethmoid bone, the sphenoid bone, and the nasal septum as shown in Fig. 5–1. The nasal bones are thicker along the midline where they articulate with each other and with the perpendicular plate of the ethmoid below. The perpendicular plate of the ethmoid is attached to the cribriform plate above and the maxillary crest below. The perpendicular plate of the ethmoid and the maxillary crest articulate with the quadrangular cartilage of the nose.[10]

The cartilaginous support structure of the nose consists of the central support structure of the septal quadrangular cartilage, the paired upper lateral cartilages, and the paired lower lateral cartilages. As mentioned above, the quadrangular cartilage has strong attachments to the maxillary crest as far anteriorly as the anterior nasal spine and provides the flexible and dynamic support of the lower two

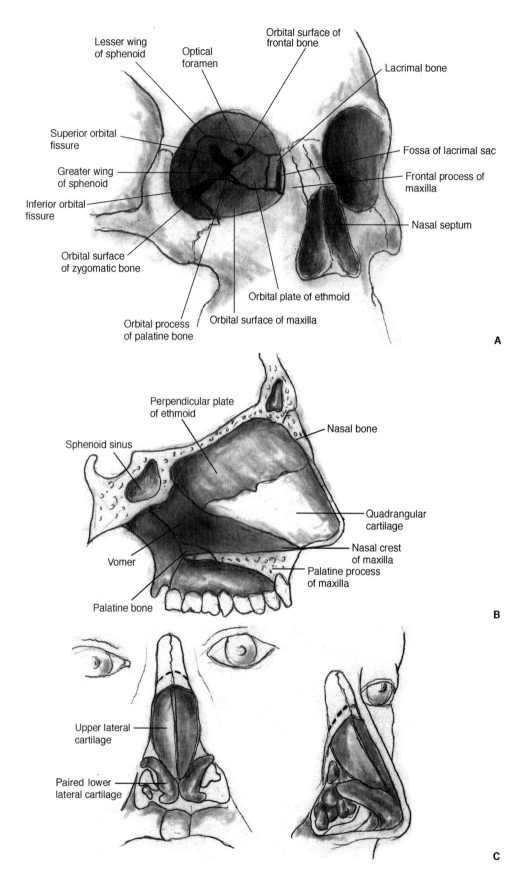

FIGURE 5–1 Anatomy of the midface region. A: The bony support structure in the midface region including the bones composing the orbit. B: The bony and cartilaginous structures composing the nasal septum. C: The external cartilaginous support structures of the nose.

thirds of the nose. The paired upper lateral cartilages have solid attachments to the caudal aspect of the nasal bones and help to maintain the midline location of the quadrangular cartilage.[10] At their caudal aspect, the upper lateral cartilages have a complex fibrous attachment with the lower lateral cartilages, which functions as the nasal valve. This valve acts to modulate the flow of inspired air.[9] Lastly, the lower lateral cartilages provide little midline structural support but are responsible for much of the aesthetics and contour of the nasal tip.[10]

Lateral to the nasal bones is the NOE region, a delicate and intricate skeletal structure that serves as the confluence of the nose, orbits, maxilla, and cranium.[11] The bones composing this region include the lacrimal and frontal bones, the lamina papyracea of the ethmoid, and the maxilla. In trauma to the midface causing posterior and inferior displacement of the entire nasal pyramid (consisting of the nasal bones and underlying ethmoid perpendicular plate), fractures of the NOE region occur.[10]

Attached to the bony structures composing the NOE region, the medial canthal tendon serves to maintain globe and eyelid support while providing an aesthetic appearance to the palpebral fissure. Disruption of the tendon results in telecanthus and rounding of the medial canthus.[10] The medial canthal tendon consists of three limbs. A fan-shaped anterior limb inserts onto the lateral surface of the anterior lacrimal crest and nasal bones. A superior limb encompasses the lacrimal sac before attaching to the suture between the frontal process of the maxilla and the internal angular process of the frontal bone. Lastly, a thin posterior limb attaches to the posterior aspect of the lacrimal fossa, the posterior lacrimal crest.[12]

Other soft tissue structures of importance in the region include the lacrimal system, the trochlea, and the nerve and blood supply. Although not managed during the initial repair of NOE fractures unless obviously transected, injuries to the lacrimal canaliculi can result in excess tearing due to the inability to clear lacrimal secretions. The treating physician should be aware of injuries to the duct so that appropriate postoperative care can be arranged.[13] The trochlea is subject to injury in NOE fractures due to its location on the internal angular process of the frontal bone. It is important redirecting the vector of pull of the superior oblique muscle. Failure to return the trochlea to its position results in diplopia on downward gaze.[14] The sensory innervation of the nose and adjacent face is supplied by the supratrochlear, infratrochlear, anterior ethmoidal,

and infraorbital nerves.[9] Care must be taken in dissecting away fractured bones from these nerves in repair of nasal and NOE fractures. Finally, the blood supply to the nasal and NOE region is rich, but hemorrhage can usually be controlled by direct pressure. The most common source of anterior epistaxis is Kiesselbach's plexus or the anteroinferior septal plexus found on the nasal septum. The plexus receives blood supply both from the internal and external carotid arteries. Posterior epistaxis, often a more severe hemorrhage but less common than anterior epistaxis, arises from branches of both the sphenopalatine and anterior ethmoidal arteries. In nasal fractures, the anterior ethmoidal artery can be injured as it passes into the nose through an aperture at the level of the crista galli.[14] In cases of particularly severe hemorrhage, when packing, Foley balloon catheterization of the nasal passage, and temporary reduction of the fracture do not result in hemostasis, interventional embolization of the maxillary or sphenopalatine arteries has been reported.[15]

NASAL FRACTURES

CLINICAL ASSESSMENT

The examination of the midface should proceed with a systematic approach to the patient. Although facial trauma is often seen as a consulting service, the examining physician should ensure that more serious injuries have first been ruled out, including intracranial and cervical spine injuries.[13] The ABCs (airway, breathing, circulation) of trauma care are just as crucial to the consulting physician as they are to the initial management team.

A complete history can provide insight into the premorbid state, the suspected type of injury, and the ability of the patient to heal. Important in the history are photographs of the individual prior to the injury and any previous midface trauma. Often the presenting injury is not the first sustained by the individual[6] and this directly affects the potential outcome. In addition, photographic documentation of the nasal fracture is an important contribution to the medical-legal record.[9] The injury that results from trauma to the midface is directly related to the age of the individual (bones become more brittle with age), the amount of force applied, and the vector of the applied force.[9] For example, with blows to the lower two thirds of the nose, the resilience of the upper and lower lateral cartilages combined with their loose association with the bony structures allows for high-energy absorptive and dissipation properties. As a result, true fractures of the cartilage are less common than dislocation, displacement, or avulsion injuries.[6] A patient's report of changes in nasal appearance or changes in the patency of the airway is a strong predictor of the presence of nasal fracture.[9]

A thorough physical exam is dependent on the proper equipment. To properly examine the nasal region, the physician needs a headlight, short and long nasal specula, decongestant spray, cotton-tipped applicators, Frazier-tipped suction, nasal packing material, and possibly a rigid endoscope.[16] Initial decongestion with topical application of phenylephrine aids in the intranasal inspection.[5] With equipment ready, examination should proceed from general to specific starting with a survey of the patient. This includes assessment of ocular function and appearance, the lacrimal system, occlusion and possible dental injuries, maxillary and mandibular stability, trigeminal and facial nerve function, and telecanthus. On nasal exam, signs of a nasal fracture include severe bleeding secondary to mucosal tears, external deviation or deformity, eyelid edema, scleral chemosis, ecchymosis, hematomas, subcutaneous emphysema, and crepitus. The presence of epistaxis is a strong predictor of the presence of nasal fracture, and mobility or crepitus is diagnostic.[9,16,17] Direct palpation for step-offs, mobility, and crepitus should be followed by bimanual palpation using a cotton-tipped applicator placed through each naris and against the septum. Palpation of the anterior nasal spine is achieved via the sublabial route. Lastly, the nasal tip should be pushed posteriorly to assess the integrity of septal support.[6,9,16,18]

Often a physical exam is accompanied with radiographic evaluation of bony structures for evidence of fractures. With nasal fractures, however, routine radiographs are now recognized as largely unnecessary. This is partially due to the difficulty and lack of uniformity in interpreting the radiographs, specifically in distinguishing sutures and old fractures from acute injury. Although computed tomographic (CT) scans are useful in evaluating NOE fractures, they play little role in most isolated nasal fractures.[5,6,9]

Finally, in the evaluation of the potential nasal fracture, the examining physician needs to be aware of the emergent situations associated with nasal fractures: severe bleeding, nasal airway obstruction in the neonate, septal hematoma, cerebrospinal fluid (CSF) rhinorrhea, and visual impairment.[6] The most serious aspect of severe epistaxis is usually secondary to airway compromise and not from exsanguination. As mentioned above, nasal packing and temporary reduction is successful in controlling bleeding in most patients but can be followed by interventional embolization in refractory cases.[15] A septal hematoma occurs with injury to the cartilaginous septum. Portions of the mucoperichondrial soft tissue are avulsed from the septum, creating a space that can fill with blood. This hematoma can produce airway obstruction, or more importantly, can lead to necrosis of the septum. The septal cartilage derives its nutrients from the perichondrium, a process prevented by the interposition of a hematoma. Atrophy or necrosis of the cartilage can occur within 3 to 4 days, leading to a saddle deformity and retraction of the nasal columella. In addition, septal hematomas are particularly susceptible to infection, again leading to cartilage loss.[6,16,17] It is important to note that septal hematomas are more likely to occur in children, possibly due to the softer cartilage.[6,19]

Cerebrospinal fluid leaks may occur with nasal fractures due to compromise of the dura, often at the cribriform plate. Even though the leak may not appear for several days, suspicion of injury to the cribriform plate should be elevated in patients complaining of anosmia or continual nasal drainage of clear fluid.[9,20,21] Many CSF leaks resolve spontaneously within a week; however, persistence of the problem may require insertion of a lumbar drain and, in the most severe cases, operative closure. Finally, up to 65% of facial fractures sustain some form of ocular injury, emphasizing the importance of a thorough ocular exam.[22]

CLASSIFICATION

Several different approaches to classification of nasal fractures have been taken. Of these, the pathologic classifications presented by Murray et al[23] provide a thorough approach to fractures resulting from both different amounts and different vectors of force. To arrive at their conclusions, 50 unembalmed fresh cadavers were subjected to various controlled traumatic insults. The results were divided into a classification of seven different patterns of injury. Several important conclusions were drawn from their work. First, the fracture pattern was not consistently predicted by the amount and vector of the applied force. The variation was thought to depend on the variability in the strength of the subjects' noses. Second, in comparison to previous studies, significant septal fractures occurred within the perpendicular plate instead of the quadrangular cartilage.[24] More significant is the demonstration of the importance of the septum in returning the nose to its preinjury position and maintaining it there. In their experiments, the authors showed that if the nose was deviated by more than half of its width from the midline, the septum, particularly the perpendicular plate of the ethmoid, was involved. If only the nasal bones are manipulated and the septal fracture not repaired, the nasal deformity is likely to recur with time.[2,23]

SURGICAL INDICATIONS

The three nasal fracture sequelae that warrant immediate surgical attention are open nasal fractures, hematoma of the nasal septum, and, airway compromise.[5] Open nasal fractures require extensive irrigation of the wound and reduction of the fracture followed by meticulous closure of the soft tissue envelope. As mentioned previously, septal hematomas can result in septal necrosis, resorption, and subsequent nasal collapse. Drainage of the hematoma can first be attempted with simple aspiration; however, any question as to complete removal should be followed with formal incision and drainage. This should be followed by placement of anterior nasal packs, absorbable mattress sutures through the septum, and bilateral Silastic splints that are left in place for several days to ensure adherence of the perichondrium to the septum.[5] As also mentioned previously, severe epistaxis resulting from a nasal fracture can result in airway compromise.

TIMING OF REPAIR

The best opportunity for successful reduction of a nasal fracture is within the first 3 hours of the injury.[1] But rarely is the patient seen within this time window. Usually several additional hours have passed, and swelling becomes a factor. Unless the above indications for immediate intervention are present or a particularly severe deformity is seen, the accepted practice is to discharge the patient with pain medications, antibiotics for any open wounds, and instructions for ice use, elevation of the head, and a follow-up appointment in 3 to 5 days. The window for repair in follow-up lies between the time needed for resolution of edema and natural fixation of the nasal bones. Most authors agree that the nasal bones become more difficult to move between 7 and 10 days from injury and are relatively fixed at 2 to 3 weeks past the injury.[16]

ANESTHESIA/ANALGESIA

The first decision to make regarding anesthesia is whether the nasal fracture will have an open or closed repair. As detailed further below, this decision depends on the complexity of the fracture, the presence of other injuries, including open wounds to the nose itself, and the presence of previous scarring or nasal injuries. If the decision for an open reduction is made, general anesthesia should be used.

For a closed reduction, local anesthesia is an option. Factors important in consideration of local versus general anesthesia include cooperativeness of the patient, patient expectations and needs, the patient's overall health, the cost difference, and the anticipated effort required to obtain an optimal reduction and stabilization. For instance, for intranasal examinations and simple reductions, topical anesthesia such as cocaine and Pontocaine often suffice. For significant manipulation of the skeleton, both topical and local infiltration might be necessary, whereas complicated reductions often require general anesthesia.[5,16]

The use of local anesthesia for simple reductions is common. Reduction of a simple nasal pyramid fracture under local anesthesia within 10 to 14 days after the traumatic injury is an accepted practice.[25] Multiple previous studies have shown that patients tolerate the manipulation under local anesthesia well and that the results with general, local, and local with sedation are similar.[26]

Local anesthesia consists of both topical and infiltration anesthetics. Topical anesthesia is important both for pain control and vasoconstriction and consists of pledgets soaked in either 4% cocaine or a 1:1 mixture of Pontocaine and oxymetazoline. With cocaine, it is important to remember to restrict the total amount to 8 mL of 4% cocaine.[27] The soaked pledgets should be placed in three places:

1. Along the dorsal aspect of the septum affecting the anterior ethmoid nerve and artery
2. Along the floor of the nose and septum affecting the nasopalatine nerve and sphenopalatine artery
3. Along the posterior edge of the middle turbinate affecting the sphenopalatine artery and nerve branches from the pterygopalatine ganglion

These pledgets should be left in place for 10 minutes to achieve maximal vasoconstriction and analgesia.

Infiltrated solutions can include 2% lidocaine with 1:100,000 epinephrine or a combination of 1% lidocaine with 1:100,000 epinephrine with 0.5% bupivacaine with 1:200,000 epinephrine. For less painful injections, the solutions can be buffered 1:10 with sodium bicarbonate. Areas for injection include:

1. The infraorbital foramen blocking the infraorbital nerve

2. Both above and below the bony nasal dorsum blocking the anterior ethmoid nerve and the infratrochlear nerve
3. The base of the columella blocking the internal nasal nerve branches
4. The nasal septum blocking the nasopalatine and anterior ethmoid nerves
5. The nasal floor blocking the palatine and superior alveolar nerve

Infiltration of these five regions provides complete anesthesia for the reduction of nasal fractures.[6,16]

REPAIR

A simplistic but worthwhile approach to nasal fracture repair is to identify the actual fracture and then reverse the force of injury.[16] The goals of management of nasal fractures that define the approach to repair include:

1. Restoration of a satisfactory appearance
2. Restoration of the nasal airway patency
3. Replacement of the bony and cartilaginous septum to the midline
4. Preservation of the nasal valve integrity
5. Prevention of complications, such as stenosis, septal perforation, columellar retraction, and saddle deformity
6. Avoidance of interference with future growth[9]

Approaches to repair include both closed and open reduction. The decision of open versus closed reduction of the nasal fracture is dependent on the timing of repair, the type of fracture, and patient expectations. As alluded to previously, closed reductions of nasal fractures should be performed within 3 to 7 days for children and within 5 to 10 days for adults from the time of injury. Difficulty in manipulating the fracture first appears 5 to 10 days postinjury and is nearly complete within 3 weeks if the patient is young and healthy.[6] Indications for closed reduction of nasal fractures include:

1. Unilateral fracture of the bony nasal pyramid with a stable nasal dorsum
2. Bilateral fracture with minor dislocation (less than half the width of the nasal bridge) without significant septal trauma
3. Disruption of an upper lateral cartilage from the nasal aperture[9,28]

Within the literature, much debate exists over outcome and patient satisfaction, especially with the long-term results. For example, in a 3-year follow-up study, Illum[29] found that 90% of the patients repaired with closed reduction were still fully satisfied with their results and that 82% had no cosmetic complaints. He concludes that closed reductions of nasal fractures affords satisfactory long-term results, and indications do not exist for a large number of open reductions.

In contrast, others have concluded that nasal bone fractures are routinely undermanaged with closed reduction procedures and should all be managed with some form of open technique. Like closed reductions, open reductions are ideally performed early, within 3 weeks of the injury. If the early window is missed, an open reduction can be performed 6 months postinjury when the bones have stabilized.[16] Indications for open reduction of nasal fractures include:

1. Extensive fracture dislocation of the nasal bones and septum
2. Nasal pyramid deviation greater than half the width of the nasal bridge
3. Fractures of the cartilaginous pyramid without dislocation of the bony nasal dorsum with or without dislocation of the upper lateral cartilages
4. An open septal fracture
5. When it is impossible to achieve optimal reduction using closed reduction[9,30]
6. Several months after a closed reduction where a defect persists[16]

It is important to approach the open technique conservatively, emphasizing reposition of the fractured elements rather the excising existing elements. Excessive excision can quickly lead to deficits in both contour and projection.[6]

CLOSED REDUCTION TECHNIQUE

The essential tools for closed reduction are adequate anesthesia, a Boies elevator, proper lighting, and the surgeon's fingers. As mentioned previously, the repair is approached by reversing the direction of force that caused the original fracture. The typical approach is to first reduce the bony nasal pyramid followed by reduction and stabilization of the septum. The bony pyramid is reduced using a combination of external digital pressure and intranasal instrument pressure to reduce the fracture. Two caveats are important. First, pressure should not be exerted too high on the nose; the bones are thick here and rarely fracture, yet the mucosa is easily torn and can result in difficult bleeding. Second, if the bones appear to be immobile, suspect a greenstick fracture that may need to be completed with an osteotome to allow for reduction. Reduction of the septum is approached by elevating the nasal pyramid followed by direct application of pressure to the displaced septal portion.[5,6,9,16] As outlined below, splinting follows reduction of the nasal fracture.

OPEN REDUCTION TECHNIQUE

Incisional approaches to open reduction of nasal fractures are dependent on the injuries present. Straightforward approaches include the traditional rhinoplasty incisions that expose the nasal skeleton. From the intranasal approach (usually an intercartilaginous incision), the dorsal nasal skin is elevated from the upper lateral cartilages in a supraperichondral plane. Further dissection in the subperiosteal plane directly exposes the nasal bone. This offers limited access if fixation of the skeleton is needed and may result in compromised blood supply due to excessive undermining of the comminuted segments. The septum is approached through an incision on the side of the dislocation with further access through the intercartilaginous incisions. For wider exposure, the open rhinoplasty approach is preferred. Although popular in the past, the "open-sky" incision (a transverse incision high on the dorsum connected to vertical incisions in the medial canthal region) is generally no longer used due to the visibility of the scars. Lastly, traumatic lacerations may be used for direct exposure.[5,6,9]

Once exposed, reduction is accomplished through both plating and wiring. Of particular use in shaping a comminuted fracture are 1-mm mesh plates.[16] Several caveats are important to remember in the open reduction. First, with the nasal bones mobilized, the incisors can serve as a midline reference.[16] Second, the base of the frontal bone or maxilla can serve as an anchor in plating, but thin small plates should be used and caution exercised in patients who wear glasses due to problems with skin erosion. If wires are used, 26- to 30-gauge is preferred; larger wires can produce palpable sharp edges. In addition, thick absorbable sutures in figure-of-eight patterns can be used in lieu of wire and will lock the bone into position.[5] Fourth, rasping should not be attempted near the fracture fragments due to a danger of devascularizing the bony segments. Fifth, the fractures should all be reduced prior to attempting repair of the soft tissue lacerations.[31] Lastly, the goal is to repair the injury and not necessarily alter the preinjury appearance.[9]

If full reduction of the bony fragments does not achieve adequate projection and support of the nasal skeleton, primary bone grafting should be considered.[6] Currently, the preferred method is a split calvarial bone graft. It is anchored to the frontal process with a small plate or a single lag screw.

Approaches to the fractured septal cartilage components are similar to that of the bony structures. Once reduced the cartilage can be held in place with small figure-of-eight sutures, transseptal mattress sutures, or septal splints sutured transseptally.[32] Healing usually results in a dense scar holding the segments within place.[5]

POSTREDUCTION SPLINTING AND PACKING

After reduction of the nasal fracture via both open and closed reduction, splinting is often required to retain the projection and dorsal support, prevent obstruction of the nasal airways, and ensure adherence of the soft tissues to the bony and cartilaginous skeleton. Nasal packing consisting of gauze with lubricating antibiotic is used only if the reduced nasal components are very unstable and prone to collapse. The packing is left in place for a maximum of 3 to 5 days due to concerns about its acting as a culture medium for bacteria, possibly resulting in toxic shock syndrome. More commonly, bilateral septal Silastic splints with transseptal sutures are used. The splints can be left in for up to 10 days but need to be monitored for erosion of the mucosa. With splinting and packing, crust formation can be minimized and patient comfort maximized with the use of normal saline nasal sprays. In addition, decongestants and steroid sprays can minimize inflammation of the nasal mucosa.[5,6,9]

Lastly, external splints can be left in place longer, provide addition support and protection, and serve as a reminder to the patient to exercise caution in regard to the nose. External splints are typically made of light pliable metal such as aluminum, plastered gauze, or thermoplastic material, and are held in place by both adhesives and tape.

NASO-ORBITAL-ETHMOID FRACTURES

CLINICAL ASSESSMENT

As with the clinical assessment of nasal fractures, the clinical assessment of a potential NOE fracture should proceed with a systematic approach to the patient. Again, of first importance in the examination of the trauma patient is the assessment of the ABCs: airway, breathing, and circulation. This should be followed by a complete head and neck examination, not just an exam for the consulted injury. Lastly, the mechanism of trauma and the history are important in determining the possible extent of injuries and help to focus the remainder of the examination. In addition, a preinjury photograph assures both the patient and physician that a preexisting deformity was not present. The photograph also allows for an estimation of the preinjury intercanthal distance.[33]

Suspicion of an NOE fracture should be increased in patients with a short and sunken nasal bridge, telecanthus, and a shortened palpebral fissure.[33] Specific examinations include measurement of the intercanthal distance. As a general rule, the intercanthal distance should be approximately one half of the interpupillary distance. A measurement of more than 35 mm suggests an NOE fracture, and more than 40 mm is diagnostic.[34] It should be mentioned that the more the nasal dorsum projects anteriorly, the smaller the intercanthal distance appears.[33]

Furthermore, physical exam should include palpation of the medial canthus using the thumb and index finger, checking for both movement and crepitus. Palpation of the nasal dorsum may reveal step-offs or incongruities. A traction test described as "grasping the margin of the lower eyelid and pulling laterally to test for asymmetry or 'give'" can identify laxity in the tendon.[10] The "gold standard" exam is the bimanual examination, in which a Kelly clamp is inserted intranasally and the tip placed against the medial orbital rim beneath the medial canthal tendon. The contralateral index finger is then placed externally over the medial orbital rim. The palpation is for instability with intranasal pressure placed over the tendon insertion site.[35]

In patients suspected of having a fracture, a CT scan with both axial and coronal images at 1.5-mm intervals is the most effective study. Plain radiographs do not provide sufficient detail.

Injuries associated with NOE fractures that need to be ruled out include frontal sinus fractures, ocular injuries, anterior cranial fossa injuries, and lacrimal injuries. Frontal sinus fractures are suggested by air-fluid levels on imaging studies, especially persistent ones.[11] As mentioned previously, every patient with facial trauma should be considered to be at risk for ocular injury. Previous studies have shown 67% of patients with facial fractures had concomitant ocular injuries.[22] A thorough ophthalmologic examination includes assessment of visual acuity, speed and symmetry of pupillary reaction, visual fields, and intraocular pressure in addition to visualization of the anterior and posterior chambers. Injury to the anterior cranial fossa is heralded by CSF rhinorrhea. Dural tears and pneumocephalus may be associated with this injury. Lastly, a laceration overlying the medial canthus should also raise the suspicion of disruption of the canalicular lacrimal system. Although not emergent, it will ultimately require repair over fine silicone tubes.[11]

CLASSIFICATION

The NOE fracture involves the lower two thirds of the medial orbital rim where the medial canthus is inserted.[30] A true NOE fracture includes five separate fractures: the lateral nose, the inferior orbital rim, the medial orbital ethmoid wall, the nasal maxillary buttress at the pyriform aperture, and the junction of the frontal process of the maxilla with the internal angular process of the frontal bone.[36]

Two major systems have been presented that attempt to classify the different NOE fractures and treatment approaches. The first by Gruss[37] in 1985 classifies NOE fractures as isolated or in combination with adjacent maxillofacial injures. The second, and more widely cited, by Markowitz et al[38] 1991, classifies NOE fractures by the various fracture patterns in relation to the attachment of the medial canthus, or central fragment.

The three patterns of NOE fractures are presented in Fig. **5–2**. As shown, type I fractures are the simplest, with a single bone fragment, the central fragment, including the medial canthal attachment. Type II NOE fractures are comminuted fractures of the bones of the NOE region; however, the fractures remain external to the attachment of the medial canthal tendon insertion. The central bone fragment remains intact. Type III NOE fractures are comminuted fractures of the NOE region, but the fractures extend into the bone bearing the medial canthal tendon insertion. The central bone fragment is fractured and the canthal tendon frequently disinserted. The method of treatment for this injury relates directly to the fracture classification.[38]

REPAIR

Immediate treatment of a NOE fracture is minimal and should focus on concomitant life-threatening injuries. Of primary importance is the treatment of associated central nervous system (CNS) and ocular injuries. This should be accompanied by closure of any lacerations once the patient is stabilized. If CSF rhinorrhea is seen, initial treatment includes elevation of the head of the patient's bed and neurosurgical consultation.[14]

Once the patient is stable and can withstand general anesthetic, repair of the NOE fracture can proceed. The two most important goals in the treatment of NOE injuries are, first, reestablishment of the intercanthal width and dorsal nasal height. Second, NOE fractures are probably better overcorrected with respect to intercanthal distance as the deformities associated with undercorrection have proven to be very difficult to treat secondarily.[33]

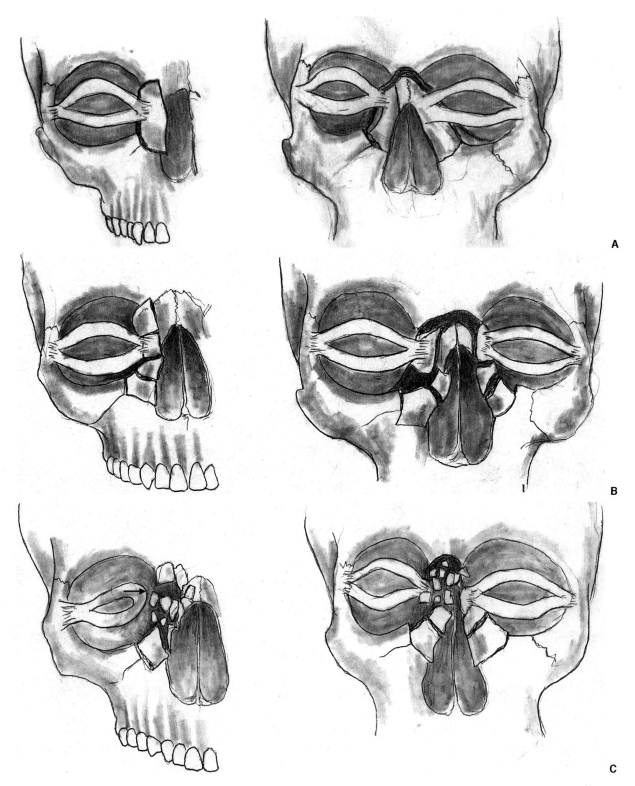

FIGURE 5–2   The three patterns of naso-orbital-ethmoid (NOE) fractures as classified by Markowitz et al[38] in 1991.
A: Type I NOE fracture with a single bone fragment, the central fragment, including the medial canthal attachment.
B: Type II NOE fracture with more comminution but the fractures remain external to the medial canthal attachment.
C: Type III NOE fracture with comminution extending into the bone bearing the medial canthal attachment.

The advent of open reduction and internal fixation (ORIF) of NOE fractures early following the injury has greatly improved on the results seen with delayed repair. In a delayed repair, extensive scar tissue must be mobilized in a thin and fragile region to release the misplaced central fragment and medial canthal tendon. This is usually associated with disappointing results.[10,11,14]

As shown in Fig. **5–3**, the approach for the repair is dictated by the fracture classification. Essentially all of these injuries require a coronal and a lower eyelid incision (preferably transconjunctival). Type I incomplete single fragment fractures are repaired by plate and screw fixation along the superior and inferior aspects of the fracture segment. The fixation is to the stable nasal process of the frontal bone and the frontal process of the maxilla. If the fragment is substantially displaced laterally, transnasal wires may be helpful in reduction.[11,13]

With a type II NOE fracture, after identifying the central fragment, transnasal (30-gauge) wires are passed through the nasal bone to exit on the side of the fracture at a point posterior and superior to the lacrimal fossa. The wire is then passed through the fracture fragment containing the canthal tendon and then back transnasally. It is secured to the region of the superomedial orbital rim either to the bone or to a microscrew. The other fracture fragments are secured using microplates. One must take great care in this dissection not to strip the canthal insertion on the fracture fragment.[11,13]

In the repair of the type III fracture, there is extensive comminution usually requiring bone grafting. Additionally the canthal tendon is detached from the bone segments. Reduction of the medial orbital wall proceeds, often requiring bone grafting to re-create a central fragment for reattachment of the canthal tendon. The preferred bone graft donor

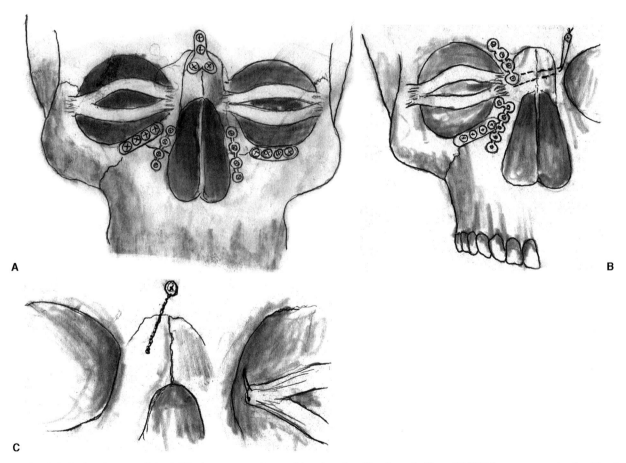

A

B

C

FIGURE 5–3 Repair of the NOE fracture as dictated by the classification. A: Type I NOE fracture repaired with plate and screw fixation along the superior and inferior aspects of the fracture segment. B: Type II NOE fracture repaired with transnasal stabilization of the central fragment bearing the medial canthal attachment and plate and screw fixation of the remaining fracture fragments. C: Transnasal wire fixation of the medial canthal tendon used in repair of a type III NOE fracture.

site is the outer table of the parietal skull. It is important to firmly fixate the graft to provide a stable anchor for medial canthal attachment. After reconstruction of the medial orbital wall, the canthus is reattached using transnasal reduction wires. The medial canthus is localized through a small vertical dermal incision over the canthus several millimeters medial to the commissure to avoid the lacrimal system. Then the wire is passed on either side of the canthal tendon through this dermal incision and the wire passed transnasally.[12]

Several considerations are important in the transnasal reduction of the medial canthus. First, symmetry is important. If one canthus is higher than the other, the literature suggests bringing the lower one higher to match.[33] Second, too anterior of a canthal position prevents the eyelid and lacrimal punctum from properly adhering to the globe. The tension placed on the wire is crucial. The wire should be tightened as much as possible to slightly overreduce the medial orbital rim.[33] As a general rule, it is hard to overcorrect the medial canthal position, whereas undercorrection (telecanthus) is frequently seen.

With the medial canthal tendon reduced, the remaining nasal fractures are approached. Loss of central nasal support is often found with NOE fractures. Reduction proceeds with the use of Asch forceps to straighten the fractured septum, centering it over the vomer and perpendicular plate of the ethmoid. This maneuver both re-creates the nasal projection and prevents airway compromise.[33]

Even with proper reduction of the nasal fractures, dorsal nasal support is frequently inadequate. This lack of support may result in a saddle nose deformity. In this setting, nasal bone grafts provide proper projection and narrowing of the nasal base. Appropriate grafts may be harvested from the outer table of the calvarium. The mostly cortical bone grafts are shaped similar to a surfboard with a width deemed appropriate for the patient's face and a length equal to the distance from the nasofrontal junction to 1 to 2 mm caudal to the cephalic end of the lower lateral cartilage. The graft is then inserted into a subcutaneous pocket below the lower lateral cartilages and secured to the nasofrontal junction using a single lag screw.[33] This increase in projection in the region of the radix also diminishes the appearance of telecanthus.

Soft tissue considerations in repair of the NOE fracture include both the skin and nasolacrimal system. After repair of lacerations and incisions, the skin is carefully redraped over the skeletal support. The adherence of the skin in the medial canthal region is also very important in obtaining a good result. Soft tissue bolsters are helpful in limiting edema and the accumulation of blood and fluid at the site of repair.[11,33] Routine exploration of the lacrimal system is not indicated in an NOE fracture unless there is obvious lacrimal system transection. Routine exploration may result in injury to the canaliculi.[11,38]

Lastly, in addition to the external splints described above, NOE fracture repairs are splinted in a similar fashion to the nasal fracture splinting described earlier. Intranasal splints protect the mucosa from synechia formation[10] and stent the corrected nasal structure during healing.

COMPLICATIONS

The most common complications in NOE fracture repair are residual cosmetic and functional defects. Inadequate treatment can result in a shortened and retruded nose, a shortened palpebral fissure, and telecanthus. These are typically difficult to correct secondarily, emphasizing the need for precise anatomic reduction at the time of primary repair. Other possible complications include epiphora and dacryocystitis resulting from lacrimal drainage problems. These are managed secondarily by reestablishing drainage into the lacrimal sac or nose.[14,38]

PEARLS: NASAL AND NASO-ORBITAL-ETHMOID FRACTURES

- Patients with nasal fracture should be carefully evaluated for the presence of septal fracture, and orbital and other midface fractures.
- Nasal fractures are usually reduced immediately after injury (if there is minimal swelling) or 5 to 10 days later, after the swelling has diminished. Indications for immediate surgical attention are open nasal fracture, nasal septal hematoma, and airway compromise.
- Closed reduction with splinting is usually adequate for nasal fractures, but open reduction is occasionally needed. Some authors argue that open reduction should be performed more frequently.
- The most important clinical feature of an NOE fracture is the position of the medial canthus of the eye. The appropriate intercanthal distance is about half of the interpupillary distance, with 30 to 35 mm being the typical distance.
- Axial CT scanning is perhaps the optimal radiologic view to assess NOE fractures.
- NOE fractures can be classified based on extent of injury, and the injury stage can direct treatment

planning. Treatment should consider the "central fragment" of bone, to which the canthal tendon is attached.

- The general principles of repair are ORIF of displaced bony fragments, with reattachment of the medial canthal tendon if needed, sometimes achieved with a transnasal wire. Undercorrection of the displaced medial canthal tendon is a common problem, so the surgeon should strive for meticulous reapproximation and perhaps attempted overcorrection.

- The surgical approach usually includes a bicoronal incision, and perhaps Lynch or inferior orbital rim incisions.

REFERENCES

1. Dingman RO, Natvig P. The nose. In: Dingman RO, Natvig P, eds. *Surgery of Facial Fractures*. Philadelphia: WB Saunders, 1969:267

2. Murray JA. Management of septal deviation with nasal fractures. Facial Plast Surg 1989;6:88–94

3. Breasted JH. Edwin Smith surgical papyrus. In: *Facsimile and Hieroglyphic Translation with Translation and Commentary*. Chicago: University of Chicago Press, 1930

4. Lascaratos JG, Segas JV, Trompoukis CC, Assimakopoulos DA. From the roots of rhinology: the reconstruction of nasal injuries by Hippocrates. Ann Otol Rhinol Laryngol 2003;112:159–162

5. Renner GJ. Management of nasal fractures. Otolaryngol Clin North Am 1991;24:195–213

6. Doerr TD, Arden RL, Mathog RH. Nasal fractures. In: Cummings CW, ed. *Otolaryngology–Head and Neck Surgery*, 3rd ed. St. Louis: Mosby, 1998:866–882

7. Murphy RX Jr, Birmingham KL, Okunski WJ, Wasser T. The influence of airbag and restraining devices on the patterns of facial trauma in motor vehicle collisions. Plast Reconstr Surg 2000;105:516–520

8. Simoni P, Ostendorf R, Cox AJ III. Effect of air bags and restraining devices on the pattern of facial fractures in motor vehicle crashes. Arch Facial Plast Surg 2003;5:113–115

9. Bailey BJ, Tan LKS. Nasal and frontal sinus fractures. In: Bailey BJ, ed. *Head and Neck Surgery–Otolaryngology*, 2nd ed. Philadelphia: Lippincott-Raven, 1998: 1007–1031

10. Vora NM, Fedok FG. Management of the central nasal support complex in naso-orbital ethmoid fractures. Facial Plast Surg 2000;16:181–191

11. Leipziger LS, Manson PN. Nasoethmoid orbital fractures. Current concepts and management principles. Clin Plast Surg 1992;19:167–193

12. Zide BM, McCarthy JG. The medial canthus revisited–an anatomical basis for canthopexy. Ann Plast Surg 1983;11:1–9

13. Hoffmann JF. Naso-orbital-ethmoid complex fracture management. Facial Plast Surg 1998;14:67–76

14. Duvall AJ, Banovetz JD. Nasoethmoidal fractures. Otolaryngol Clin North Am 1976;9:507–515

15. Shimoyama T, Kaneko T, Horie N. Initial management of massive oral bleeding after midfacial fracture. J Trauma 2003;54:332–336

16. Cox AJ III. Nasal fractures–the details. Facial Plast Surg 2000;16:87–94

17. Jordan LW. The management of acute injuries of the nasal septum. Laryngoscope 1967;77:1121–1129

18. Clark WD. Nasal and nasal septal fractures. Ear Nose Throat J 1983;62:352–356

19. Hinderer KH. Nasal problems in children. Pediatr Ann 1976;5:499–509

20. Colton JJ, Beekhuis GJ. Management of nasal fractures. Otolaryngol Clin North Am 1986;19:73–85

21. Holt GR. Nasal septal fractures. In: English GM, ed. *Otolaryngology*, rev. ed. Philadelphia: JB Lippincott, 1989

22. Holt GR, Holt JE. Incidence of eye injuries in facial fractures: an analysis of 727 cases. Otolaryngol Head Neck Surg 1983;91:276–279

23. Murray JA, Maran AG, Busuttil A, Vaughan G. A pathological classification of nasal fractures. Injury 1986;17:338–344

24. Harrison DH. Nasal injuries: their pathogenesis and treatment. Br J Plast Surg 1979;32:57–64

25. Jones TM, Nandapalan V. Manipulation of the fractured nose: a comparison of local infiltration anaesthesia and topical local anaesthesia. Clin Otolaryngol 1999;24:443–446

26. Green KM. Reduction of nasal fractures under local anaesthetic. Rhinology 2001;39:43–46

27. Mathog RH. Acute nasal fractures. In: Cummings CW, Fredrickson JM, Harker LA, Krause CJ, Schuller DE, eds. *Otolaryngology–Head and Neck Surgery*, vol 4. St. Louis: Mosby, 1986:xxxix, 3102, 3456

28. Verwoerd CD. Present day treatment of nasal fractures: closed versus open reduction. Facial Plast Surg 1992;8:220–223

29. Illum P. Long-term results after treatment of nasal fractures. J Laryngol Otol 1986;100:273–277

30. Weerda H, Siegert R. Stable fixation of the nasal complex. Facial Plast Surg 1990;7:185–188

31. Martinez SA. Nasal fractures. What to do for a successful outcome. Postgrad Med 1987;82:71–74

32. Farrior R. Management of late sequelae of nasal fractures. In: Mathog RH, ed. *Maxillofacial Trauma*. Baltimore: Williams & Wilkins, 1984:266–279

33. Ellis E III. Sequencing treatment for naso-orbito-ethmoid fractures. J Oral Maxillofac Surg 1993;51: 543–558

34. Paskert JP, Manson PN, Iliff NT. Nasoethmoidal and orbital fractures. Clin Plast Surg 1988;15:209–223

35. Paskert JP, Manson PN. The bimanual examination for assessing instability in naso-orbitoethmoidal injuries. Plast Reconstr Surg 1989;83:165–167

36. Evans GR, Clark N, Manson PN. Identification and management of minimally displaced nasoethmoidal orbital fractures. Ann Plast Surg 1995;35:469–473

37. Gruss JS. Naso-ethmoid-orbital fractures: classification and role of primary bone grafting. Plast Reconstr Surg 1985;75:303–317

38. Markowitz BL, Manson PN, Sargent L, et al. Management of the medial canthal tendon in nasoethmoid orbital fractures: the importance of the central fragment in classification and treatment. Plast Reconstr Surg 1991;87:843–853

Chapter 6

Ophthalmic and Optic Nerve Trauma

Charles N.S. Soparkar

Ophthalmic injuries are common in patients with facial trauma. Although reported incidences vary widely, most large series indicate serious, vision-threatening sequelae in the range of 15 to 20% of injuries.[1-7]

Early recognition of eye trauma is important for three reasons. First, many ophthalmic injuries have a better prognosis if managed urgently. Second, unrecognized, many such injuries can be exacerbated by periocular manipulations during facial fracture repair. Finally, ophthalmic deficits not recognized and documented before surgical intervention may be interpreted in this current age of rampant litigation as postsurgical complications. Thus, all physicians treating patients with midface trauma should have an appreciation of the fundamental principles of ophthalmic evaluation and emergency management. This chapter offers a simplified, practical guide for nonophthalmologists managing trauma, but it should not be viewed as a substitute for consultation by a qualified eye care provider if ocular injury is identified or strongly suspected. On the other hand, routinely requesting unnecessary ophthalmic consultation can slow down patient triage and care, add extra financial burden to the health care system, and strain relations with non–hospital-based consultants.

The Eye Examination

Visual Acuity

Effective eye evaluation requires a basic understanding of ocular function. The main purpose of the eye is to focus either parallel or divergent light rays onto the retina at the back of the eye, providing not only light perception, but also fine two-point discrimination, so-called *visual acuity*. In general, we record normal visual acuity as 20/20. This means the person being tested can see at 20 feet what the "average" person can see at this same distance. Decreased visual acuity of 20/50 indicates the individual being tested can see at 20 feet what the average person can see at 50 feet, whereas someone with spectacular 20/10 vision can see at 20 feet what the average person must be 10 feet away to see.

Combined, the tear film and the corneal curvature provide roughly 60% of the eye's convergent refractive power. The remaining 40% of the eye's light-bending power is found mainly in the intraocular lens, which in youth is able to thicken and increase refractive power, allowing the eye to focus on objects closer to us than 6 m (European infinity equivalent) or 20 feet (U.S. infinity equivalent). The ability to focus on objects closer than 20 feet away is part of a complex process called *accommodation* that starts to diminish (so-called *presbyopia*) in most people ($\sim$ 60%) over the age of 40 years, hence the need for reading glasses. Clearly, then, the majority of people screened in emergency departments over the age of 40 using a "near-vision card" without corrective lenses will test as having diminished vision, even though their distance vision is perfectly normal. In addition, a near-vision card is standardized for use at exactly 33 cm from the subject's eyes. If the card is held closer, the numbers will be larger than they should be, and more accommodation will be required. Likewise, if a presbyopic individual holds the card farther away than 33 cm to bring it into focus, the numbers will appear smaller and decreased vision may be recorded.

To further complicate matters, swelling of the upper eyelid or in the orbit can minutely deform the eye, temporarily altering the patient's refractive needs and leading to spuriously low vision testing. Alternatively, serious ocular injuries, such as a

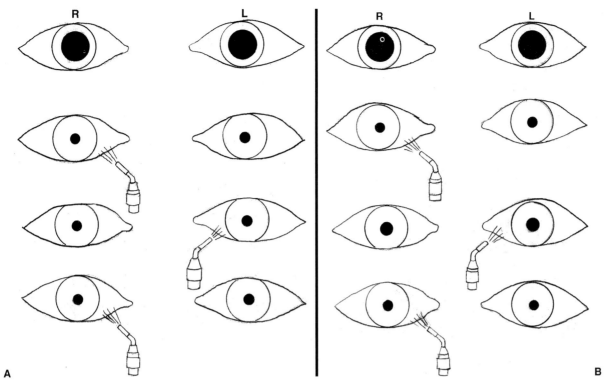

FIGURE 6–1   Evaluation for an afferent papillary defect. A: A normal examination. B: A relative afferent pupillary defect in the left eye.

penetrating scleral laceration or a peripheral retinal tear may have no immediate effect on central visual acuity. Therefore, although visual acuity is perhaps the best single test of overall ocular function and integrity, accurate testing is often very difficult (if not impossible) in the emergency room setting, and "good" vision should provide no more reassurance than "bad" vision creates concern. Bad vision often results from such innocuous things as lack of appropriate spectacle correction, blood or mucus in the tear film, and poor effort due to anxiety, pain, or intoxication.

Importantly, an eye that can see no light at all is a clear indication of severe ophthalmic injury, unless, of course, the patient is malingering—a complicated topic that is beyond the scope of this chapter. Because vision testing in the setting of trauma can be an unreliable measure of ophthalmic status, there are nine additional examination steps commonly performed, as described in the following subsections.

EXTERNAL EXAMINATION

Gross inspection of the eye and ocular adnexa is very important. Lacerations and contusions over the lateral eyebrow or in the mid-glabella are worrisome for the association with *posttraumatic optic neuropathy* (discussed below). Eyelid lacerations are also

concerning, as they may be full-thickness with underlying globe injury. Remember that forced closure of the eye, such as often occurs in anticipation of a blow, creates upward rotation of the globe behind the closed eyelids, known as *Bell's phenomenon*. Therefore, when exploring a through-and-through upper eyelid injury, don't forget to look at the inferior corneal limbus, often hidden beneath the margin of the lower eyelid. Fat prolapsing through an eyelid cut is strongly suggestive of orbital penetration, and foreign bodies are often difficult to identify in the billowing adipose.

Blunt trauma to the eyelids often results in a medial, full-thickness defect involving the eyelid margin. In most cases, due to a relative, focal weakness in the medial canthal tendon, this occurs medial to the punctum, creating a laceration in the canaliculus that should be repaired under magnification and stented with Silastic tubing. Conversely, posttraumatic telecanthus is almost never the result of the medial canthal tendon pulling off the lacrimal bone. Instead, the nasal side wall is fractured, and the bone fragment moves laterally with the still-attached canthal tendon insertion.

General surveillance of the eyelids, ocular surface, and ocular adnexa should include palpation of the orbital rims, as well as assessment of cranial nerve V and VII function.

OPTIC NERVE FUNCTION ASSESSMENT

In the verbal, cooperative patient, two of the best tests of overall optic nerve function are subjective red color saturation and light intensity. In the former test, a red object (such as a very bright penlight shined through a finger) is presented to one eye at a time. The patient is asked whether the color is of equal color and intensity in both eyes. If an optic nerve has suffered significant injury, the ipsilateral color perception will be altered. The red object will appear more "dull," "orange," or "brown" than it does with the contralateral eye. Even patients with color appreciation deficiencies (8% of males in the U.S.), but not the most severe, rare forms of true color blindness, will be able to tell a difference. The light intensity test is similar, but is performed with a bright white light and in general is less sensitive although more useful if there has been trauma within the eye. For example, an eye filled with blood will still see about the same light intensity as an eye that is not. Additionally, eyes with unequal-sized pupils may appreciate differences in the low illumination of a red color test, whereas a brighter stimulus of a white light will look more similar. Because the bright white light can temporarily "bleach" the retina, the red color test should be performed first. Importantly, both tests yield a falsely normal result if there is equal compromise of both optic nerves. This is more likely to occur from ischemic optic neuropathy associated with low blood pressure and severe anemia than from traumatic injury.

PUPIL EVALUATION

Although the tests described above for optic nerve function are usually considerably more sensitive than a pupil evaluation, in the nonverbal or uncooperative patient the pupil examination may be the only measure of total ocular function available.

There are three parts to a pupil exam. First, the appearance of the pupils should be recorded. This includes both the shape and size of each pupil. An irregularly shaped pupil (corectopia), especially a teardrop-shaped pupil, should raise concern about an anterior penetrating injury to the eye. The point of the teardrop may point toward a laceration, where the iris has become incarcerated and sealed the wound.

Pupil size has no relationship to optic nerve function or visual potential. Instead, pupil size is determined by sympathetic fibers traveling along cranial nerve (CN) V and parasympathetic fibers traveling along the inferior division of CN III, whereas vision is dependent on CN II, the optic nerve. A totally blind eye is likely to have a normal-sized pupil, and an eye with a "blown" dilated pupil may have totally normal vision. Remember also that many systemic medications, such as narcotics and recreational drugs, can affect pupil size.

The second part of the pupil examination is determination of the reactivity of the pupils to bright light. View each pupil independently and record the degree of reactivity. A good grading system understood by all nonophthalmologists is "trace," "sluggish," and "brisk." Then swing the light from one eye to the other and back to determine whether there is a relative afferent pupillary defect (Fig. **6–1**). An easy way to test this is to watch just one pupil, say the left. Shine the light in the left eye and watch the degree of constriction. Then, while still watching the left pupil, shine the light into the right eye. The left pupil should minimally dilate in the time it takes to move the light from one eye to the next and should then constrict to the same degree as when the light was shined in the left eye. If the left pupil did not constrict as well or even dilated with the light shined in the left eye as compared with when the light was shined in the right eye, then there is a serious problem somewhere along the left visual pathway (retina, optic nerve, optic chiasm, or optic tract).

The third and final part of the pupil examination is assessment of miosis during near synkinesis, often erroneously referred to as pupillary accommodation. This test, in fact, is of little value when evaluating eye trauma, especially if the remainder of the pupil examination is normal, and more properly belongs as part of a complex neurologic evaluation.

In the setting of trauma, carefully performing and recording a pupil examination is always critical. Too often "PERRLA" (pupils equal, round, react to light and accommodation) is jotted on the chart. Not only is this notation nonsensical, as explained above, but it also doesn't effectively convey the status of the visual and neurologic systems, an error that can have profound consequences if disorders are missed. A better description might be "Pupils: 4 mm, round, briskly and equally reactive to light."

VISUAL FIELD DETERMINATION

In the trauma setting, visual field testing in an awake and fully cooperative patient can be more revealing than visual acuity determination. There are three parts to the visual field analysis. The first, central visual field, evaluates overall macular function. There are several formal testing mechanisms, such as the Amsler grid, but a simplified test is to stand roughly 2 feet from the patient, cover one of the patient's eyes, ask the patient to focus on your nose, and while doing so, the patient should be able to appreciate all the features of your face, including your ears, without any "dark" or "blurry" spots. Repeat this test for the patient's second eye.

To assess peripheral visual field, position yourself 2 to 3 feet in front of the patient with both you and the patient covering one eye. If the patient covers the left eye, you should cover your right eye. Then, with your contralateral hand equidistant between your two heads, bring a wiggling finger in from the far periphery. Have the patient tell you when the moving finger is first visible. You and the patient should see the finger at about the same time.

The third part of visual field analysis, double simultaneous confrontation, more properly belongs as part of a complex neurologic evaluation.

Penlight Examination

With a penlight, an assessment should be made of the conjunctiva, the cornea, the anterior chamber, and the lens. The conjunctiva, the thin mucous membrane covering the eye, runs from the edge of the cornea, across the surface of the eye, and up the insides of the eyelids almost to the eyelashes in the upper and lower eyelids. Vascular hyperemia of the conjunctiva gives a "red eye" or "pink eye" appearance that is nonspecific for ocular surface inflammation and irritation. The conjunctival examination should focus on identifying any foreign bodies, tears in the conjunctiva, and chemosis (conjunctival swelling, either pale or hemorrhagic). Although most subconjunctival blood is simply indicative of a bruise to the eye, more worrisome injuries must be ruled out, such as focal globe penetration with intraocular contents extrusion below the blood. Further, pale (nonhemorrhagic) chemosis (conjunctival swelling) may represent an occult globe rupture and subconjunctival accumulation of ocular aqueous fluid that belongs in the anterior chamber.

The cornea and lens should appear clear with intact red reflex through both. Clouding of the cornea most likely suggests either old scar or acute microbial keratitis (corneal infection), and clouding of the lens is generally a cataract. Some types of posttraumatic cataracts can develop acutely.

The anterior chamber is the area between the cornea and the iris or lens. This space should be totally clear, and there should be an appreciable depth to the eye. If the anterior chamber is "flat," and there is no space between the cornea and the iris, an occult globe rupture must be suspected. Red blood cells filling the anterior chamber are called a *hyphema*, and white pus in the anterior chamber is called a *hypopyon*.

Intraocular Pressure Measurement

A globe rupture must be excluded before performing any manipulation of the eye itself. Most techniques for evaluating the intraocular pressure are not amenable to being performed by a casual and infrequent examiner. Two exceptions are Shiötz and Tonopen tonometry, the latter being simpler. Both of these are hand-held contact devices that require prior administration of a local anesthetic to the eye. Specific, detailed directions for using these devices are generally included with the packaging of the instruments. Note that contrary to frequently published recommendations in trauma and ophthalmic texts, very high intraocular pressure created by increasing orbital volume, as might occur with orbital hemorrhage, should *not* be managed by passing a needle into the anterior chamber. This does not significantly lower intraocular pressure and it results in a flat anterior chamber, possibly creating even higher intraocular pressure by occluding the trabecular meshwork and blocking aqueous outflow.

Motility

There are essentially two parts to a motility examination. The first is to determine whether the eyes work together while the patient is looking straight ahead, the so-called primary gaze position. If there is sufficient vision to see an object, such as a finger held at 3 feet, and the vision is roughly equal in both eyes, it is adequate to ask cooperative patients whether or not they see two images and have double vision. The finger should be held first vertically and then horizontally to check for diplopia in both primary meridians. If present, the type of diplopia should be recorded (e.g., vertical, horizontal, torsional, or a combination at 3 feet). More complex testing and data interpretation are beyond the scope of an emergency room, posttraumatic evaluation.

The second part of the motility examination tests eye movement in each of the six major gaze positions off of primary: left, right, up and in, up and out, down and out, and down and in. Most significant movement disorders are picked up with an even more simplified examination testing just up, down, left, and right gaze. If "normal" movement is detected, it is imperative that the test used be clearly noted in the medical record. For example, if only four positions of movement are tested, a "+" should be entered, as opposed to an "H" if six positions are examined. Trained eye care providers carefully quantify and denote underacting and overacting movements in each eye, but for the uninitiated, simply writing "the left eye has trouble in upgaze" is probably adequate.

Although we are recommending a truncated examination, when evaluating midface trauma, especially orbital fractures, a carefully performed and documented ocular motility assessment is critical. Globally restricted movement suggests significant orbital swelling, whereas limited movement much worse in one meridian (e.g., vertical, up and down gaze), is worrisome for an inferior rectus muscle entrapment requiring correlation with computed tomographic (CT) imaging and perhaps urgent fracture repair.

Children under the age of 12 years, and certainly under the age of 6 years, are at risk for developing amblyopia if they do not use their eyes together. Therefore, children with likely muscle entrapment should undergo surgical repair urgently.

Fundus Examination

Examination of the retina, optic nerve, and retinal vessels is the most technically difficult part of an eye evaluation, especially through an undilated pupil and using a direct ophthalmoscope. Nevertheless, it should be performed. Dilating the pupil with 1% Mydriacyl and 2.5% phenylephrine can greatly facilitate the examination. If there is any question about vision, optic nerve injury, or visual field, pupil-altering drops should not be placed in both eyes until thorough assessment by an eye-care provider has been completed. However, one eye can usually be dilated without problem, but be sure to mark clearly in the chart and advise nursing personnel that one pupil has been dilated.

If an accomplished observer finds that there is a good red reflex, but no view of the retina or a portion of the retina is possible, then perhaps the posterior (vitreous) chamber is filled with blood. If there is a large white or pale area instead of a continuous red retina, retinal ischemia (many hours old) or ocular contusion are possible. A retinal detachment may be most easily recognized by large undulating folds in a pale-appearing retina or by finding that while holding the power correction constant in the direct ophthalmoscope, different parts of the retina are out of focus as compared with others, indicating that the retina is sitting at different levels.

Imaging

Important information regarding the eye may be gained by magnetic resonance imaging (MRI), plain film radiography, ultrasonography, traditional angiography, and fluorescein angiography, but the single most useful imaging study in the setting of trauma is probably a CT scan. Relative to the CT, plain films are often not as sensitive, and their evaluation is becoming a lost art, especially among younger radiologists often on-call in the middle of the night. MRI is contraindicated in the potential presence of metal foreign bodies, more expensive, often more difficult to obtain quickly, and does not show bone as well. Finally, other CT imaging of the brain and midface is often being performed anyway to rule out other injuries. For the orbit, 3-mm sections are usually sufficient, unless a small foreign body is being sought. Coronal images are preferred over axials, although the combination is most helpful.

Eye Exam Summary

With a little practice, careful evaluation of all of the above parts of the eye examination can be rapidly performed and will identify the vast majority of ophthalmic difficulties. If an eye problem is uncovered, then formal consultation by a trained eye care provider is warranted.

True Ophthalmic Emergencies

Although there are many ocular insults that require rapid attention, the two ophthalmic emergencies where every minute may count are chemical exposure (in particular alkaline substances) and a stroke to the eye.

Industrial chemicals are more likely to be acid, whereas solutions found in the home are more likely to be alkaline, and the latter is generally more dangerous for the eye. The treatment in either case is copious irrigation with any neutral irrigant such as water, normal or half-normal saline, or even lactated Ringer's. First placing a topical anesthetic in the eye will greatly facilitate the process. The use of irrigating contact lenses should be avoided, as these can trap chemical particles within the ocular fornices and continue to release injurious substances. If there is evidence of cutaneous eyelid injury, a white appearance to the eye is a bad prognostic sign, indicating severe ocular surface ischemia. In the presence of severe chemical exposure, 10 to 20 L of irrigation may be appropriate. The best way to determine when enough irrigation has been performed is to check for a pH of 7 in the inferior ocular fornix, wait 10 minutes and check again. In the absence of narrow-range pH paper, a urine dipstick (trimmed if necessary) provides at least some indication.

Based on monkey studies, the best hope for vision return after a stroke to the eye comes with intervention implemented within 94 minutes of the insult.

In an ophthalmic stroke, the patient reports sudden vision loss, and the only objective finding is an afferent pupillary defect. Other things, such as posttraumatic optic neuropathy, can present in this fashion, but a vascular accident must always be considered. Intervention should be individualized and directed by someone trained in managing this emergency.

ORBITAL COMPARTMENT SYNDROME

Orbital compartment syndrome warrants special discussion because it can develop in the setting of trauma and lead to rapidly blinding ophthalmic stroke. Any sudden increase in orbital pressure can create a compartment syndrome, and the two most common offenders after trauma are air (orbital emphysema) and blood.

Sneezing with the mouth closed can generate wind velocities over 200 mph. If there is an orbital fracture with sinus communication, the air may be forced into the orbit. As the pressure head finally drops, orbital fat falls back into the bone defect, acting as a ball valve and trapping the large volume of air. Nose blowing to evacuate blood can have the same effect. Sudden increases in orbital pressure may lead to arterial spasm or true compression, resulting in ophthalmic stroke. Treatment in vision-compromised patients consists of expeditious air evacuation, either through open surgical technique or CT-guided needle aspiration.

Alternatively, lysis of the lateral canthal tendon (inferior crus, superior crus, or both) can rapidly decrease orbital pressure. This requires very little skin incision and fully releases the eyelid when done correctly. In the setting of an active orbital hemorrhage, cantholysis must be performed with caution, as continued bleeding with growing posterior pressure can lead to progressive proptosis and stretch optic neuropathy (or even very rarely partial optic nerve avulsion). The most likely culprit of such heavy bleeding is the infraorbital artery, although the anterior and/or posterior ethmoidal arteries may also contribute. The treatment then is emergent orbital exploration to obtain artery control.

POSTTRAUMATIC OPTIC NEUROPATHY

Posttraumatic optic neuropathy (PTON) is vision loss of any degree from optic nerve injury following head trauma. Causes of PTON include direct optic nerve injury, bone impingement on the nerve, nerve ischemia, and nerve compression from intrinsic or extrinsic hematoma or edema. Often, more than one mechanism is involved. In the most common scenario, PTON develops following a blow to the lateral eyebrow, mid-glabella, or sometimes even the occiput. Bone vibrations are transmitted to the optic canal where the optic nerve sheath is rigidly fixated to the periosteum. Although optic canal fractures (with or without displacement of bone fragments) and blood in the sphenoid sinus are strongly associated with the development of PTON, optic nerve injury may arise from surprisingly little trauma and in the absence of any fractures.

Optic neuropathy may affect any or all of the following: visual acuity, visual field, pupillary response, and color perception. Yet, in our experience, red color desaturation is perhaps the most sensitive indicator of PTON in the emergency room, posttraumatic setting.

The management of PTON remains highly controversial, and a thorough discussion of the issues surrounding PTON treatment are beyond the scope of this chapter, but in our practice we take an aggressive approach and have seen remarkable vision recoveries with combined intravenous corticosteroid therapy and optic canal surgical decompression. Vision improvement may be obtained months after injury, but we continue to believe that the best visual prognosis is achieved with the introduction of intervention as early as possible.

CORNEAL EXPOSURE

Many head trauma patients suffer from multiple medical problems and are unable to protect their eyes due to cranial nerve VII injuries, gross exophthalmos, periocular lacerations or tissue loss, or deficient blink rate or eyelid excursion. Although a suture tarsorrhaphy can be temporarily curative, the eye becomes hidden, and any complications will go unnoticed. Instead, we advocate the frequent use of thick, lubricating ointment. Pure petroleum jelly (Vaseline) is an inexpensive option. Alternatively, a clear adhesive dressing, as is used to dress intravenous line sites, can be applied directly over the eye. It does not stick to the wet eye itself, but adheres strongly to the surrounding skin and forms an effective moisture chamber.

SUMMARY

Being able to recognize ophthalmic injury is an essential skill for all physicians managing patients with head and face trauma. Not only do many eye injuries require timely intervention for sight preservation, but the globe manipulation and increased orbital pressure that occur during normal orbital fracture repair may dramatically exacerbate any occult visual pathway problems, leading to postoperative vision loss.

Pearls: Ophthalmic and Optic Nerve Trauma

- In the emergency room setting, the single best indicators of overall visual pathway function are the red color saturation test in a cooperative patient and the pupillary examination in a nonverbal patient.
- A patient-appropriate, 10-step ophthalmic examination can be rapidly performed and will identify the vast majority of eye injuries.
- Three-millimeter coronal section CT imaging is an appropriate screening study for suspected orbital trauma.
- Globally decreased ocular motility is less suggestive of muscle entrapment than decreased eye movement within a single gaze position or gaze meridian.
- The diagnosis of muscle entrapment within an orbital fracture requires a correlation of clinical and radiographic findings. Truly entrapped muscles should be rapidly surgically released.
- Alkali exposure and ophthalmic vascular accidents are two eye insults in which every minute may count.
- Nose blowing in the presence of an orbital fracture may lead to orbital emphysema and blindness.

- Orbital compartment syndrome, from whatever cause, is often effectively managed emergently by a skillful lateral canthotomy and cantholysis.
- Posttraumatic optic neuropathy is common in head and face trauma and requires rapid recognition and intervention.
- Corneal exposure can be avoided using Vaseline or clear intravenous adhesive dressings applied directly over the eye.

References

1. al-Qurainy IA, Stassen LF, Dutton GN, Moos KF, el-Attar A. The characteristics of midfacial fractures and the association with ocular injury: a prospective study. Br J Oral Maxillofac Surg 1991;29:291–301
2. al-Qurainy IA, Stassen LF, Dutton GN, Moos KF, el-Attar A. Midfacial fractures and the eye: the development of a system for detecting patients at risk of eye injury. Br J Oral Maxillofac Surg 1991;29:363–367
3. Brown MS, Ky W, Lisman RD. Concomitant ocular injuries with orbital fractures. J Craniomaxillofac Trauma 1999;5:41–46
4. Cook T. Ocular and periocular injuries from orbital fractures. J Am Coll Surg 2002;195:831–834
5. Holt GR, Holt JE. Incidence of eye injuries in facial fractures: an analysis of 727 cases. Otolaryngol Head Neck Surg 1983;91:276–279
6. Manolidis S, Weeks BH, Kirby M, Scarlett M, Hollier L. Classification and surgical management of orbital fractures: experience with 111 orbital reconstructions. J Craniofac Surg 2002;13:726–737
7. Poon A, McCluskey PJ, Jill DA. Eye injuries in patients with major trauma. J Trauma 1999;46:494–499

Chapter 7

ORBITAL FRACTURES

Michael G. Stewart and Charles N.S. Soparkar

The orbit is composed of seven bones: ethmoid, maxilla, zygoma, lacrimal, palatine, sphenoid, and frontal (Fig. **7–1**). The anterior projection of the orbit, the orbital rim, is relatively thick and acts as part of the facial structural buttress system, whereas the orbital walls are relatively thin, fracture more easily, and thus act as "shock absorbers" for injurious forces downloaded around the globe. In the deepest portion of the orbit, the bony walls thicken again, providing further protection for the middle cranial fossa. The orbital periosteum lining the walls is usually called the periorbita.

The orbit is shaped something like a cross between a pyramid and an egg (Fig. **7–2**), with the largest cross-sectional area behind the orbital rim, as the orbital roof curves slightly upward, and the floor slopes gently downward. The equator of the globe usually lies at this position of maximum orbital diameter. The medial orbital rim is discontinuous around the lacrimal fossa, so that the orbital rim actually creates a spiral.

The optic canal, located within the lesser wing of the sphenoid, enters the orbit at the orbital apex and contains the optic nerve and the ophthalmic artery. The orbit does not form a symmetrical cone, and the optic canal is relatively medial and superior to the "geometric" apex. The superior orbital fissure separates the greater and lesser wings of the sphenoid, and contains cranial nerves III, IV, and VI; V_1, the ophthalmic division of the trigeminal nerve; and sometimes the supraorbital vein draining the superior orbit and sub-brow region. The inferior orbital fissure contains the infraorbital nerve and more venous drainage from the orbit. The anterior and posterior ethmoid arteries enter the orbit through small foramina in the medial wall, and a line through these arteries and the optic canal essentially defines the position of the skull base along the medial orbital wall. The infraorbital nerve also travels in a canal in the orbital floor and is frequently impinged upon by orbital floor fractures.

The intraorbital soft tissue anatomy is also important. The globe forms the base of a cone defined by the extraocular muscles. The apex of this cone (called the muscle cone) is the annulus of Zinn that surrounds the optic canal and straddles the middle portion of the superior orbital fissure. Orbital fat both fills and surrounds the muscle cone, cushioning the posterior aspect of the globe. A fine network of ligaments runs throughout the orbital fat, setting up a scaffold and interconnecting the extraocular muscles and the periorbita.[1] Because all the orbital soft tissue is so interconnected, herniation and partial entrapment of the orbital fat can result in decreased globe mobility and diplopia, even if the extraocular muscles themselves are not directly entrapped.

IMAGING

The orbital rims and orbital floor are best imaged by computed tomography (CT) scan. The coronal view is best for the orbital roof and floor, and axial views often provide the most information about the medial and lateral orbital walls. The orbit is often well visualized on plain facial x-rays; the rims are best seen with a Caldwell view, and the orbital floor is best visualized with a Waters view. Unfortunately, interpretation of plain facial x-rays is a vanishing skill, and many clinically significant orbital fractures (especially small fractures of the orbital floor) can be missed when plain x-rays are used as a screening tool. Therefore, if there is a clinical suspicion of an orbital fracture, CT imaging should be obtained. In the absence of a horizontal gaze problem, 3-mm coronal sections usually provide adequate screening.

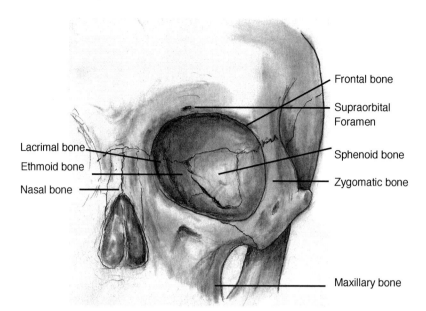

Frontal bone

Supraorbital
Foramen

Sphenoid bone

Zygomatic bone

Lacrimal bone

Ethmoid bone

Nasal bone

Maxillary bone

FIGURE 7–1 Orbital bony anatomy: frontal view.

The patient's exposure to ionizing radiation and the institutional cost of this approach is usually not significantly different from obtaining a plain film series. If the coronal images indicate an abnormality, axial images can then be obtained.

CLINICAL ASSESSMENT

With any orbital fracture, the patient should be evaluated for possible eye and optic nerve injury;

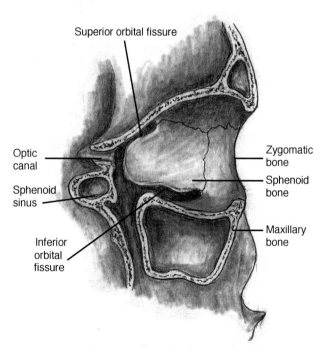

Superior orbital fissure

Optic
canal

Sphenoid
sinus

Inferior
orbital
fissure

Zygomatic
bone

Sphenoid
bone

Maxillary
bone

FIGURE 7–2 Orbital bony anatomy: lateral wall view.

this is discussed in Chapter 6. Fortunately, blinding ocular injuries are infrequent, but more minor injuries are fairly common and must be recognized and managed.

Aside from potential injuries to the eye and optic nerve, the important clinical sequelae of orbital fractures are globe malposition (most commonly enophthalmos and hypoglobus), extraocular muscle entrapment with diplopia, and infraorbital nerve hypesthesia. Orbital fractures are sometimes missed on physical examination when patients are evaluated early, because the periorbital and intraorbital edema can obscure the rim deformities and enophthalmos, which present later as the edema resolves. Conversely, orbital edema caused by trauma can cause reduced extraocular motility and diplopia, which resolves as edema diminishes. Although not always true, a good rule of thumb is that edema globally reduces motility, whereas entrapment usually presents with decreased movement in only one or two directions. Recognizing muscle entrapment in the face of considerable orbital edema can be very challenging, especially when the CT scan shows prolapse of a muscle belly into a sinus, but it is unclear whether or not there is actual muscle entrapment. Thus, physical examination is important, but physical findings, clinical history, and radiologic evaluation must all be integrated in evaluating a patient with suspected orbital fractures.

Isolated orbital rim fractures are rare, but they can have important clinical effects. Some rim fractures are palpable and bothersome to the patient, but even a palpable rim step-off is usually not visible. However, an orbital rim fracture can cause apparent enophthalmos by two mechanisms. First, a relatively small outward displacement in the orbital rim can create large volume changes within the pyramid-shaped orbit. Second, orbital rim fractures involving the lateral wall can change the position of the lateral canthal tendon, creating an apparent enophthalmos.

Fractures limited to the walls behind the orbital rim may result from either blunt or penetrating trauma. Blunt trauma causing a pure orbital wall blowout fracture most commonly involves an object larger than the opening of the orbit, such as a fist. Forces downloaded onto the orbital rim are spread broadly and create either a buckling effect on deeper orbital bones or an increase in orbital pressure as the globe is forced backward and the thin orbital bones are fractured outward. Trauma with thinner objects, such as a steering wheel, will often cause tremendous localized force, resulting in a combined orbital rim and wall fracture.

INJURY PATTERNS

Orbital wall fractures are usually called "blowout" fractures because the typical pattern is distraction of the orbital wall fragments outside the orbit—into the maxillary sinus for floor fractures, or the ethmoid sinus for medial wall fractures. In this way, the orbital walls serve as effective shock absorbers for forces around the globe, fracturing away from the orbit and absorbing the force of blunt trauma, thus protecting the eye.

"Blow-in" fractures of the orbital walls occur less commonly, but can result in exophthalmos as well as medialization (from lateral injuries) or hypoglobus (from a superior blow-in). The most common location of a blow-in fracture is the orbital roof in young children (with the floor of the frontal sinus buckling in adolescents after a blow to the brow), and the lateral wall in adults (especially associated with zygomatic-maxillary fractures).

Although the medial wall is the thinnest orbital wall, the orbital floor is more frequently fractured. This is probably because the thin septa between the ethmoid air cells act as supporting struts for the medial wall. Nevertheless, orbital floor, medial wall, as well as combined fractures are all common.

Medial wall, orbital floor, and some orbital roof fractures communicate with the paranasal sinuses. In these cases, patients should be carefully counseled about preoperative and postoperative nose blowing. Sneezing (which can generate wind velocities in excess of 200 mph) should be performed with the mouth open. Increased pressure in the nose or sinuses can cause forced air entry into the orbit. As pressure falls in the sinuses, the orbital fat may fall back into the bone defect, acting as a ball valve and

maintaining high pressure within the orbit. Significant orbital emphysema can lead to ophthalmic artery occlusion and total blindness.

Lateral orbital wall and rim fractures are most frequently associated with zygomatic complex fractures (and sometimes LeFort fractures) and with frequent associated injuries to the inferior orbital rims and orbital floors. Orbital roof fractures usually occur along with frontal sinus and/or skull fractures. Superior orbital rim fractures are associated with frontal sinus, nasal, and naso-orbital ethmoid fractures. Medial orbital rim fractures are often associated with nasal or naso-orbital-ethmoid complex fractures.

SURGICAL INDICATIONS

Orbital injuries are frequently seen in patients with other facial trauma, such as zygomatic complex fractures. The management of orbital issues related to these more extensive injury patterns is discussed in Chapter 8, whereas here we limit our discussion to isolated orbital fractures. However, when treating the orbital component of any facial fracture, the same principles apply.

As in any trauma patient, timing of surgical intervention may depend on other injuries and the overall condition of the patient. Additionally, considerable controversy has surrounded recommendations for the timing and indications of orbital surgery, but in the last two decades, most surgeons have now reached a management consensus. In general, late fracture repair is more difficult than earlier repair because of soft tissue scarring (especially if the extraocular muscles are involved) and bones healing in abnormal positions. Therefore, if orbital fracture repair is indicated (Table 7–1), the sooner it is performed after the initial swelling has subsided, the better.

ORBITAL RIM FRACTURES

If not causing facial instability or cosmetic deformity, isolated orbital rim fractures do not always require reduction or fixation. Because the rims lie under such a thin layer of skin, even the smallest plates can still be palpable and sometimes visible. However, open reduction and internal fixation for isolated fractures is relatively straightforward. When an orbital rim fracture is identified, the patient should be carefully evaluated for associated injuries.

TABLE 7–1 INDICATIONS FOR ORBITAL WALL FRACTURE REPAIR

Indications for early (urgent) intervention

- Persistent, activated oculocardiac reflex in the presence of tissue entrapment demonstrated by CT scan
- Brain herniating into the orbit
- Bone fragments impinging upon the globe or extraocular muscles
- Evidence of extraocular muscle belly entrapment by *both* CT scan and clinical examination
- "White-eyed" trapdoor blowout fracture in children

Indications for routine (within 1 to 4 weeks after trauma) intervention

- Greater than 50% of area of orbital floor fractured
- Enophthalmos > 2 mm relative to the contralateral eye
- Persistent diplopia due to restriction of ocular motility, or extraocular muscle entrapment
- Hypoglobus > 2 mm
- Total medial wall fracture combined with > 33% of the orbital floor
- Orbital fractures in the presence of other facial fractures, such as zygomaticomaxillary complex (ZMC) or naso-orbital-ethmoid (NOE) fractures
- Lacrimal bone fracture with telecanthus
- Significantly displaced orbital rim or lateral wall fractures

Indications for delaying repair until 4 to 6 weeks

- Ruptured globe
- Intraocular injury with retinal detachment (unless performed at the same time as retinal detachment repair)
- Intraocular injury with acute angle closure glaucoma
- Posttraumatic optic neuropathy
- Recent (within past month) ocular-penetrating surgery
- Increased orbital pressure (orbital compartment syndrome) from either air (orbital emphysema) or blood with vision loss from globe or nerve ischemia is an indication for emergent orbital decompression, followed by *late* orbital fracture repair

ORBITAL WALL FRACTURES

Concerning the timing of exploration and repair of orbital wall fractures, much of the historical debate originated from the lack of adequate radiologic imaging of the orbit in the pre-CT era, and the only way to fully assess the extent of a floor fracture was surgical exploration. For decades, there was debate concerning the benefits of early exploration and intervention, versus the benefits of prolonged observation with eventual surgical intervention in selected patients. Proponents of early intervention argued that leaving the soft tissue herniated or the globe enophthalmic for prolonged periods resulted in scarring and tissue loss, so that even when the floor fracture was eventually repaired, diplopia or enophthalmos could still result, and the delayed repair could be more difficult. Proponents of delayed intervention argued that even with sizable floor fractures, many patients did not develop eventual diplopia or enophthalmos, and that some surgeries

and their potential complications could be avoided by waiting.

The wide availability of CT scanning changed that debate, as it became more possible to estimate the size and extent of orbital wall fractures. Clinicians were able to predict which fractures would almost certainly develop sequelae and require repair, and which could be observed.[1,2] In addition, if impingement of a bony fragment on the inferior rectus muscle was identified, there was a high probability of persistent diplopia, and if both the medial wall and floor were significantly fractured, there was a high probability of eventual enophthalmos or globe malposition.[3] In isolated medial wall fractures, neither enophthalmos nor diplopia seemed to routinely occur, even with a fairly large area of wall fractured.

ORBITAL FLOOR

The relative indications for orbital floor repair are shown in Table 7–1. Immediate repair is indicated for entrapped periorbital tissue with a nonresolving oculocardiac reflex, and in children under the age of 6 years with the "white-eyed" trapdoor fracture. In children and young adults, the orbital floor is softer and more pliable than in older adults. During a downloaded force to the orbital rim in the young, the orbital floor may buckle and crack, and then spring back into place, sometimes tightly entrapping orbital tissues. This can lead to a relatively bland-appearing eye without bruising, but with significant vertical-gaze double vision. Rapid intervention is indicated to avoid compromised blood supply to entrapped orbital fat or extraocular muscle with resultant scarring, especially in young children where severe ocular dysmotility may lead to amblyopia (permanently decreased vision in the affected eye).[4] Routine repair of orbital fractures, performed within 1 to 4 weeks of injury, is indicated when there is a high probability of developing enophthalmos, hypoglobus, or ocular dysmotility. If none of those indications are present, then the patient can be observed for a period of weeks, and a decision on delayed repair made at that time.

MEDIAL WALL

The indications for surgical repair of a medial orbital blowout fracture are enophthalmos, globe medialization (rare), or diplopia. However, many medial blowout fractures do not require surgical repair. This makes sense when one considers both the history and the anatomy. For decades, the surgical approach to the ethmoid sinus was through an external ethmoidectomy, involving removal of a portion of the lamina papyracea. Everyone who underwent external ethmoidectomy thus had a medial orbital wall fracture, but enophthalmos and diplopia were rarely encountered in those patients. In addition, considering the anatomy of the orbital walls and the forces of gravity, the orbital contents tend to prolapse down into floor defects, but medial defects (and by extension lateral and superior defects) are less likely to result in prolapse of orbital contents. Thus, even fairly large defects in orbital walls other than the floor may not result in significant globe malposition.

SURGICAL TECHNIQUES

In all orbital fracture repairs in which an implant, plate, or screw is used, perioperative intravenous antibiotics should be administered. Consideration should also be given to corticosteroid use to minimize the potentially blinding effects of orbital swelling.

ORBITAL RIM

Camouflaged approaches to the orbital rim are usually possible, such as a transconjunctival or subciliary incision for the inferior rim, upper blepharoplasty or eyebrow incision for the superior rim, and simple cantholysis for the lateral rim. Because there is no structural weakness associated with isolated rim fractures, the smallest possible plates and screws should be used to minimize palpability and visibility; simple bony approximation with adaptational healing usually suffices. Likewise, suture fixation using drill holes is often adequate for an isolated rim fracture.

ORBITAL FLOOR

The approach to the orbital floor can be accomplished using a transconjunctival or trans-eyelid (i.e., subciliary) incision. In the transconjunctival approach, a lateral canthotomy may be used to improve exposure if necessary. At the level of the orbital rim, care should be taken to divide the orbital periosteum exactly at the level of the rim, for later reapproximation. Additionally, the infraorbital neurovascular bundle lies just below the orbital rim in children, so periosteal incisions below the rim margin may lead to infraorbital numbness.

The periorbita of the orbital floor is carefully elevated, along with intraorbital fat and other orbital contents. There are usually two perforating vessels that enter the orbit from the infraorbital neurovascular bundle. In floor blowout fractures, the periorbita is inevitably torn so that it cannot be elevated in one piece, and orbital fat has usually herniated into the maxillary sinus. All herniated orbital contents should be reduced back into the orbit without also pulling any sinus mucosa into the orbit; displaced mucosa may lead to orbital mucocele formation much later. Meticulous orbital dissection can be tedious, but is necessary, as damage to the infraorbital neurovascular bundle and inferior rectus and oblique muscles may occur.

Vasoconstrictive agents, such as epinephrine, and thrombotic agents, such as thrombin, should never be used in the posterior orbit, as they may lead to ophthalmic artery or posterior ciliary artery spasm and occlusion. Likewise, monopolar cautery in the posterior orbit can theoretically lead to unilateral blindness, and current carried along the optic nerve might be transmitted via the chiasm to the contralateral optic nerve as well. Surgicel, a highly acidic clotting scaffold, should also not be placed in the posterior orbit, as it may expand as a rigid mass and compress the optic nerve or ophthalmic artery.

Once the orbital floor is visualized and the limits of the fracture are seen, the surgeon should evaluate the stability of the bordering bone and the amount of orbital tissue loss and volume expansion and then decide which type of implant to use. The implant rests on the solid bone around the fractured portion, and is usually fixed into position. It is important to recognize the upward slope of the floor toward the orbital apex, and to identify a firm shelf of bone posteriorly on which to rest the implant. This posterior aspect of the orbit is fairly thick bone, and even in large fractures there is usually a shelf of stable posterior bone remaining. If it is difficult to identify that posterior shelf, a surgical pearl is to pass an elevator through the floor fracture into the maxillary sinus, identify the posterior wall of the sinus, and then slide the elevator up that wall until the posterior lip of the orbital floor is identified. The relatively superior position of that posterior edge of the orbital floor can be surprising, even to an experienced surgeon. If the entire posterior floor has been fractured or destabilized, the surgeon needs to create a rigid implant to reestablish the contour of the floor, remembering its superior slope.

An important distance to remember in the orbit is that the orbital apex is 4.5 to 5 cm posterior to the inferior orbital rim; however, this is a guideline only and can be quite variable. Other anatomic clues that the orbital apex is being approached are a rise of the orbital floor, a thickening of the medial wall, and the position of the inferior orbital fissure. When fashioning an implant, you can either make the implant custom-sized to the patient's defect, or you can support the entire orbital floor with the implant, being careful to avoid overcorrection from vaulting over the lateral recess. When creating a custom-sized implant however, most turn out to be about the size of a standard guitar pick. So, creating an implant that is the same shape but slightly larger than a guitar pick is a reasonable starting point.

The materials used to repair orbital floor fractures are (1) autologous material such as cartilage or bone; (2) permanent alloplastic materials such as Gelfilm, porous polyethylene, Silastic, Teflon, Marlex mesh, hydroxyapatite, titanium plate or mesh; (3) dissolvable alloplastic materials such as Gelfilm or Lactosorb; and (4) allogenic materials such as banked bone or lyophilized cartilage.[5] There are advantages and disadvantages to each implant material.

Dissolvable implant materials such as Gelfilm have been reported for use in small fractures, but delayed proptosis due to cystic degeneration of Gelfilm has been reported.[6] Furthermore, this material has no rigidity after it comes in contact with moist tissue and provides essentially no support. Lactosorb, on the other hand, offers sufficient rigidity and may be used successfully in cases where a permanent implant is not desired.

Permanent alloplastic implants have been successfully used for many years and have been quite popular due to their ready availability and the fact that a second (donor) surgical site is not needed. These implants are inert, and can be easily cut into exactly the size needed for floor repair. Teflon sheets were popular for many years. Their major disadvantage, however, was delayed extrusion in roughly 5 to 10% of cases.[7] Nevertheless, the dense fibrous capsules formed around these smooth implants usually function as adequate orbital support after extrusion. But the capsules themselves also have a disadvantage. A fine vascular network travels through these capsules, and sometimes the fragile vessels break, creating spontaneous hemorrhage within the capsule and sudden proptosis years or decades after the orbital repair. Other permanent implant materials such as Marlex and Silastic have also been used successfully over many years; however, delayed infection and extrusion can also occur.

More recently, porous polyethylene (Medpor, Porex Surgical, Newnan, GA) has emerged as a particularly useful alloplastic implant, because it allows tissue ingrowth and has a very low rate of extrusion, infection, and other short-term or long-term complications. It is also very easy to manipulate and cut to size.

Another alloplastic option is the use of a metallic orbital floor plate or mesh. There are several orbital floor plates included in most commercial plating systems; some are more solid and shaped like an orbital floor with wings that can be removed or trimmed as needed, whereas others are made of a thinner and lighter material and are usually fan-shaped for easy trimming down to the needed size.

To help prevent extrusion and migration, many surgeons recommend fixing the alloplastic material in place.[8] This can be accomplished by drilling a small hole in the stable bone of the floor or rim, and then passing a small screw or suture through the implant, or by suturing the implant to an orbital rim plate (if present). If no rim plate is present, a small plate can be bent into a right-angle shape and attached to the rim and the implant to fix it into position. Another option is to cut and bend a small portion of the anterior rim of an alloplastic implant into a small inferiorly directed tab, which then fits into the anterior edge of the floor defect. Care should be taken with anterior fixation techniques, in particular the tab technique, as it can cause the implant to cant upward posteriorly, putting pressure on the optic nerve.

Autologous materials have the theoretical advantage of decreased rejection. In many ways, autologous implants are the standard against which other techniques have historically been measured. However, autologous materials almost invariably require a second surgical donor site. Septal and ear cartilage have been reported, but there is some concern with buckling and long-term instability when cartilage is used. Bone grafts work very nicely, and there are several potential sources of bone. Split calvarium is a popular choice, particularly if a bicoronal or craniotomy incision is needed for another reason. Iliac crest bone, split into a single piece of cortex, is another option, because the incision is well hidden under clothing, and because there are very few significant sequelae of the technique, except for pain in the immediate post-operative period. Rib is another option, but the incision may be visible, and there are potential sequelae such as pneumothorax. For smaller floor fractures, bone can be harvested from the anterior wall of the maxilla, being careful to leave the medial and lateral buttresses undisturbed. The antral bone is very thin, and is itself easily fractured during harvest and manipulation. Whichever donor bone is used, once the free graft is put into position, it receives blood supply from the elevated periorbita that is laid back on top of the graft. With non-enchondral bone graft sources, there is some resorption, so slight overcorrection is a good idea. Because calvarium is enchondral bone, very little resorption occurs when it is used.

Allogenic materials, such as banked bone, are the final option. There is little written about these materials, and there are obvious concerns about the transmission of disease (both those currently recognized as well as those that may be identified in decades to come).

There are very few comparative studies using different types of implants. Most reports are case series where the authors' technique of choice was consistently used. Interestingly, most case series show overall good results, indicating that several different techniques seem to have equal efficacy in skilled hands. One recent report did compare outcomes (orbital volume, position of implant, accuracy of reconstruction) between cranial bone grafts and titanium mesh.[9] Using a rigorous CT-based analysis, the authors found that titanium mesh created a more accurate orbital floor reconstruction than bone graft. This is likely because metal implants can be shaped more easily to approximate the missing floor.

After the implant has been placed, the position of the globe should be inspected for symmetry with the opposite side. Some swelling associated with the surgery is expected, so slight proptosis seen intraoperatively usually does not persist. Next, forced ductions of the globe should be performed to demonstrate no motion restriction, ensuring that no intraorbital tissue was entrapped by the implant or other surgical materials. Forced duction testing should be performed routinely three times during orbital reconstructions: at the start of the case, after implant placement, and at final wound closure. This ensures that the inferior oblique was not inadvertently captured during periosteal closure, and that the final orbital volume is not so great as to impede globe movement.

Even when the globe has been removed as a result of trauma, if the floor defect is large enough, it is still important to reconstruct the orbital floor, otherwise the ocular prosthesis may not be maintained in correct position.

MEDIAL ORBITAL WALL

The medial wall can be approached using an extended transconjunctival approach, but this can be difficult because of the intervening lacrimal sac and origin of the inferior oblique muscle. If the floor and medial orbital wall both require repair, then extension of this approach is probably most appropriate. An alternative approach, particularly useful in isolated medial blow-out fractures, is using a standard external ethmoidectomy (Lynch-type) incision, although it does leave a cutaneous scar. The medial canthal tendon is carefully divided, being careful to leave a remnant attached to the lacrimal bone for easy reapproximation with permanent suture during closure. Careful dissection and attention to detail during this dissection is important because if the tendon is detached from the bone, then holes will need to be drilled in the bone for refixation of the tendon, and even a subtle malposition of the medial canthus is unfortunately quite visible. Similarly, if the tendon is not reattached firmly, then rounding of the canthus can result, which is also cosmetically unattractive. Once the fracture is identified and the periorbita and orbital contents have been carefully reduced from the ethmoid sinus and replaced into the orbit, the medial wall is reconstructed using a thin bone graft or alloplastic material. This graft can be fixed into place using similar techniques as used for floor implants.

An alternative technique, but one that requires more experience and the ability to work within a tighter space, is the subcaruncular, transconjunctival approach, which avoids tendon disruption and does not leave a visible scar.

Orbital Roof

If the floor of the frontal sinus is involved, the orbital roof can be approached through the frontal sinus itself. If there is no frontal sinus or the fracture extends beyond its limits, neurosurgical assistance for a frontal craniotomy will probably be needed. Alternatively a superior orbitotomy approach through an eyelid crease incision could be used, although it is very difficult to reduce and fixate roof fractures from below. Again, the orbital contents and periorbita are carefully preserved and replaced into the orbit. If a frontal sinus is present, care is taken to avoid displacing sinus mucosa into the orbit. The orbital roof is reconstructed with a bone graft or alloplastic material, but this reconstruction can be difficult. As discussed previously, the orbital roof has a concave shape facing inferiorly, so if the roof is reconstructed with a perfectly straight graft from rim to posterior edge, the globe can be pushed inferiorly, resulting in hypoglobus. The roof also slopes inferiorly as it courses posteriorly, so if the graft is placed too horizontal, orbital volume might be too large. However, this rarely results in enophthalmos because gravity does not pull the orbital contents upward.

Complications

The most dreaded complication of orbital surgery is visual loss, which is best avoided by knowing the orbital anatomy and appropriate distances from the orbital rim to the orbital apex, and avoiding surgical manipulation or implant placement in the deepest portion of the orbital apex. Other more common complications are enophthalmos or exophthalmos, diplopia and impaired globe mobility, infraorbital nerve hypesthesia, and sinus mucosa ingrowth.

Enophthalmos occurs because of inadequate wall repair (i.e., the orbital volume is too large) or significant loss of intraorbital tissue. Exophthalmos is a result of overcorrection of wall repair or undercorrection of an impinging fracture, such as an imploded lateral wall fracture, creating an orbital volume that is too small. Careful assessment of globe position after implant placement is helpful. Less than a 2-mm difference in globe position with the contralateral eye is usually undetectable to the casual observer. We recommend purposeful overcorrection in the anterior-posterior direction of ~1 to 2 mm at the conclusion of surgery, because orbital edema must be considered. In cases when orbital fat atrophy is expected, as might occur with tremendous traumatic forces or where a large amount of orbital fat has been devitalized, then even more overcorrection is strongly considered. Plates shaped to rest slightly higher than the original floor or seemingly thicker-than-needed alloplastic implants or bone grafts are helpful to create overcorrection.

Diplopia and impaired globe mobility are typically caused by tissue entrapment, either from an inadequately reduced wall fracture, or an iatrogenic entrapment caused during repair, which is most commonly due to entrapment of the inferior rectus or adjacent tethering fat at the posterior orbit. Postoperative diplopia can also be caused by edema, so careful radiologic evaluation and clinical observation is important to avoid unnecessary reexplorations for diplopia that will resolve spontaneously in days to weeks.

Infraorbital nerve hypesthesia is caused by the orbital fracture in most cases, and as such is not really a "complication." It is often a traction or bruise injury, and sensory function will return over time. However, in some cases hypesthesia or dysesthesia will persist, particularly if the fracture is not repaired. Actually, surgical repair tends to make the hypesthesia worse temporarily, but in our experience, by 9 months after surgery more than 90% of patients have achieved full recovery of sensory function, compared with ~60% with full recovery if no surgery is performed.

Sinus mucosal ingrowth and mucocele formation can be caused by inadequate closure of connections between the surrounding sinuses and the orbit or by pulling sinus mucosa into the orbit during repair. These rare complications usually present months to years after the initial injury.

Summary

Orbital fractures are challenging to evaluate and treat, as the symmetry of the eyes is an important aesthetic feature. In addition, the orbits are surrounded by important anatomic structures. Nevertheless, a systematic approach to evaluation and treatment can yield reliable aesthetic and functional results.

PEARLS: ORBITAL FRACTURES

- To visualize the orbital rims and walls, the best imaging study is the CT scan.
- The possibility of ocular or optic nerve injury should be carefully considered in all orbital fractures.
- The most common sequelae of orbital fractures are globe malposition, diplopia, and infraorbital nerve hypesthesia.
- The orbital floor is the most commonly fractured wall and usually fractures in a "blowout" fashion, with distraction of the wall fragments outside the orbit.
- Not all orbital wall fractures require surgical reduction; the indications for surgery are detailed in Table **7–1**.
- Orbital wall fractures can be repaired using autologous materials, permanent or dissolvable alloplastic materials, and allogenic materials; each has advantages and disadvantages.
- Orbital fractures are frequently associated with other midface fractures, such as zygomatic complex fractures, and nasal-orbital-ethmoid fractures.

REFERENCES

1. Manson PN, Iliff N. Early repair for selected injuries. Surv Ophthalmol 1991;35:280–292
2. Brady SM, McMann MA, Mazzoli RA, et al. The diagnosis and management of orbital blowout fractures: update 2001. Am J Emerg Med 2001;19:147–154
3. Nolasco FP, Mathog RH. Medial orbital wall fractures: classification and clinical profile. Otolaryngol Head Neck Surg 1995;112:549–556
4. Burnstine MA. Clinical recommendations for repair of isolated orbital floor fractures; an evidence-based analysis. Ophthalmology 2002;109:1207–1213
5. Chowdhury K, Krause GE. Selection of materials for orbital floor reconstruction. Arch Otolaryngol Head Neck Surg 1998;124:1398–1401
6. Stewart MG, Patrinely JR, Appling WD, Jordan DR. Late proptosis following orbital floor fracture repair. Arch Otolaryngol Head Neck Surg 1995;121:649–652
7. Jordan DR, Stonge P, Anderson RL, et al. Complications associated with alloplastic implants used in orbital fracture repair. Ophthalmology 1992;99:1600–1608
8. Rubin PAD, Shore JW, Yaremchuk MJ. Complex orbital fracture repair using rigid fixation of the internal orbital skeleton. Ophthalmology 1992;99:553–559
9. Ellis E, Tan Y. Assessment of internal orbital reconstructions for pure blowout fractures: cranial bone grafts versus titanium mesh. J Oral Maxillofac Surg 2003;61:442–453

Chapter 8

ZYGOMATIC COMPLEX FRACTURES

Michael G. Stewart

Zygomatic complex fractures are relatively common injuries. They have been given several different names, such as trimalar, tripod, malar complex, tetrapod, maxillary complex, and orbitozygomatico-maxillary fractures. The term *trimalar fracture* is perhaps most commonly used, but is a misnomer, because there are actually four components in most cases. This chapter uses the term *zygomatic complex fracture*.

ANATOMY

The bony anatomy of the zygomatic region is shown in Fig. 8–1. The zygomatic bone itself has four projections, which give it a quadrilateral shape; it projects medially and creates the lateral portion of the infraorbital rim, inferiorly to the alveolus of the maxilla, superiorly articulating with the frontal bone, and posteriorly forming the anterior portion of the zygomatic arch. Similarly, the zygoma articulates with four other bones: frontal, maxilla, temporal, and greater wing of sphenoid. The zygoma creates the malar prominence, which is an important aesthetic facial landmark. In addition, the zygomatic arch sets the width of the face and is prominent in the oblique facial profile.

In addition to its aesthetic importance, the zygomatic-maxillary region represents the convergence of the midface buttresses and the orbit. The midfacial *buttress* system refers to areas of thicker bone that provide support and stability to the midface and also protection to the orbit. There are three horizontal buttresses: (1) the superior orbital rims and frontal bone; (2) the inferior orbital rims and nasal bones; and (3) the maxillary alveolus. In addition, there are medial and lateral vertical buttresses on each side of the face; the lateral buttress is called the zygomati-comaxillary (ZM) buttress and the medial buttress the nasomaxillary buttress; these buttresses are shown in Fig. 8–2. The most important buttress from the standpoint of strength and stability during mastication is the lateral (ZM) buttress. The anterior, lateral, and medial bony walls of the maxillary sinus may also be fractured in zygomatic complex fractures, but their thin bone provides little facial stability or aesthetic projection.

Surrounding the bones of the ZM region are important soft tissues. The masseter muscle attaches to the zygoma, and its pull is partially responsible for the typical downward and inward rotation of the malar process after zygomatic complex fractures. The temporalis muscle travels under the zygomatic arch and attaches superiorly to the squamous portion of the temporal bone. Depressed arch fractures can press on that muscle and on the coronoid process of the mandible causing significant pain on mouth opening and chewing. The lower eyelid sits in front of the inferior orbital rim, and is suspended by the medial and lateral canthal tendons; the lateral canthal tendon attaches to the zygoma at Whitnall's tubercle, which is located just inside the lateral orbital rim. In addition, the horizontal position of the globe is maintained by the suspensory ligament of Lockwood, which attaches to the lacrimal bone medially and to Whitnall's tubercle laterally.

Importantly, the facial nerve travels through the lateral facial soft tissue, and the area of concern in zygomatic complex fractures is the area where the frontal branch crosses over the zygomatic arch. This is usually near the midpoint of the arch, where the nerve travels in a plane deep to the superficial temporal fascia and lateral to the zygomatic periosteum. This anatomic relationship has significant implications if exposure and plating of the zygomatic arch are required.

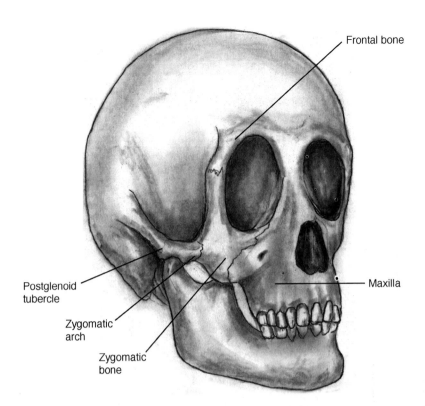

Frontal bone

Postglenoid
tubercle

Zygomatic
arch

Zygomatic
bone

Maxilla

FIGURE 8–1   Bony anatomy of the zygomatic region.

The typical fracture pattern of a zygomatic complex fracture is shown in Fig. **8–3**. There are usually four external components that are fractured: the frontozygomatic (FZ) suture, the zygomatic arch, the lateral (ZM) buttress, and the inferior orbital (IO) rim. The ZM buttress and IO rim fractures are usually connected through an anterior maxillary wall fracture. This anterior portion of the fracture usually passes through or near the infraorbital foramen, with associated trauma to the infraorbital nerve. In addition, the fracture almost always involves the orbit, with both lateral orbital wall and orbital floor fractures. The zygoma usually moves as a unit, and is displaced inferomedially. However, the zygoma can also be fractured into pieces. Unusual fracture patterns can be seen, which involve a "partial" zygomatic complex fracture, for example, without a zygomatic arch fracture, or without an FZ suture fracture. Nondisplaced fractures are also seen; however, the continued action of the masseter muscle can displace the zygoma, so patients with nondisplaced fractures should be followed to make sure that the fracture does not become displaced in a delayed fashion.

IMAGING

The facial series of plain x-rays can be helpful in identifying the presence of a zygomatic complex fracture; there are several key findings, particularly on the Waters view, including asymmetry of the malar processes, opacification of the maxillary sinus, or visible fracture of the FZ suture, IO rim, or zygomatic arch. The submental-vertex ("bucket handle") view can also show the displaced zygomatic

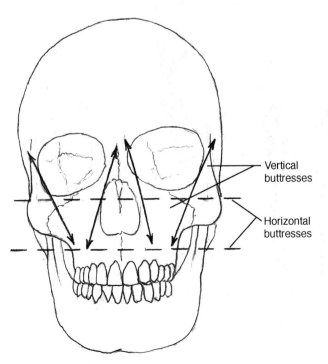

Vertical
buttresses

Horizontal
buttresses

FIGURE 8–2   Midfacial buttresses.

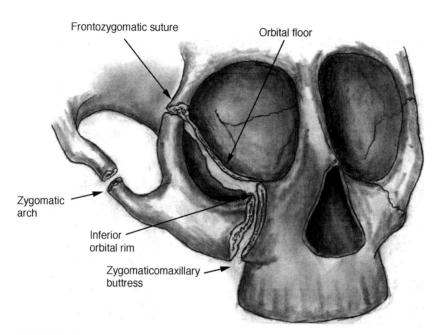

Frontozygomatic suture

Orbital floor

Zygomatic arch

Inferior orbital rim

Zygomaticomaxillary buttress

FIGURE 8–3 Typical fracture pattern of the zygomatic complex fracture.

arch and occasionally the displaced malar process. However, if a fracture is present, a computed tomography (CT) scan is needed for complete evaluation. Both coronal and axial views are helpful. The coronal CT views demonstrate the FZ suture, the IO rim, and the ZM buttress, and also show the orbital floor. Axial views demonstrate the lateral orbital wall, the zygomatic arch, and the position of the malar process. Example CT scans are shown in Fig. 8–4 and Fig. 8–5. Three-dimensional computerized reconstructions of CT scans may be helpful, but are usually needed only in complicated injuries involving multiple facial bones because a straightforward zygomatic complex fracture can be evaluated

and understood using the axial and coronal CT views.

CLINICAL ASSESSMENT

The clinical assessment of the injured patient can be difficult because of soft tissue swelling that can obscure the cosmetic deformity. Even in the presence of swelling, however, a zygomatic complex fracture can sometimes be identified by inferior rotation or posterior displacement of the lateral canthus of the

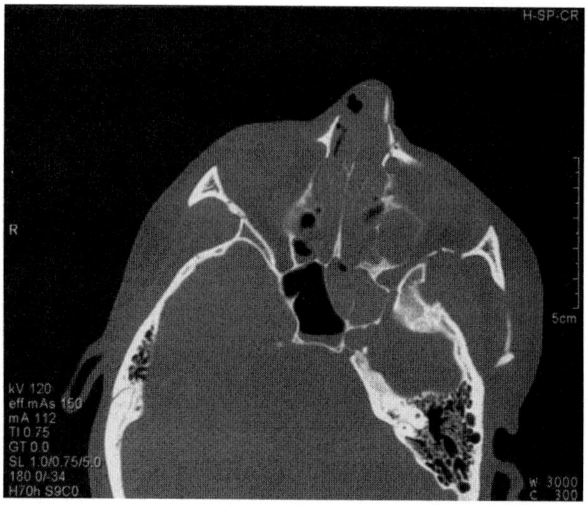

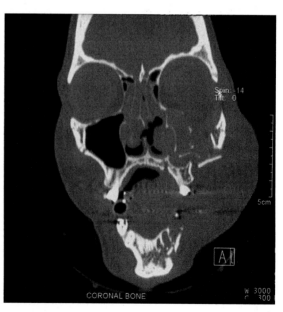

FIGURE 8–4 Axial computed tomography scan showing typical pattern of zygomatic complex fracture.

FIGURE 8–5 Coronal computed tomography scan showing typical pattern of zygomatic complex fracture.

eye. The inferior rotation of the palpebral fissure is also called an antimongoloid rotation. Once the swelling decreases somewhat, a flattening of the malar eminence is usually noted, as well as depression over the zygomatic arch. Palpable step-offs at the IO rim and the FZ suture can usually be appreciated on examination even in the presence of swelling. The ZM buttress, however, is beneath a thick layer of soft tissue, making palpation difficult. Although evaluation with physical examination is important, the external physical findings can often be predicted by the CT scan findings; bony displacement of more than 2 mm usually results in visible aesthetic deformity.

Although orbital wall fractures are usually seen in zygomatic complex fractures, significant displacement does not always occur. Enophthalmos, diplopia, or entrapment usually indicates a displaced orbital floor fracture. In addition, the globe itself can be injured by the trauma. Ophthalmology consultation is recommended in all patients with an orbital wall fracture, to document the vision as well as ocular motility, and to identify other potential traumatic injuries. The minimal preoperative evaluation should include visual acuity, pupillary function, ocular motility, inspection for hyphema, and examination of the fundus for gross disruption.[1]

Evaluation of the dental occlusion is also important. Fractures through the alveolar portion of the maxilla can result in malocclusion. In addition, pain on mouth opening or chewing can be an indication of an inwardly displaced zygomatic arch fracture. Also, most patients have some numbness in the infraorbital nerve distribution due to nerve injury commonly associated with the zygomatic complex fracture.

Associated injuries include nasal fracture, mandible fracture, LeFort midface fracture, and sagittal palate fracture. These other potential injuries should be considered during the evaluation process.

SURGICAL INDICATIONS

Visible displacement of the zygomatic complex is an indication for fracture reduction. Rarely, the fracture can be reduced without fixation. However, in most fractures open reduction and internal fixation is needed. The indications for open reduction (with possible internal fixation) of the zygomatic complex are cosmetic deformity, trismus, pain with chewing, diplopia, gaze restriction, or globe malposition.[2]

In the isolated zygomatic arch fracture, the indications for reduction are cosmetic deformity, trismus, or painful chewing. A nondisplaced arch fracture does not require reduction, because there is no loss of stability and most patients are asymptomatic.

SURGICAL APPROACHES

Several components of the zygomatic complex fracture should be exposed for visualization during reduction and fixation. If the patient has existing lacerations over the fractures, they can be opened for fracture exposure and repair. In fact, use of existing lacerations or old scars is preferred when they are present, because second incisions near existing lacerations can endanger the blood supply of the intervening skin. If there are no existing lacerations, then hidden incisions are preferred and usually provide very adequate exposure.

The IO rim and orbital floor can be approached using a transconjunctival incision or a subciliary skin incision. The transconjunctival approach has been shown to have a lower risk of ectropion in comparison to the subciliary approach.[3,4] Using either incision, but particularly with the transconjunctival approach, performing a lateral canthotomy at the same time gives added exposure and access to the entire orbital rim and floor, and allows extended dissection to the lateral orbital rim and wall if needed. However, the lateral canthotomy does require meticulous reapproximation during closure, and there may be an increased risk of ectropion, compared with the same incision performed without a canthotomy. For those reasons, some surgeons prefer not to perform a lateral canthotomy. However, I routinely use the transconjunctival approach with a lateral canthotomy, and have not seen additional complications caused by the canthotomy.

The FZ suture can be approached using either an upper blepharoplasty incision extended laterally or a curvilinear skin incision partially hidden in the lateral eyebrow. The FZ suture can also be approached using an extended hemicoronal incision and approach, but that amount of additional dissection is not usually necessary because both options for adjacent incisions are very well camouflaged, and give nearly direct access to the fracture site. However, if the patient is undergoing a coronal approach for another reason (i.e., frontal sinus fracture or naso-orbital-ethmoid fracture), then that dissection can be extended to include exposure and fixation at the FZ suture. The ZM buttress can be approached using a sublabial incision without difficulty. That incision allows access to the medial midface buttress and the anterior maxillary sinus wall as well.

When part of a zygomatic complex fracture, a fractured zygomatic arch seldom requires direct visualization or internal fixation; palpation and indirect open reduction are usually adequate. For indirect reduction, the approach is either through a Gillies incision or sublabial incision. Because of the presence of the frontal branch of the facial nerve overlying the arch, direct incision near the arch is not advisable, so if *direct* visualization and internal fixation are needed, then a hemicoronal incision with extended dissection to the arch should be used.

SURGICAL TECHNIQUES

ISOLATED ZYGOMATIC ARCH FRACTURE

In the *isolated* arch fracture, open indirect reduction is usually adequate and internal fixation is seldom required. Using either a Gillies or intraoral approach, the tissue planes are followed bluntly to reach the zygomatic arch. In the Gillies approach, maintaining the dissection deep to the temporalis fascia and along the surface of the temporalis muscle protects the frontal branch of the facial nerve. In the intraoral approach, a subcutaneous plane just lateral to the lateral aspect of the maxilla is followed, being careful to avoid penetration or exposure of the buccal fat pad. Once the arch is reached, the depressed portion can be elevated using any heavy instrument: there is a flat-sided angled elevator called the Gillies elevator that is useful, and other options are a long blunt-tip curved clamp, or a heavy urethral sound. The arch usually snaps or pops into position and remains there after reduction; the tension of the bony contact and the natural shape of the arch tend to hold the bones into position. This snap into position can be palpated with the surgeon's other hand through the skin overlying the arch, but the surgeon should take care that during the external palpation the arch is not pushed back out of anatomic position. The procedure using either approach can be performed under local anesthesia, and the patient can then confirm the resolution of pain on mouth opening after the arch is reduced. Another technique for reduction is to use a towel clamp directly through the skin to elevate the arch; however, this method is risky because of the potential for injury to the facial nerve branch with the sharp tips of the clamp.

It is important to keep in mind that the zygomatic "arch" is not actually arch-shaped, but is fairly flat in its midportion. Review of axial CT scans demonstrates this point. If during reduction the surgeon attempts to re-create the shape of an arch, the bone will be overcorrected with a resultant aesthetic asymmetry between sides.

After reduction, some sort of external protection over the arch may be helpful, to prevent inadvertent contact pushing the arch back out of reduction. A metal eye patch or a bent aluminum finger splint can be taped or sutured over the arch and left there for about a week. Others have recommended placing some soft material beneath the arch such as a folded Penrose drain or an inflated Foley balloon catheter, which is then removed in about a week.[5] Another approach is to pass one or two heavy sutures under the arch, and suspend the arch into position using those sutures with an overlying metal eye patch or gauze bolster, although again care should be taken with the facial nerve branch.

If the arch cannot be reduced using the indirect technique, then open direct reduction with internal fixation is needed. The arch is fixed into position using very small plates and screws, maintaining the normal flat shape of the arch.

Reduction is confirmed clinically by elimination of the soft tissue depression and elimination of pain on chewing or mouth opening. Reduction can be confirmed radiologically using the submental-vertex plain x-ray, or a CT scan. If the arch has been reduced adequately but the patient still has pain on chewing or mouth opening, then an unrecognized fracture of the mandibular coronoid should be considered.

ZYGOMATIC COMPLEX FRACTURE

Some zygomatic complex fractures are nondisplaced and do not require reduction. In addition, some fractures can be treated with closed reduction only, although there is controversy about how frequently this can be adequately achieved[5]; although some have reported that ~60% of zygomatic complex fractures remain stable after reduction alone without fixation, others have reported that only 15% of fractures can be treated using reduction alone. Most authors agree that displaced zygomatic complex fractures usually require open reduction and internal fixation.

To perform adequate internal fixation of the zygomatic complex fracture, there are a few helpful concepts to keep in mind: (1) expose and reduce all appropriate fractures before beginning plating; (2) consider the anterior, horizontal, and vertical projections of the zygoma during reduction; and (3) secure the ZM complex to stable bone. Although it might seem easier to expose, reduce, and plate each fracture site one at a time, sequentially moving to the next site, it is very difficult to achieve the appropriate reduction and orientation of the zygoma if that is done.

The important fractures that always should be exposed are the FZ suture and the ZM buttress. Many times the IO rim requires exposure as well, particularly if the orbital floor is also displaced and fractured; however, the skin overlying the rim is very thin, and the bone can be easily palpated. So, in selected cases not requiring orbital floor exploration, if reduction at the orbital rim can be palpated, then the rim does not have to be visualized. Alternatively, the IO rim can be exposed by following the anterior wall of the maxilla up to the rim; care should be taken to avoid iatrogenic damage to the infraorbital nerve. The rim can be exposed and palpated through a sublabial approach to confirm appropriate fracture rotation and reduction, but that limited exposure does not allow direct fixation of the rim fragments. If plate or wire fixation of the rim is required, then a transconjunctival or subciliary incision is usually needed.

The zygomatic arch is rarely exposed and visualized in the uncomplicated zygomatic complex fracture; reduction of the arch is either achieved by rotation of the zygoma back into position, with correct position confirmed by palpation, or the arch can be elevated and reduced after the zygoma has been secured into position. In one series of 813 patients treated successfully with open reduction and internal fixation, the arch never required direct fixation with a plate.[4]

After the involved fracture sites have all been exposed, the zygoma should be reduced into position. This usually requires a pull both upward and outward, as well as rotation in the superomedial direction. A useful technique for achieving this reduction is to use a large bone hook placed transcutaneously through a small stab incision in the cheek.[2,4] The hook is placed under the inferolateral aspect of the zygoma, and is used to pull and rotate the bone into position; the hook in place is shown in Fig. 8–6. It is important to seat the hook around the solid lateral edge of the zygoma, and

avoid the thinner bones of the lateral wall of the maxillary sinus and lateral orbital wall. As the zygoma is reduced, the fracture sites are each checked to make sure that reduction is adequate. If the fracture is several days old and there has been some fibrosis and soft tissue healing in addition to masseter contraction, it may require several sequential attempts at mobilization and reduction of the bone before finally achieving adequate rotation and reduction. As an alternative to the bone hook, some surgeons use a heavy elevator placed through a Gillies temporal incision and under the malar eminence. Lifting on that elevator restores the zygoma to its anatomic position, and the fractures are fixed with the zygoma held in reduction.

During reduction, in addition to achieving fracture edge contact at each fracture site, the surgeon should keep in mind the projections of the zygoma. The zygoma projects anteriorly, mainly through the shape and continuity of the zygomatic arch. It is also projects horizontally, primarily through the orbital rim and malar eminence, but also through the relationship with the arch. Finally, the zygoma has a vertical component through the ZM buttress and the FZ suture. So, in addition to achieving apposition of the bony edges at fracture sites, the surgeon should orient the zygoma so that there is adequate projection in the three dimensions discussed. If the fracture is unilateral, then symmetry with the opposite side is an excellent guide. In bilateral fractures, the surgeon must depend on knowledge of normal three-dimensional anatomic relationships in the region.

Also, the surgeon needs to consider the stability of the adjacent bony structures before completing fixation of the zygomatic complex. For example, if

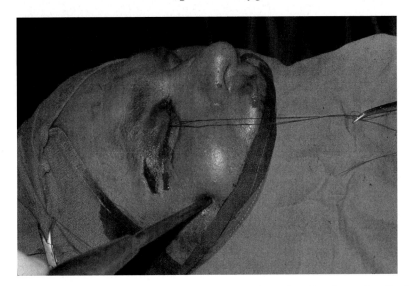

FIGURE 8–6 Bone hook in place; a superolateral pull reduces the displaced zygoma.

the patient has a medial maxillary buttress fracture or a significant nasal fracture, the medial portion of the IO rim may be displaced from its normal anatomic position and also be unstable. If the surgeon does not recognize that, the lateral aspect of the rim can be plated to unstable malpositioned bone, which will establish the rim in an incorrect position, jeopardizing the other anatomic relationships and the eventual position of the zygoma. Similarly, in a palatal fracture with malocclusion, if the ZM buttress is anatomically plated to the alveolar portion of the maxilla, the zygoma may be malpositioned, and malocclusion could persist. So, although the surgeon must start somewhere, because the anatomic position of the malar eminence is such an important aesthetic facial feature, it is prudent to establish all *surrounding* bony structures appropriately, for example, using intermaxillary fixation (IMF) or open reduction and internal fixation, before attempting to reduce the zygoma into position. If indicated, establishment of occlusion using IMF is of critical importance; even if the bite is only off by a few millimeters, that will be very noticeable to the patient, so the extra time spent establishing occlusion prior to fracture fixation is well worth it in favorable patient outcomes.

After the zygoma has been reduced, then internal fixation is performed. The number of plates needed for adequate fixation has been studied using skulls with artificially created fractures and measurement of the rotational force required for displacement after some combination of plate and wire fixation.[6] Those laboratory experiments found that two-point fixation, preferably involving at least one miniplate, provided acceptable stability. If one plate and one wire were placed, the strongest fixation was achieved by placing the plate at the ZM buttress and the wire at the FZ suture. In that study, three-point fixation provided the strongest repair; however, the additional stability measured in the laboratory was probably not clinically necessary to achieve a stable repair. Interestingly, those authors found that three-point fixation (IO rim, FZ suture, ZM buttress) using wire osteosynthesis provided fixation almost as strong as three-point fixation using miniplates. Overall in several different varieties of plates and wires, the most important site for placement of a *single* plate was the FZ suture. Of course, that study involved skulls and force measurements, and did not account for bone healing or the variety of real-life forces on the face and maxilla.

Clinical studies tend to agree that as long as the fracture is adequately reduced, two-point fixation is usually clinically sufficient,[4,7] and the FZ suture and ZM buttress are typically preferred. In some cases,

fixation of the IO rim may be necessary; wire fixation is preferred by some authors over very small microplates because the plates may be palpable and visible postoperatively through the thin skin overlying the rim.[4] However, the current generation of low-profile microplates (using 1.0-mm screws) remain remarkably camouflaged even under the thinnest skin. In many cases, however, two-point fixation at the FZ suture and ZM buttress is adequate, and the IO rim does not require fixation.

As mentioned previously, it is important to reduce the zygoma into position at all fracture sites before beginning to plate individual fracture components. However, it can be technically difficult to hold the zygoma into position while simultaneously beginning to cut, adapt, and apply plates to an individual fracture, all while the bone is still mobile. So, one recommendation is to use a single wire for fixation at the FZ suture that will hold the zygoma in position temporarily while other fractures are plated.[4] Once the zygoma is held by at least one plate, the wire can be removed and replaced with a miniplate.

The size of plates needed for fixation of a zygomatic complex fracture are much smaller than those required for fixation of a mandible fracture because there is significantly less force applied to the zygoma. The larger midface plates (using 1.5- to 2.0-mm screws) are usually applied to the ZM buttress, with a smaller plate applied to the FZ suture, and the smallest plate (or wire) used at the IO rim. Studies have shown that when drilling into the skull, intracranial penetration can be achieved at a depth of 12 mm; this is important to keep in mind when drilling into the frontal bone at the FZ suture.

If the bone is comminuted, then a single long plate or multiple plates can be used to reapproximate the individual pieces. Occasionally, a single plate needs to be fashioned, bridging from the frontal bone to the maxillary alveolus, and the pieces of the zygoma are then pulled up and attached to that plate. In addition, if there is a gap of missing bone, a heavier plate can be used to span that gap, maintaining the normal bony relationships. However, if that bony gap is significant, then placement of a bone graft should be considered. There is no rule on how large is too large, but some recommend that if the gap is larger than 5 mm, then a bone graft is indicated.[5] However, the clinical experience of others demonstrates that gaps larger than 5 mm have been treated with plate fixation only, with good success.

The orbital floor should be explored and repaired *after* the zygoma has been reduced into position. Unless there is significant comminution or depression of the floor, reduction of the zygoma into position might adequately reduce the orbital floor and lateral orbital wall fractures. So, direct repair of the orbital floor is not always necessary. However, in many zygomatic complex fractures the force of injury will also result in additional fracture displacement of the orbital floor. The stronger bone of the lateral wall usually does not shatter, however, but fractures in a straight line, so rotation and reduction of the zygoma is usually sufficient to address the lateral wall.

The final position of the zygoma is confirmed by evaluating its projection in the directions described previously, and by checking for reduction at the key fracture sites of the FZ suture, ZM buttress, and IO rim. Another helpful tip during reduction is to check reduction along the lateral orbital wall. Axial CT scans demonstrate that this wall is almost always displaced in zygomatic complex fractures, so to confirm adequate reduction, a thin elevator can be used to gently palpate that wall after minimal dissection. If the zygomatic fracture is well reduced, the lateral wall should be continuous with no step-off; if not, then the zygoma needs to be further rotated to complete the reduction.

There is a single report on the use of *intraoperative* CT scan in the repair of zygomatic complex fractures.[8] Of course, in such a pilot study, the use of the scanner was cumbersome and time-consuming, but at least one important benefit was identified. Although the intraoperative CT scan was not particularly helpful in the reduction of the fracture itself, it was found to be very useful for the positioning of large bone grafts when needed, such as along the orbital floor. The author found that when a large portion of bone was missing and a bone graft was placed, achieving the optimal orientation of the graft was difficult. The CT scan was very helpful in those cases.

POSTOPERATIVE CARE

As in all patients with facial fractures, perioperative antibiotics should be used. In addition, head elevation helps minimize edema. Eye care should be meticulous and include moisturizing drops and patching as needed. Taping and suspension of the lower eyelid and midfacial skin can help reduce edema, ectropion, and other soft tissue problems.

COMPLICATIONS

The complications of zygomatic complex fractures can be categorized as eye, cosmetic, healing, and functional complications. These complications can be due to the initial injury itself, or can be iatrogenic resulting from the surgical reduction.

Eye complications include globe injuries such as corneal abrasion, hyphema, and retinal or other intraocular injuries. Retrobulbar hemorrhage and superior orbital fissure syndrome have also been reported.[5] The most common eye-related complications are enophthalmos and diplopia due to inadequate reduction of the orbital walls. Some reports have stated that *measurable* enophthalmos can be identified after zygomatic complex fracture repair in up to 80% of patients, although others report that complication rate as 5 to 25%.[5] In addition, enophthalmos of 2 mm or less is usually not visibly detectable. Persistent diplopia is usually due to entrapment of periorbital tissue or muscle in an orbital wall fracture; this can be minimized by performing forced ductions of the eye to confirm adequate mobility before and after manipulation of the orbital walls.

Cosmetic complications are almost entirely due to a missed component of the fracture, inadequate reduction, or inadequate fixation with subsequent rotation back out of position. Of these, the most common problem is inadequate reduction prior to fixation.

Healing complications include infection, malunion, plate exposure, and oroantral fistula; these are quite uncommon in zygomatic fractures, and are usually due to technical errors at the time of surgery. Another important cosmetic complication is lower lid malposition, including ectropion or entropion. Any asymmetry in the amount of scleral show is quite noticeable, so meticulous care should be taken to ensure that the lower eyelid and lateral canthus are restored into good anatomic position.

Functional complications include sensory deficits, usually in the infraorbital nerve distribution, and are mostly due to the fracture itself. Adequate fracture reduction may "untrap" the nerve and allow eventual recovery of some sensory function. Nevertheless, despite adequate reduction, numbness, dysesthesia, or hypesthesia can persist in the infraorbital nerve distribution. Another functional neurologic complication is facial nerve weakness, usually in the frontal branch. This weakness is rarely caused by the injury itself, but if so it will obviously be present prior to surgery. If weakness presents after surgical reduction, it is likely iatrogenic from the surgical approach or repair. Other functional complications include trismus and malocclusion. Trismus usually occurs from inadequate reduction of the zygomatic arch with impingement on the mandibular coronoid, or from an unrecognized coronoid fracture. In addition, trismus can occur secondary to fibrosis or ankylosis of the coronoid to the arch. Malocclusion usually occurs because of an unrecognized displacement of the maxillary alveolus that is not reduced prior to fixation of the zygoma.

PEARLS: KEY CLINICAL POINTS IN ZYGOMATIC COMPLEX FRACTURES

- The zygoma articulates with four other facial bones, the midface buttresses, and the orbit.
- The malar process is an important aesthetic facial landmark.
- An isolated zygomatic arch fracture should be reduced — usually fixation is not required — if the patient has a significant cosmetic deformity, trismus, or pain with chewing.
- Indications for surgical reduction and fixation of a zygomatic complex fracture are cosmetic deformity, trismus, pain with chewing, enophthalmos, diplopia, or gaze restriction.
- At surgery, at least two fracture sites should be exposed before the zygoma is reduced.
- Stable repair requires fixation of at least two fracture sites, usually the FZ suture and ZM buttress.
- Orbital floor and lateral wall fractures are associated with zygomatic complex fractures, and may require additional exploration or repair.
- Complications of zygomatic complex fractures are categorized as eye, cosmetic, healing, and func-

tional complications such as infraorbital hypesthesia or trismus.

REFERENCES

1. Stanley RB Jr. Maxillary and periorbital fractures. In: Bailey BJ, ed. *Head and Neck Surgery–Otolaryngology*, 3rd ed. Philadelphia: Lippincott-Raven, 2001:777–792
2. Appling WD, Stewart MG. Zygomatic fracture. In: Gates GA, ed. *Current Therapy in Otolaryngology-Head and Neck Surgery*, 6th ed. St. Louis: Mosby, 1998:125–138
3. Appling WD, Patrinely JR, Salter TA. Transconjunctival approach versus subciliary skin-muscle flap approach for orbital fracture repair. Arch Otolaryngol Head Neck Surg 1993;119:1000–1007
4. Zingg M, Chowdhury K, Ladrach K, Vuillemin T, Sutter F, Raveh J. Treatment of 813 zygoma-lateral orbital complex fractures. Arch Otolaryngol Head Neck Surg 1991;117:611–622
5. Perrott DH, Kaban LB. Acute management of orbito-zygomatic fractures. Oral and Maxillofacial Surgery Clinics of North America 1993;5:475–492
6. Davidson J, Nickerson D, Nickerson B. Zygomatic fractures: comparison of methods of internal fixation. Plast Reconstr Surg 1990;86:25–32
7. Holmes KD, Matthews BL. Three-point alignment of zygoma fractures with miniplate fixation. Arch Otolaryngol Head Neck Surg 1989;115:961–963
8. Stanley RB Jr. Use of intraoperative computed tomography during repair of orbitozygomatic fractures. Arch Facial Plast Surg 1999;1:19–24

Chapter 9

LE FORT AND PALATAL FRACTURES

Jose M. Marchena and James V. Johnson

This chapter discusses the pertinent anatomy, diagnosis, and contemporary management of palatal and Le Fort fractures. Emphasis is placed on fracture patterns and the importance of recognizing and addressing the altered maxillary position in these fractures. Appropriate airway management and sequencing of treatment in the presence of coexisting non-Le Fort fractures is also discussed. Specifics on orbital, zygomatic, frontal sinus, and naso-orbital-ethmoidal (NOE) injuries not causing a change in maxillary position and occlusion are discussed elsewhere in this text.

ANATOMIC CONSIDERATIONS AND FRACTURE PATTERNS

The midface lies between a line drawn through the zygomaticofrontal sutures tangential to the base of the skull and a line corresponding with the maxillary occlusal plane. It contains the orbits, NOE complex, zygomatic bones, and maxilla. Developmental suture lines between these structures are areas of weakness and are common fracture sites. Examples of such common fracture sites include the frontozygomatic, zygomaticomaxillary, zygomaticosphenoid, nasofrontal, and midpalatal sutures. Other areas of bony weakness include those containing a neurovascular bundle such as the medial orbital rim at the level of the infraorbital foramen, and bones containing sinus air cells such as the maxilla, ethmoid bones, and the frontal bone.

The maxilla and midface are suspended from the cranium by three supporting and strengthening buttresses that absorb and distribute masticatory forces from the teeth to the cranium. From anterior to posterior these vertical buttresses are (1) the anterior maxillary buttress formed by the frontal

process of the maxilla and pyriform rims; (2) the zygomaticomaxillary buttress and its extension through the body of the zygoma to the zygomaticofrontal suture; and 3) the pterygomaxillary buttress (Fig. 9–1). Reconstruction of the anterior maxillary and zygomaticomaxillary buttresses is critical to anatomically reduce the maxilla in relation to the cranium, restore facial vertical height, and provide resistance against masticatory forces.[1]

The Le Fort classification of facial fractures represents three common fracture patterns observed from a single impact on cadaver skulls.[2] Pure Le Fort fractures are therefore not very common in clinical practice. Conceptually, the distinguishing feature between Le Fort fractures and other midface fractures is that the relationship between the maxilla and the mandible, and therefore the occlusion, is always altered in Le Fort fractures in the presence of displacement. The only exception is a palatal fracture, which would obviously cause an alteration in the occlusion and has been shown to be present in up to 15% of Le Fort fractures.[3]

A Le Fort I fracture is a horizontal fracture of the maxilla through the midportion of the pyriform rims and nasomaxillary suture anteriorly and posteriorly below the zygomatic buttresses and through the pterygoid plates (Fig. 9–2A). There is separation and mobility of the body of the maxilla separate from the remainder of the midface. A Le Fort II fracture causes separation at the nasofrontal junction and medial orbital walls. The fracture line continues inferiorly and posteriorly through the medial orbital rims, the zygomaticomaxillary sutures, and pterygoid plates. In contrast to a Le Fort I, in a Le Fort II fracture, the mobile segment consists of the body of the maxilla, as well as its frontal and zygomatic processes and the nasal bones. Le Fort II fractures are also referred to as pyramidal fractures because of

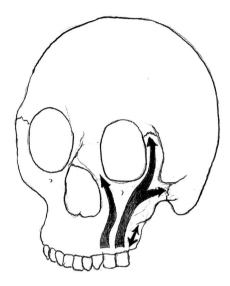

FIGURE 9–1 Diagrammatic representation of the vertical maxillary buttresses. These are areas of thicker bone and provide support against vertical masticatory and traumatic forces.

the triangular shape of the mobile portion of the midface (Fig. **9–2B**). A Le Fort III fracture causes mobility and complete separation of the entire midface from the cranium through the nasofrontal suture, inner orbits, zygomaticofrontal sutures, zygomatic arches, and pterygoid plates (Fig. **9–2C**).

Modern maxillofacial fractures secondary to high-velocity motor vehicle accidents tend to be more complex than those described by Le Fort. Pure Le Fort fractures tend to occur in less than 50% of midface fractures.[4,5] Pure Le Fort fractures are by definition bilateral, and this classification should be used only when a bilateral Le Fort level fracture exists requiring fixation at that level bilaterally. For example, a horizontal separation of the maxilla

combined with a unilateral zygomatic complex fracture should be described as a Le Fort I fracture combined with a zygomatic complex fracture. Similarly a Le Fort II fracture with a unilateral zygomatic complex fracture should be described as such. Describing such fracture as a hemi-Le Fort II and hemi-Le Fort III would be misleading in that it would imply that fixation at the zygomaticomaxillary junction on one side is not necessary as would be the case in a true Le Fort III fracture.

INITIAL EXAMINATION

All facial trauma patients should be evaluated according to the Advanced Trauma Life Support (ATLS) protocol. Special attention should be paid to the airway and cervical spine. Patients with panfacial fractures are at risk for airway obstruction secondary to soft tissue edema or displacement of the facial fractures. In addition, oral and nasopharyngeal bleeding may also lead to airway obstruction and aspiration. Early endotracheal intubation or a surgical airway must be considered for these reasons. Maxillofacial examination and manipulation should be performed with strict cervical spine precaution protocol, because the incidence of cervical spine injuries in patients with maxillofacial trauma has been reported to be up to 3%.[6]

Once the airway has been addressed and hemodynamic and neurologic stability confirmed, a detailed maxillofacial examination is conducted. The examination is initiated with evaluation of the facial skin and scalp for lacerations that may be repaired acutely and for areas of ecchymosis that may indicate underlying fractures. A detailed examination of the cranial nerves, eye, and ear is then conducted. Intraoral examination should include

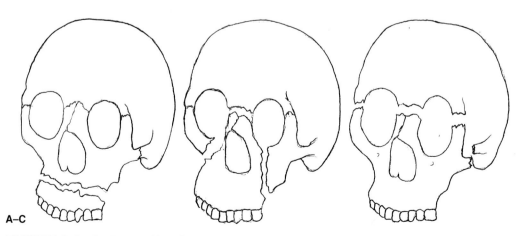

A–C

FIGURE 9–2 Le Fort midface fractures. A: Le Fort I fracture separating the inferior body of the maxilla horizontally. B: Le Fort II fracture causing separation of the entire maxilla and nasal complex from the cranial base. C: Le Fort III fracture causing a complete separation of the entire midface from the cranial base.

assessment for the presence of dentoalveolar injuries, malocclusion, ecchymosis of the floor of the mouth (may indicate a mandibular fracture), ecchymosis on the palate (may indicate a palatal fracture), and fractured or missing teeth. Chest and abdominal films should be obtained to account for missing teeth or teeth fragments that may have been aspirated or swallowed. Midface mobility in Le Fort fractures is assessed by placing one's thumb and index fingers on the anterior maxillary alveolus and the opposite hand on the forehead. The maxilla is then rocked forward and downward.

CLINICAL FINDINGS IN LE FORT FRACTURES AND PALATAL FRACTURES

Patients with Le Fort I fractures may have minimal external signs. Intraorally, there may be ecchymosis of the maxillary vestibule and palpable bony steps in the area of the buttress accompanied by tenderness. Displacement usually occurs in a posterior and inferior direction causing an anterior open bite with the molars contacting prematurely. Unless the fractured maxilla is firmly impacted, mobility should be palpable at the pyriform rims and buttresses intraorally. A similar malocclusion may be present as the result of a widened palatal fracture, and the palatal mucosa should be inspected for the presence of a laceration or bruising. Palatal fractures usually occur at or adjacent to the midline longitudinally dividing the palate. Dentoalveolar fractures of the palate also occur. These fractures are commonly displaced causing an asymmetric malocclusion and separate mobile segments (Fig. 9–3).

Le Fort II fractures produce more obvious external findings because they involve the orbits and nasal bridge, and because they may be associated with significant NOE complex injuries. Patients may have an obvious nasal deformity along with subconjunctival and periorbital ecchymosis and edema (Fig. 9–4). Infraorbital nerve paresthesia is usually present. In severely displaced fractures, restriction of globe movement and other forms of orbital trauma may be present and ophthalmologic consultation is imperative. The malocclusion seen with Le Fort II fractures is similar to that of a Le Fort I. With manipulation of the maxilla, however, mobility can be felt at the nasofrontal junction and medial aspects of the infraorbital rims. Cerebrospinal fluid (CSF) rhinorrhea may also be present if the cribriform plate is fractured.

Le Fort III fractures involve a separation of the midface from the cranial base. Dural tears in the

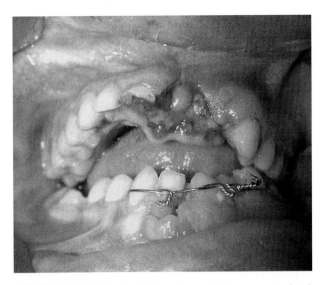

FIGURE 9–3 Le Fort I fracture with separate palatal and dentoalveolar fractures.

areas of the cribriform plate or the roof of the auditory canal may lead to CSF rhinorrhea or otorrhea respectively. Bleeding from basilar skull fractures near the stylomastoid foramen may track superficially and create an area of ecchymosis over the mastoid process and occiput (Battle's sign). Because Le Fort III fractures involve separation at the nasofrontal suture, inner orbits, and zygomaticofrontal sutures, significant clinical findings may be found. Bilateral periorbital edema and ecchymosis, and nasal bridge flattening may be present. In addition, there may be a significant increase in orbital volume from fracture displacement and orbital floor blow-out fractures resulting into enophthalmos and soft tissue entrapment. With manipulation of the maxilla, mobility should be felt at

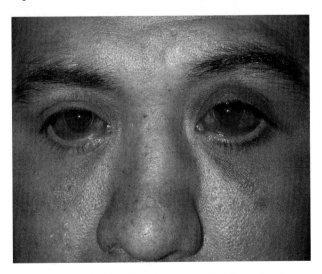

FIGURE 9–4 Nasal deformity and bilateral subconjunctival and periorbital ecchymosis in a patient with a Le Fort II fracture.

the nasofrontal junction and zygomaticofrontal sutures.

Imaging

Computed Tomography (CT) remains the gold standard modality for the evaluation of facial fractures. Facial CT should be ordered in both the axial and coronal planes and printed as separate bone and soft tissue windows. Additional 1.5-mm cuts through the orbits should be obtained in the presence of orbital trauma requiring reconstruction. Three-dimensional images of the skull and face can also be reconstructed from two-dimensional CT images, but should not be used for accurate diagnosis of fractures because details are lost from volume averaging and processing of the digital data. They should be obtained to elicit additional information on the displacement and spatial relationship of the midface with the mandible and orbits. Plain radiographs such as frontal, lateral, submental vertex, and occipitomental views are useful but infrequently obtained since the advent of CT.

Initial Management

The initial management should be aimed at securing the airway, controlling bleeding, and closing lacerations. Bleeding from the greater palatine and internal maxillary arteries may be extensive, requiring regional packing and expeditious maxillary reduction and immobilization. Immobilization with intermaxillary fixation is useful in that it stabilizes fractures and fully or partially reduces the maxilla when used in conjunction with elastic traction. Immobilization with intermaxillary fixation also reduces patient discomfort. If the occlusal relationship is questionable or if a palatal fracture is present, alginate impressions should be made for the fabrication of study models and stabilizing palatal splints. Ophthalmologic consultation should be obtained in the presence of orbital or ocular trauma.

Management of the Airway

Surgical management of Le Fort fractures requires correction of the occlusion and therefore intraoperative intermaxillary fixation. The choice of endotracheal intubation should not interfere with maxillomandibular fixation. Nasal intubation and tracheotomy are the preferred approaches. A tracheotomy is especially beneficial in the presence of nasal fractures and when access and plating through

a coronal approach is needed. In the past, nasal intubation was contraindicated in patients with midface fractures involving the cribriform plate because of the concern about an increased risk of meningitis or that the tube could enter the cranial fossa. In a study of 160 patients with midface fractures with CSF rhinorrhea, Bahr and Stoll[7] reported no such complications from nasal intubation. A similar finding was reported by Rhee et al.[8] Nasal intubation with fiberoptic guidance, therefore, is a sensible alternative to a tracheotomy in the absence of fractures of the frontal sinus and NOE structures. Another approach in panfacial fractures would be to first intubate the patient nasally to rigidly fix the maxillary, zygomatic, and mandibular fractures and then switch to an oral tube to address fractures of the frontal sinus and NOE complex. In patients who are missing teeth, oral intubation with a noncollapsible steel-reinforced tube exiting through the edentulous space is another viable alternative. Airway options in patients with facial fractures are summarized in Fig. **9–5**.

Reduction and Fixation

Reduction and fixation of Le Fort fractures should be performed as soon the general condition of the patient is stable. Facial edema alone should not preclude early treatment because facial fractures should be reduced and fixated anatomically under direct vision. Delay in treatment may result in difficulty with reducing the midface due to soft tissue fibrosis and contraction. Soft tissue scarring and fibrosis may also lead to malposition of the soft tissue envelope of the facial bones even if these were anatomically reduced and fixated.

After intubation and surgical exposure, the maxilla is disimpacted and mobilized with Rowe's forceps. During disimpaction, it is recommended to overreduce the maxilla anteriorly relative to the mandible to the point where passive repositioning of the midface results in anatomic realignment upon release. Failure to accomplish this may result in long-term relapse because dynamic forces from muscle pull and soft tissue contraction may overcome the stability provided by plate fixation. This is especially important when smaller miniplates are used. If an acrylic splint is needed for a coexisting palatal fracture, it is secured at this point (Fig. **9–6**). Although plate fixation of palatal fractures has been described,[9] the use of custom-made stabilizing splints in conjunction with intermaxillary fixation gives the most accurate results. After reduction and stabilization of the palate, the jaws are placed into intermaxillary fixation while assuring that any

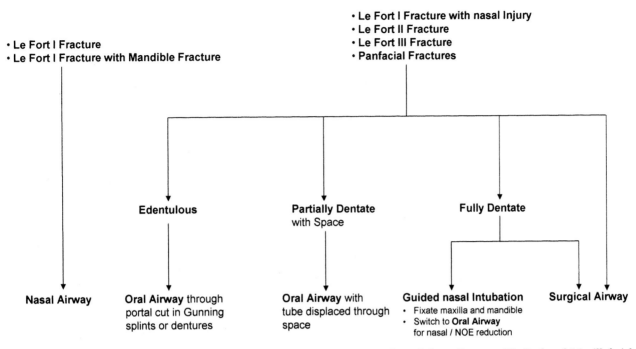

FIGURE 9–5 Airway options in patients with midface fractures. (Adapted from Fonseca RJ. *Oral and Maxillofacial Surgery,* vol 3. Philadelphia: WB Saunders, 2000:266, with permission.)

widening of the palate has been reduced and that the upper and lower teeth come in the appropriate occlusal relationship. Appropriate seating of the mandibular condyles in the glenoid fossae at the time of intermaxillary fixation is mandatory (Fig. 9–7). Failure to do so will lead to fixation of the maxilla, and in panfacial fractures, the remainder of the midface in an incorrect position. This results in an open-bite deformity and facial lengthening. After

placement into intermaxillary fixation, the remainder of the fractures should be exposed. These initial steps are essential in the treatment of any Le Fort fractures, including panfacial injuries involving the mandible. Critical steps in treatment of palatal and Le Fort fractures are summarized below.

PALATAL FRACTURES

- A custom-made reducing splint is constructed in the laboratory from stone models.
- Palatal segments are loosened and mobilized.
- The splint is adapted to the palate and wired to the maxillary teeth.
- Intermaxillary fixation is applied and the occlusion assessed.

LE FORT I FRACTURES

- Exposure of bilateral zygomaticomaxillary and pyriform buttresses is obtained through an intraoral vestibular incision.
- The maxilla is mobilized and intermaxillary fixation is applied.
- Comminuted bony fragments in the area of the buttresses are anatomically repositioned to reestablish the vertical height of the maxilla and midface.

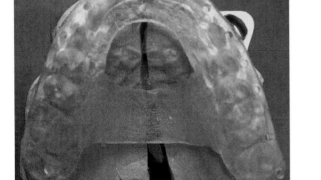

FIGURE 9–6 Custom-made acrylic palatal splint with extension over the occlusal surfaces for the reduction and stabilization of palatal fractures.

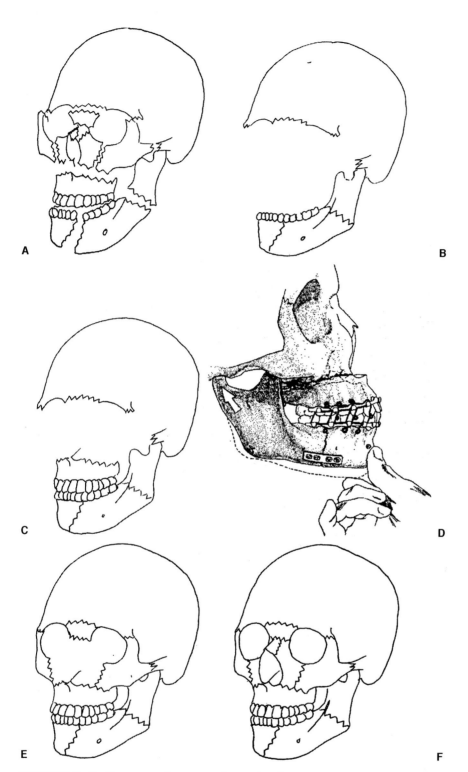

FIGURE 9–7 Sequence of treatment in panfacial trauma. A: Extensive panfacial trauma. B: Mandibular reconstruction. C: Positioning of the maxilla in relation to the mandible using intermaxillary fixation. D: Appropriate seating of the mandibular condyles into the fossa. E: Reduction of zygomatic complexes and reconstruction of the nasofrontal junction. F: Reconstruction of the naso-orbital-ethmoid (NOE) complex (frontal sinus is addressed first). Fixation at the infraorbital rims is performed next, followed by fixation at the Le Fort I level. Bone grafting of orbital and nasal defects is performed last. (Adapted from Fonseca RJ. *Oral and Maxillofacial Surgery,* vol 3. Philadelphia: WB Saunders, 2000:268, with permission.)

- The zygomaticomaxillary and pyriform buttresses are fixated.
- Comminuted areas and defects of the buttresses are spanned with bone plates and bone grafted if necessary to prevent midface collapse.
- Loose bony fragments and any torn sinus membrane are removed from the sinus cavity to prevent sinus infection.
- Anterior maxillary wall defects may be covered with titanium mesh or bone grafted to prevent soft tissue collapse.

LE FORT II FRACTURES

- Exposure is obtained through an intraoral vestibular, bilateral transconjunctival, and coronal incisions.
- The maxilla is mobilized and intermaxillary fixation is applied.
- The zygomaticomaxillary buttresses, the inferior orbital rims, and the frontonasal junction are plated.
- Medial orbital floor or wall defects, if present, are reconstructed with titanium mesh, high-molecular polyethylene sheets, or bone grafts.

LE FORT III FRACTURES

- Exposure is obtained through coronal and vestibular incisions.
- The maxilla is mobilized and intermaxillary fixation is applied.
- The zygomatic arches, zygomaticofrontal sutures, frontonasal junction, and zygomaticomaxillary buttresses are plated.
- Orbital defects are accessed through transconjunctival incisions and reconstructed with titanium mesh or bone grafts.

Isolated Le Fort fractures occur infrequently and the Le Fort classification is useful only for approximate description of midface fractures. Most patients with extensive facial injuries have components of Le Fort fractures concurrent with separate palatal, zygomatic, or NOE complex fractures. Mandibular fractures may also be present. Appropriate sequencing of reduction and fixation of multiple facial fractures becomes crucial for an optimal outcome in terms of occlusion and facial proportions.

SPECIAL CONSIDERATIONS AND SEQUENCING IN PANFACIAL FRACTURES

In patients with panfacial fractures, the mandible becomes an excellent reference for the reconstruction of the midface. This is especially the case when an adequate dentition is present and posterior ramus height has been preserved with at least one intact or reconstructed mandibular ramus-condyle unit. Reconstruction of the mandible is performed first and must include reconstruction of the ramus-condyle unit and tooth-bearing areas with the patient in intermaxillary fixation. This initial step reestablishes lower facial height and reduces the maxilla. A partial or complete reduction of the Le Fort component could have been obtained at this point on. Because in most instances separate zygomatic or NOE complex injuries are present, sequencing of treatment becomes crucial at this point.

After mandibular reconstruction and reduction of the Le Fort component with intermaxillary fixation, the outer frame of the upper midface is addressed. This involves reconstruction of the zygomatic arches with the zygomatic body correctly oriented to the cranial vault and posterior root of the zygoma. Verification of alignment at the zygomatico-sphenoid junction is critical for proper orientation of the zygoma. The fracture at the zygomaticomaxillary buttress is assessed at this point and should be close to anatomic alignment. The zygomatic bones are then plated at the zygomaticofrontal sutures, the arch, and zygomaticomaxillary buttress, and in the absence of NOE fractures, the orbital rims. Fixation of the maxilla at the Le Fort I level is then completed. If NOE fractures are present, these must be addressed before fixation at the pyriform rims in Le Fort I fractures and medial orbital rims in Le Fort II fractures. The bones of the nasal vault are fixated to the frontal bone (after addressing the frontal sinus), followed by fixation at the central portion of the NOE complex, and then the orbital rims. Fixation of the orbital or pyriform rims in Le Fort fractures prior to reducing the NOE complex may prevent alignment of the frontal process of the maxilla with the frontal bone. Grafting of orbital defects or the nasal dorsum is performed last if indicated (Fig. 9–7).

CHOICE OF PLATE SYSTEMS

A strong 2.0-mm system should be used at the vertical pillars of the face to resist masticatory forces. In areas of thin skin such as the orbital rims, smaller plates are preferred to prevent excessive palpability and visible appreciation of the plate through the skin. Thin-skinned individuals require special consideration and often benefit from smaller plates to avoid such problems.

RECOMMENDED PLATE SYSTEMS FOR SPECIFIC SITES

- A 2.0-mm system at the zygomaticomaxillary buttresses and pyriform areas (vertical buttresses) to withstand masticatory forces and prevent vertical collapse.
- A 1.5- or 1.3-mm system at the zygomaticofrontal junctions and nasal root.
- A 1.5- or 1.3-mm system at the zygomatic arches.
- A 1.3-mm system at the orbital rims.
- A 1.0-mm system is reserved for areas of small comminuted fragments and thin bone.

COMPLICATIONS

Common complications resulting from midface fractures and their treatment include malocclusion, cranial nerve injuries, and secondary facial deformities. Complications related to associated orbital, frontal sinus, or NOE injuries are discussed elsewhere in the text. In a review of 100 patients with midface fractures, Haug et al[10] reported postoperative malocclusions in 12% of patients treated with rigid fixation and 4% in patients treated with intermaxillary fixation.

Malocclusion may result from fixation of improperly reduced fractures or insufficient fixation. Inadequate fracture reduction may result from improper seating of the condyles when applying intermaxillary fixation or failure to reduce coexisting palatal fractures. The malocclusion in these instances will be appreciated in the immediate postoperative period and require immediate attention, especially if rigid fixation was used.

Significant occlusal discrepancies require prompt surgical intervention or orthodontics followed by orthognathic surgery after 3 to 6 months. Minor occlusal problems may respond to gradual elastic traction and intermaxillary fixation.[11] Whether such correction occurs from skeletal movement or dental compensation is unknown. Progressive development of a postoperative malocclusion usually indicates improper fixation leading to skeletal relapse. This should be managed with a liquid diet and elastic traction or full intermaxillary fixation. In the presence of severe fracture comminution requiring bone grafting or the use of smaller than recommended plates, postoperative intermaxillary fixation for 4 weeks is recommended. This prevents skeletal relapse resulting from masticatory forces and allows for adequate bone graft incorporation. Intermaxillary fixation for at least 4 weeks is also recommended in the presence of palatal or alveolar ridge fractures.

Facial deformities usually result from improperly treated nasal, zygomatic, or orbital components. Secondary nasal deformities after Le Fort II and III fractures are common and result from inadequate reduction and stabilization of the nasal bones. Nasal deformities have been reported in 13 to 33% of patients with upper midface fractures.[12–14] Improper orientation of coexisting zygomatic fractures leads to facial and orbital asymmetry. Failure to appropriately reconstruct internal orbital defects may lead to hypoglobus and diplopia. Management of these posttraumatic deformities is beyond the scope of this chapter but generally require surgical procedures such as a septorhinoplasty, orbitozygomatic osteotomies, and grafting procedures to bridge bony defects or for contour augmentation.

The incidence of an immediate postoperative infraorbital nerve deficit from Le Fort I and II fractures has been reported at 65% and was directly related to fracture displacement of greater than 1 mm.[15] Patients with less than 1 mm of displacement in that study regained normal sensation after 3 months. Thirty percent of those with displacement of greater than 1 mm had a persistent sensory deficit at 1-year follow-up. In a review on the subject, Thurmuller et al[16] found that coexisting orbitozygomatic fractures may lead to a persistent sensory disturbance of up to 46%. They also found that a delay in treatment of greater than 1 week resulted in a higher incidence of a persistent sensory disturbance.

PEARLS: LE FORT AND PALATAL FRACTURES

- Proper reestablishment of maxillary position and the occlusion is imperative in the treatment of all Le Fort fractures.
- Airway management should not interfere with the application of intermaxillary fixation and often requires special techniques or a surgical airway.
- Facial fractures should be treated within 2 weeks to achieve optimal and stable bony and soft tissue results.
- Adequate disimpaction and immobilization of the maxilla is imperative prior to fixation.

- Appropriate condylar seating and reduction of palatal fractures prior to the application of intermaxillary fixation reduces the incidence of postoperative malocclusions.
- Proper reduction and stabilization of the vertical pillars of the face are essential to reestablish vertical height and to prevent relapse resulting from masticatory forces.
- Postoperative intermaxillary fixation or elastic guidance may increase stability and correct minor occlusal problems, especially in the presence of palatal fractures.
- Early reduction and fixation of midface fractures reduces the incidence of a persistent infraorbital nerve deficit.
- Treatment of Le Fort fractures should be appropriately sequenced in the presence of multiple facial fractures.

REFERENCES

1. Manson PN, Hoopes JE, Su CT. Structural pillars of the facial skeleton: an approach to the management of Le Fort fractures. Plast Reconstr Surg 1980;66:54–62

2. Tessier P. The classic reprint: experimental study of fractures of the upper jaw. 3. Rene Le Fort, M.D., Lille, France. Plast Reconstr Surg 1972;50:600–607

3. Manson PN, Shack RB, Leonard LG, et al. Sagittal fractures of the maxilla and palate. Plast Reconstr Surg 1983;72:484–489

4. Klotch DW, Gilliland R. Internal fixation vs. conventional therapy in midface fractures. J Trauma 1987;27:1136–1145

5. Marciani RD. Management of midface fractures: fifty years later. J Oral Maxillofac Surg 1993;51:960–968

6. Haug RH, Savage JD, Likavec MJ, et al. A review of 100 closed head injuries associated with facial fractures. J Oral Maxillofac Surg 1992;50:218–222

7. Bahr W, Stoll P. Nasal intubation in the presence of frontobasal fractures: a retrospective study. J Oral Maxillofac Surg 1992;50:445–447

8. Rhee KJ, Muntz CB, Donald PJ, et al. Does nasotracheal intubation increase complications in patients with skull base fractures? Ann Emerg Med 1993;22:1145–1147

9. Manson PN, Glassman D, Vanderkolk C, et al. Rigid stabilization of sagittal fractures of the maxilla and palate. Plast Reconstr Surg 1990;85:711–717

10. Haug RH, Adams JM, Jordan RB. Comparison of the morbidity associated with maxillary fractures treated by maxillomandibular and rigid internal fixation. Oral Surg Oral Med Oral Pathol Oral Radiol Endod 1995;80:629–637

11. Jensen J, Sindet-Pedersen S, Christensen L. Rigid fixation in reconstruction of craniofacial fractures. J Oral Maxillofac Surg 1992;50:550–554

12. Morgan BD, Madan DK, Bergerot JP. Fractures of the middle third of the face—a review of 300 cases. Br J Plast Surg 1972;25:147–151

13. Sofferman RA, Danielson PA, Quatela V, et al. Retrospective analysis of surgically treated Le Fort fractures. Arch Otolaryngol 1983;109:446–448

14. Heimgartner-Candinas B, Heimgartner M, Jonutis A. Results of treatment of midfacial fractures. Indications for exploration and drainage of the maxillary sinuses. J Maxillofac Surg 1978;6:293–301

15. Schultze-Mosgau S, Erbe M, Rudolph D, et al. Prospective study on post-traumatic and postoperative sensory disturbances of the inferior alveolar nerve and infraorbital nerve in mandibular and midfacial fractures. J Craniomaxillofac Surg 1999;27:86–93

16. Thurmuller P, Dodson TB, Kaban LB. Nerve injuries associated with facial trauma: natural history, management, and outcomes of repair. Oral Maxillofac Surg Clin North Am 2001;13:283–293

Chapter 10

Basic Principles in the Treatment of Mandibular Fractures

Jaime Gateno

At birth, the mandible consists of two halves, which are united in the median plane by a fibrous symphysis. This articulation becomes ossified during the first year of life, after which, the mandible is considered a single bone. Each mandibular half consists of a horizontal portion, the body, and a vertical portion, the ramus. The body contains the teeth and extends from the midline to the last molar. Clinically, the parasymphysis comprises the area of the mandible that extends from the symphysis to the canine tooth. The ramus of the mandible is flat, and has four borders and two processes. The junction of the inferior border and the posterior border make the angle of the mandible. The two processes are the anterior coronoid process and the posterior condylar process.[1]

The inferior alveolar nerve, a branch of the third division of the trigeminal nerve, enters the mandible through the mandibular foramen in the medial aspect of the ramus. It runs through the mandibular canal, which ends at the mental foramen. The nerve has two terminal branches: the incisive branch gives sensory innervation to the lower incisors, and the mental nerve provides sensation to the lower lip and the chin.[1] Fractures of the mandible crossing through the canal can produce trauma to the nerve, causing temporary or permanent altered sensation in the chin and lip.

To avoid damage to the inferior alveolar nerve, surgeons should be familiar with the three-dimensional anatomy of the mandibular canal. This canal begins at the mandibular foramen. In this area the canal is the furthest away from the inferior border of the mandible. From here, it runs anteriorly and inferiorly following a gentle curve. It gets closest to the inferior border of the mandible in the area of the first molar before it curves back up to exit at the mental foramen, which is in close proximity to the second premolar.[2]

While in the vicinity of the nerve, the placement of bicortical screws should be limited to the area between the mandibular canal and the inferior border of the mandible. Table 10–1 provides the mean distances from the inferior border to this canal.[2] As shown, the nerve is at the highest risk of injury at the first and second molar regions, where the mean distances between the canal and the inferior border are only 7.3 and 7.5 mm, respectively. The distances presented in Table 10–1 can be used to direct the placement of screws in this area. However, caution is advised before these mean distances are used clinically. If, for example, in a large group of patients, screws were to be placed in the first molar area at 7.3 mm from the inferior border, statistically the nerve would be injured in 50% of cases. However, if the screws were to be placed at 4.5 mm, which is the mean distance (7.3 mm) minus two standard deviations (2.8 mm), the nerve would be injured in only 2.5% of patients.

Surgeons should be familiar with the mean thickness of the buccal cortical plate as well as the mean transverse distances between the buccal cortex and the mandibular canal.[2] This information is helpful to prevent injuries to the nerve during the placement of monocortical screws. The mandibular canal is closest to the buccal plate in the areas of the second premolar and third molar (Table 10–1). It should also be noted that the distances between the canal and the buccal surface of the mandible are fairly small and that the nerve is at risk even with the use of 6-mm screws. Therefore, we recommend placing these screws either above or below the canal.

TABLE 10-1   MANDIBULAR ANTHROPOMETRIC MEASUREMENTS

	2nd premolar	1st molar	2nd molar	Retromolar trigone	Mandibular foramen
Distance from inferior border of the mandible to mandibular canal	8.2 ± 1.5 mm	7.3 ± 1.4 mm	7.5 ± 1.7 mm	10.5 ± 2.5 mm	18.5 ± 3.7 mm
Thickness of the buccal cortex	1.8 ± 0.5 mm	1.9 ± 0.4 mm	2.3 ± 0.7 mm	1.8 ± 0.4 mm	1.5 ± 0.4 mm
Distance from the buccal cortex to the mandibular canal	3.2 ± 1.7 mm	5.9 ± 1.5 mm	5.9 ± 1.9 mm	3.5 ± 1.5 mm	5.5 ± 1.6 mm

BIOMECHANICS

Understanding of the fundamental concepts of mandibular biomechanics is important for the successful treatment of mandibular fractures. Biomechanics connotes the study of the mechanics of biologic structures. The study of mechanics is devoted to the evaluation and description of the behavior of structures acted upon by forces.[3] During function, the mandible is subjected to forces produced by the muscles of mastication and by reaction forces applied to the temporomandibular joints (TMJs) and the teeth.[4] As a result, *stresses* and *strains* are produced in the mandible. Stress is the resisting force set up in a body as a result of an externally applied force.[5] This force is equal in magnitude but opposite in direction to the external force.[6] It is measured as the ratio of force to unit of area of the material.[4] The unit of stress is the Pascal (Pa). One pascal = 1 newton/m^2, 1 Mpa = 10^{6}N/m^2, and 1 Gpa = 10^9 N/m^2. Depending on how the load is applied, stress can be classified as compressive, tensile, or shear. *Compressive stress* is developed if the material becomes shorter, *tensile stress* if it becomes longer, and *shear stress* if one region of the material moves parallel relative to the adjacent region. *Strain* is the change in shape that a body undergoes when acted upon by an external force.[5] Strain is dimensionless and is measured as the ratio of the change in length to the original length. A strain of 0.01 is equal to a 1% deformation.

The models that have been used to study the mandible have evolved from two-dimensional beam models to more realistic three-dimensional models. Much of our understanding of the biomechanics of the mandible has been derived from the study of beam models. The simplest beam model that has been compared with the mandible is a cantilever beam.[3,4] A cantilever beam is a projecting beam that is supported at only one end as it is anchored to a wall. When a downward vertical load is applied to the free end of the beam, the beam deforms so its upper surface becomes convex and its lower surface concave. Concomitantly, stresses develop within the structure. The stresses in the convex (upper) side are tensile, whereas the stresses in the concave (lower) side are compressive. Between the zones of tension and compression there is a line of zero stress. The magnitude of the stresses within the beam increases from the line of zero stress toward the surface (Fig. **10-1A**).

The addition of a new force into this system changes the stresses in the structure. An example of this is illustrated in Fig. **10-1B**, in which an upward force is inserted in the middle of the beam. If this force is of sufficient magnitude, it will bend the proximal end of the cantilever beam upward and a reversal of stresses will occur in the most proximal part of the beam. In this area, the upper surface will be under compression whereas the lower surface will be under tension.[3] Moreover, if the point of application of the downward force is moved to a point located halfway between the upward force and the beam support, the configuration of the tension-compression stress regions will change again (Fig. **10-1C**). In the proximal half of the beam, the upper surface will be under compression while the lower surface will be under tension. Additionally, the distal half of the beam will be unloaded. These examples illustrate a basic concept of beam mechanics: the configuration of the tension-compression stress regions depends on the point of application and magnitude of the force applied.[3]

Initial biomechanical studies of the mandible modeled this bone as a straight cantilever beam. From these models, it was concluded that during function the alveolar border of the mandible was under tension while the inferior border was under compression (Fig. **10-1D**). This information has been used to formulate many of the current recommendations regarding treatment; however, the use of a cantilever beam to model the mandible is technically inaccurate.

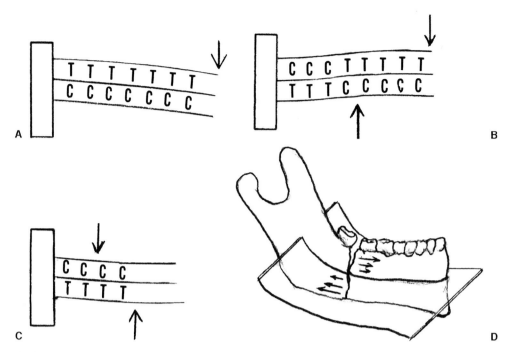

FIGURE 10–1 A: A downward vertical load is applied to the free end of the beam. The beam deforms so its upper surface becomes convex and its lower surface concave. The stresses in the convex (upper) side are tensile, whereas the stresses in the concave (lower) side are compressive. B: An upward force is inserted in the middle of the beam. This force bends the proximal end of the cantilever beam upward. A reversal of stresses occurs in the most proximal part of the beam. In this area, the upper surface is under compression while the lower surface is under tension. C: If the point of application of the downward force is moved to a point located halfway between the upward force and the beam support, the configuration of the tension-compression stress regions changes. In the proximal half of the beam, the upper surface is under compression, whereas the lower surface is under tension. Additionally, the distal half of the beam is unloaded. D: Mandible modeled as a straight cantilever beam. Red arrows, zone of tension. Black arrows, zone of compression. Plane, zone of zero stress.

The mandible is not attached at one end but is actually suspended from each end at the TMJs. A suspended beam, therefore, is a more accurate mandibular model. In this model the mandible is simulated as a straight beam that is suspended at each end by the TMJ attachments. The beam represents the whole unwrapped mandible as it is seen in a Panorex. Single force vectors acting at the coronoid processes represent the muscles of mastication, and a vertical force is used to represent the biting force (Fig. **10–2**).[3,4] The use of only one muscular force per side was derived from the summation of the separate muscle vectors, resulting in a muscular force vector directed mainly perpendicular to the occlusal plane and inserted in the region of the of the mandibular ramus.[7] When the biting force is applied, an interesting effect is noted. The lower part of the beam under the biting force becomes the zone of tension (Fig. **10–2**), and as the biting force is moved from side to side this zone of stress reversal moves through the beam.

A suspended beam model is superior to a cantilever model, but still ignores the three-dimensional nature of the mandible.[3] The mandible is not a

simple beam but a free parabolic body, upon which a variety of forces act.[8] The use of three-dimensional models has allowed investigators to study the

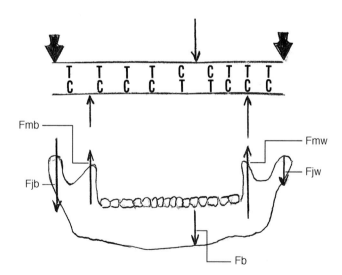

FIGURE 10–2 Mandible modeled as a suspended beam. Fjb, joint force balance side; Fjw, joint force working side; Fmb, muscle force balance side; Fmw, muscle force working side; Fb, bite force; C, compression; T, tension.

biomechanics of the mandible in a more realistic way.[3,4,9] One the main advantages of these models is that they can demonstrate the tension, compression, as well as shear stresses in the x, y, and z axes.[3]

A finite element model of the mandible has demonstrated that when the mandible is loaded on one side at the molar region, the superior border of the mandible under the load is under compression while its inferior border is under tension. This zone of compression extends anteriorly across the midline to the area of the contralateral canine. In the contralateral side of the mandible, the superior border is under tension while the inferior border is under compression. The largest compression stresses occur in the same side of the force application. Also, the zones of attachment of the pterygomasseteric sling are under compression. The results of this study are similar to other three-dimensional studies but differ remarkably from those of traditional two-dimensional models; however, it is noteworthy that the pattern of stress distribution observed in the more complex three-dimensional model is similar to that observed in the suspended beam model.

BASIC PRINCIPLES OF FRACTURE TREATMENT

To treat a fracture, the surgeon usually completes two basic and sequential steps: reduction followed by stabilization. By definition, fracture reduction is not necessary in nondisplaced fractures. Methods of fracture reduction can be indirect or direct. In indirect or closed reduction, the fracture is reduced without surgically exposing the fracture site. This can be accomplished by reestablishment of the occlusion using maxillomandibular fixation (MMF), by manual manipulation, or by a combination of both methods. In direct or open reduction, the fracture is reduced under direct visualization after the site has been exposed surgically. Direct fracture reduction is indicated when adequate reduction is impossible using indirect methods or when the fracture site will be exposed anyway for placement of internal fixation.

Once a fracture has been reduced, it should be stabilized for an appropriate length of time for healing to occur. Stabilization of mandibular fractures can be accomplished using different methods including MMF, intraosseous wiring, external pin fixation, and internal fixation.

MAXILLOMANDIBULAR FIXATION

Maxillomandibular fixation is the standard method used for both reduction as well as stabilization. The skeletal stabilization of the fracture segments is provided indirectly by fixing the lower teeth in their correct relationship to the corresponding upper teeth.[10] This method produces relative stability of the fracture, and healing will occur by callus formation.

Maxillomandibular fixation alone is sufficient for the management of many simple fractures. It is also often used in conjunction with other methods. However, MMF has several disadvantages related to the need for the patient's mouth to remain closed for an extended period of time. When general anesthesia is used, the patient is at risk for airway problems immediately following extubation. Patients in MMF experience more weight loss than patients not in MMF. Also, these patients have more difficulties with speech and oral hygiene. Finally, 6 weeks of MMF is difficult for patients to accept.

EXTERNAL FIXATION

External fixation is a method of skeletal immobilization in which bony fragments are interconnected by external stabilizing frames that are attached to the bone by percutaneously inserted pins. Its rigidity is associated with certain instability; therefore, healing occurs by callus formation. This method has an important but limited role in the treatment of mandibular fractures. The main limitation of this technique is that patients find it objectionable, not only for cosmetic reasons, but also because it interferes with natural head movements, rest, and sleep. In spite of this, its use may be preferable over other modalities of stabilization in certain patients. The main advantages of external fixation are that it can be applied with no periosteal stripping and minimal soft tissue disruption. Additionally, it leaves a minimal amount of implanted material, it is associated with decreased operative time, and the surgeon has the ability to make adjustments during treatment. Finally, the hardware is easily removed at the end of the treatment. Because of these advantages, its use should be considered in fractures of the atrophic edentulous mandible, extensive soft tissue injuries, severe comminution, and with infected fractures.

External fixation systems have three basic components: fixation pins, connecting bar, and clamps. The fixation pins are inserted percutaneously into bone. The connecting bar is used to splint the screws together, and the clamps connect the fixation pins to the connecting bar. The most significant parameter that affects the stability of an external fixation system is the radius of the pin.[11] The stiffness of the pins is proportional to the fourth power of its radius. Therefore, a small increase in diameter results in a large increase in stiffness.[11,12] Other pin-related factors that affect frame rigidity are the number, separation, and plane of insertion. To prevent the rotation of a bone fragment around a single pin, a minimum of two pins should be used to fix each major bone fragment. Generally these pins are inserted in the same plane and offer a reasonable resistance to any motion of the bone fragments in that plane. However, they are less able to resist motion perpendicular to the plane of the pins. This resistance can be improved by utilizing the widest possible separation of the two pins in the bone fragment. Resistance to bending is increased slightly by the addition of a third pin, but subsequent pins provide only negligible increase in rigidity.

In addition to the diameter, the rigidity of an individual external fixation pin is affected by its working length (i.e., the distance between the bone and the bar). Because the rigidity is inversely proportional to the square of the working length, fastening the bar close to the bone markedly increases the rigidity of fixation. Bars must be far enough away, however, to permit room for soft tissue swelling and wound access.[11,12]

The stability of external fixation is also enhanced when major bone fragments can be held together under compression. When sufficient bone stock is preserved, the frame should be applied with tension in the longitudinal connecting rods to produce static compression at the interface between the main fragments. However, in many cases, comminution or bone loss prevents fixation of main bone fragments under compression. External fixation must then be used to maintain length and alignment.

INTERNAL FIXATION

Internal fixation refers to the application of fixation devices right at the fracture site. The devices used for this purpose include wires, screws, and plates. These devices can be used to provide either absolute or relative stability of the fracture. *Rigid internal fixation* refers to the use of lag screws, compression plates, and the tension band principle to attain absolute stability of the fracture. Other techniques of internal fixation attain relative stability; they include *bridging*, *biologic fixation*, and the *Champy technique*.

RIGID INTERNAL FIXATION

Rigid internal fixation is a method of fracture treatment that was introduced by the AO-ASIF group in 1958. Plates and screws are used to stabilize the fracture with the goal of absolute stability of the bony fragments. Absolute stability is defined as the absence of relative motion between the implant and the bone and between the bony ends. Obtaining *absolute stability* requires the clear understanding of the basic principles of rigid internal fixation, the use of specialized hardware, and the rigorous adherence to a procedure protocol. In 1975, Perren et al[13] completed a series of experiments that illustrated the causes and consequences of relative motion and how it can be eliminated. In the first experiment, a compression plate was attached to the intact tibia of a live sheep. One end of the plate was installed on the bone using two screws while the other end was left free (Fig. **10–3A**). When the tibia was loaded during gait, the investigators observed *relative motion* between the free end of the plate and the bone. They concluded that the loading of the extremity had caused shortening of the relatively elastic bone in relation to the more rigid implant producing relative motion between the bone and the implant (Fig. **10–3A**).

To illustrate the consequences of relative motion, the investigators inserted a single screw in the free-end of the plate (Fig. **10–3B**). When the bone was intermittently loaded during gait, the investigators were able to document relative motion between the bone and the plate. The micro-motion between the plate and the bone produced resorption of the bone adjacent to the screw threads. The resorbed bone was replaced by connective and granulation tissue. After a while, the process of *motion-induced osteolysis* caused loosening of the screw (Fig. **10–3B**). It is interesting to note that even in the intact bone the functional loading of the bone was capable of producing loosening of the screws. This occurred because of the different elasticities of bone and the plate.

Later, the investigators were able to prevent relative motion and achieve absolute stability by fixing the free end of the plate to the bone with a single screw that was inserted eccentrically to produce tension in the plate and reciprocal compression of the bone. This technique known as prestressing or preloading (Fig. **10–3C**). It produces *primary stresses* within the plate and the bone. The primary stress in the plate is tensile, whereas the primary stress in the bone is compressive. Relative motion is eliminated because the primary stress in the bone is larger than the axial load exerted on the extremity, that is, *secondary stress*. During

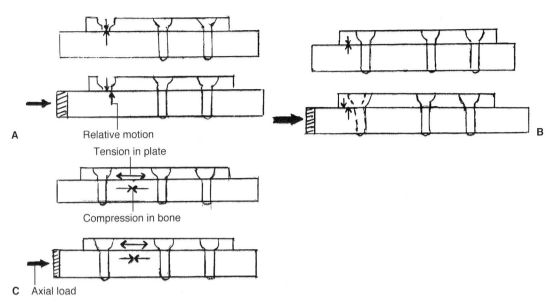

FIGURE 10–3 A: Relative motion between the bone and the plate. B: Relative motion produces loosening of the screw. C: Single screw inserted under tension. There is tension in the plate and reciprocal compression of the bone. Relative motion is eliminated because the primary stress in the bone is larger than the axial load exerted on the extremity.

loading, the primary tensile stress in the plate diminishes but retains a positive value (Fig. **10–3C**). On the whole, these experiments demonstrate an elemental law of the biomechanics of rigid internal fixation: *Relative motion will not occur at the metal–bone interface as long as the preload is greater than the functional load. If this condition is met, a state of absolute stability exists.*[14]

In practice, rigid internal fixation of the mandible is accomplished by compression of the fracture edges known as interfragmentary compression. Interfragmentary compression can be achieved in two ways, by static compression or by dynamic compression. *Static compression* refers to the establishment of constant interfragmentary compression that is not dependent on loading. *Dynamic compression* refers to the generation of interfragmentary compression during functional loading.[15]

Static compression of a fracture can be achieved using either a self-compressing plate or a lag screw. The prototypical self-compressing plate is the dynamic compression plate (DCP) designed by the AO-ASIF group. This is a misnomer, however, as this is actually a means of producing *static* compression. The DCP is able to generate axial compression at the fracture site due to the special geometry of its screw holes. The profile of the screw hole permits the downward and horizontal movement of the screw head during insertion. When the screw is placed eccentrically (i.e., in the outer side of the screw hole), as the screw head approximates the outer rim of the screw hole it meets an incline plane. As the screw continues to be inserted, it contacts the incline plane

and glides horizontally toward the inner aspect of the hole (Fig. **10–4**). Because the screw is also engaging the bone, it moves the bone inward toward the fracture line. Only one screw on each side of the fracture side should be placed eccentrically.[14,16]

A disadvantage of self-compressing plates is that they produce an asymmetric distribution of the compressive forces across the fracture. This is due to the fact that the plate can only be applied on the surface of the bone. This causes a complete closure of the fracture gap immediately underneath the plate while on the opposite side a gap may form (Fig. **10–5A**). This may be counteracted by over-bending the plate slightly just over the fracture or by using an additional lag screw across the fracture (Fig. **10–5B,C**).[14,16]

Achieving static compression may also be accomplished by using lag screws, though their application in the mandible is limited. In the mandible, they can be used in the treatment of oblique fractures, chin fractures, or as an adjunct to plate fixation.[17]

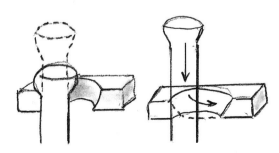

FIGURE 10–4 Gliding hole of the dynamic compression plate (DCP).

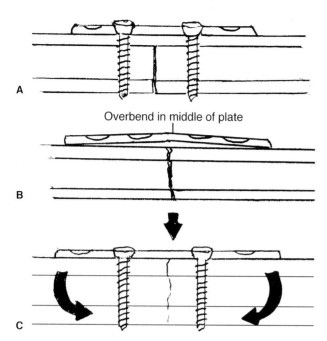

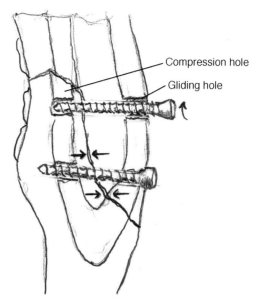

A

Overbend in middle of plate

B

C

FIGURE 10–5 A dynamic compression plate produces compression of the edge closest to the plate and a gap in the opposite edge (A), which can be prevented by over-bending the plate just over the fracture side (B,C).

FIGURE 10–6 Lag screw.

This technique was first described by Danis[18] in 1949 for the fixation of oblique fractures of long bones. By definition, a lag screw is a screw that first glides through the outer cortex of one of the bony fragments and then engages the inner cortex of the opposite fragment. When tightened, a lag screw draws the fragments together, producing interfragmentary compression (Fig. **10–6**). When placing a lag screw, several technical points should be followed: (1) The gliding hole and the threaded hole should be in the same axis. (2) The diameter of the gliding hole should match the outer diameter of the thread. (3) The diameter of the threaded hole should match the diameter of the core of the screw. (4) The screw should be oriented perpendicular to the fracture plane (Fig. **10–6**).[19] Using lag screws is the most efficient way of producing interfragmentary compression and therefore stability, but they do not provide much strength.[15] When lag screws are used, a minimum of two, but ideally three, screws are needed. Also, when a lag screw is used through a plate, it is essential that all other screws be placed in neutral position; otherwise, the fragments may shift.[15]

As mentioned previously, to achieve absolute stability it is necessary to produce compression across the whole fracture. If a bone were not loaded, the methods of static compression discussed above (i.e., self-compressing plate) would be enough, but functional loading is capable of separating the

fracture edges despite the presence of a self-compressing plate. To prevent this, methods that create compression across the whole fracture during functional loading (i.e., dynamic compression) are also utilized. In practice, dynamic compression is achieved by using the tension band principle.[14,16,17]

This principle is illustrated by observing a straight cantilever beam that has been fractured and repaired with a plate (Fig. **10–7**). If the plate is placed in the compression (concave) side of the beam, the functional load produces a gap in the tension (convex) side of the beam. Additionally, the plate takes the entire load. However, if the plate is placed in the tension (convex) side, the entire fracture is under compression and the bone shares the load with the plate.

The plate placed on the tension side of the fracture (i.e., tension band) is capable of absorbing the tensile forces and transforming them into compressive forces that act across the whole fracture. In this scenario, the bone shares the load with the plate. It is important to note that the bone is only able to share the load if the fracture edges are in close proximity (i.e., well reduced) and are capable of withstanding the compression. The bone is unable to withstand the compression in cases of comminuted fractures.[20]

In long bones, rigid internal fixation is accomplished by placing a self-compressing plate in the tension side of the fracture. In this fashion, the plate is able to generate both static and dynamic compression. Static compression is generated by the plate itself, whereas dynamic compression is produced by the position of the plate, which in this location acts as a tension band.[16,17] Unfortunately, in the

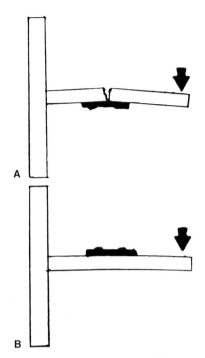

FIGURE 10–7 A: Plate installed in the compression side. Functional forces produce a separation of the fracture in the tension side. The plate takes the entire load. B: Plate installed in the tension side (tension band). The plate absorbs the tension and converts the tensile forces into compressive forces that act through the fracture. The plate shares the load with the bone.

mandible this arrangement is impossible. Because of anatomic constraints, the placement of a DCP is limited to the area of the inferior border of the mandible, an area that in many cases corresponds to the zone of compression. Therefore, to avoid separation of the fracture ends in the tension zone that is frequently located in the alveolar border of the mandible, the placement of a separate tension band is necessary. Arch bars, dental splints, or osteosynthesis plates may function as tension bands.[14] The use of rigid internal fixation is only possible in noncomminuted simple fractures. Other types of fractures are usually treated by bridging.

BRIDGING

Bridging implies the creation of a stable connection between the bone ends in cases where a bony buttress is either deficient or absent.[14] A bone buttress is deficient in comminuted fractures and absent in fractures with continuity defects. In these scenarios interfragmentary compression and load sharing are impossible; therefore, it is impossible to attain absolute stability. The goal of bridging is the creation of relative stability and the restoration of the form and function of the mandible. It is important to

emphasize that absolute stability is not a precondition to healing. Fractures treated by bridging are expected to heal if certain basic principles are followed. The plates used for bridging are expected to absorb the whole load. For this reason, the use of large reconstruction plates is recommended. In addition, to permit immediate function, a minimum of three or four screws per side should be used.[14,15]

BIOLOGIC INTERNAL FIXATION

In the middle of the 20th century, the introduction of rigid internal fixation revolutionized the treatment of fractures. Rigid internal fixation allowed fractures to unite while maintaining function. At that time, precise reduction of the fracture and absolute stability of the fixation were considered to be essential preconditions for success. For this reason, early investigators focused their work on the mechanical aspects of fixation.[21,23] However, fracture healing is ultimately a biologic event; thus investigators in the last decade have shifted their focus from the mechanical to the biologic. Recent advances have aimed at creating the best biologic environment for healing. These efforts have produced a new concept in fracture treatment called biologic internal fixation.[21,22,24]

The normal biologic mechanism of fracture healing (indirect healing) involves sequential steps of tissue differentiation, resorption of the fractured surfaces, callus formation, and remodeling. However, this normal biologic mechanism is not set off when a fracture is rigidly fixed. Instead, a different type of healing, called direct healing, occurs. This process skips the intermediate steps of tissue differentiation, bone resorption, and callus formation, and progresses directly to the final remodeling of the haversian system.

Until recently, direct bone healing without callus formation was thought to be superior to indirect bone healing, but this is no longer true. Direct bone healing is not faster than indirect bone healing. Moreover, fractures that have healed by direct healing remain mechanically weaker for up to 2 years longer than those that have healed by callus formation.[24] It is now accepted that callus formation is desirable because it provides faster recovery and a more solid union. Therefore, one of the goals of biologic fixation has been to stimulate callus formation. This has been accomplished by allowing some degree of flexibility at the fracture site (flexible fixation). To have flexibility at the fracture site, interfragmentary compression has to be avoided. But this created a technical problem because it was known that the use of conventional plates and screws without interfragmentary compression leads to premature loosening of the hardware. Therefore, new hardware had to be developed. The new hardware developed for this purpose is known as a "locked internal fixator." It resembles a plate but functions more like an external fixator that has been fully implanted.

The screws of a conventional plate stabilize the plate by compressing the plate to the bone surface, creating friction at the interface between the plate and the bone. In contrast, the locking screws of the internal fixator do not press the plate against the bone. The heads of the screws as well as the holes in the plate are threaded; thus, during insertion the threaded screw heads lock to the plate (Fig. **10-8**). In this system, the force transmission between the screw and the plate does not depend on axial preloading of the screw.

Another advantage of not pressing the plate against the bone has been the prevention of early temporary porosity. After the placement of a conventional bone plate, investigators were able to document the appearance of bone porosity within the cortical bone adjacent to the plate. This porosity appeared between 2 and 5 months after the placement of the plate. For years, it was generally accepted that unloading or stress shielding of the bone by the plate caused this porosity. This hypothesis was supported by Wolff's law, which states that bone loss occurs under conditions of unloading. There were two problems with this hypothesis. The first was that the shape of the area of porosity did not correlate with the shape of the area of unloading, and the second was that the porosity disappeared over time while the implant was still in place. Because of this, further investigations into this phenomenon were conducted.

Because it had been demonstrated that the porosity occurred only below the plate and that the shape of the area of porosity correlated with the shape of the plate, the investigators hypothesized

that the plate had caused the porosity by disrupting the blood supply to the cortical bone. To test this hypothesis, investigators first tested plates that had been modified to reduce the amount of contact between the undersurface of the plate and the bone [i.e., limited contact dynamic compression plate (LC-DCP)]. These experiments proved that these plates produced less bone porosity. Additionally, they tested plates made of soft plastic, which produced less unloading but had a tighter contact between the implant and the bone. Contrary to what was expected according to Wolff's Law, these plates did not reduce but rather enhanced the porosity.[21]

It is now understood that early temporary porosity is caused by a disruption in the cortical blood supply. As a result, the bone immediately underneath the plate becomes necrotic. Necrotic bone then stimulates internal remodeling of the surrounding bone. The first stage in this remodeling is the opening of tunnels by osteoclasts, which results in porosity. The second stage is the filling of these tunnels with newly formed bone that is laid down by osteoblasts. Over time, the porosity disappears as this area is replaced by living bone.

This temporary porosity may be viewed as a phenomenon with no clinical consequences because the bone plate can protect the temporary weakening. However, when any irritation of the bone occurs such as an infection, the increased remodeling may lead to the development of a band of confluent pores. This may result in lost of continuity and the development of sequestra beneath the plate, which in turn may support an infection.[21]

When rigid fixation is applied, even a small amount of instability may produce hardware failure and nonunion. However, the same degree of instability is usually well tolerated by bridge plating or biologic (flexible) fixation. This difference can be explained by the different strains to which the tissues within the fracture gaps are subjected. As previously stated, strain is the ratio of the change in length to the original length. A simple fracture treated by interfragmentary compression has a very small fracture gap, $\sim 10~\mu m$, which is large enough to accommodate one cell. If this gap is elongated by $10~\mu m$, a minute deformation, the cell is subjected to a strain of 1.0 (100% deformation), which is incompatible with cell survival. In a fracture treated by bridging without compression, a larger fracture gap is produced (i.e., $30~\mu m$), enough to accommodate three cells. If this fracture is then elongated by the same $10~\mu m$, the cells in this gap would be subjected to a strain of only 0.3 (30% deformation). This degree of strain is actually beneficial to fracture healing because it stimulates callus formation. Mechanical

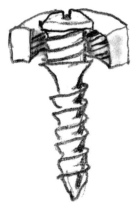

FIGURE 10-8 Locking screw of the locked internal fixator.

deformation at the cellular level appears to be a prerequisite for callus formation because a callus is not formed in the presence of complete stability.

THE CHAMPY TECHNIQUE

This technique of fracture stabilization was developed by Champy et al[25] in the mid-1970s. The biomechanical principles of this method were based on mathematical and experimental models performed in Strasbourg at the Ecole National Supérieure des Arts et Industries. It includes the exclusive use of noncompression monocortical miniplates that are applied as tension bands. The biomechanical studies completed at Strasbourg predicted tensile stresses in the upper border of the mandible and compressive stresses in the lower border. They also found that through the body of the mandible, the forces acting on it produced mainly bending moments. They also noted that in the region of the symphysis and parasymphysis, torsional forces rather than bending moments predominated.

Based on this model, Champy et al created the "ideal osteosynthesis line." It corresponds to the course of a line of tension at the base of the alveolar process. Behind the mental foramen, a plate is applied immediately below the dental roots and above the inferior alveolar nerve. At the angle of the mandible, the plate is placed on the broad surface of the external oblique line. In the anterior region between the mental foramina, in addition to the subapical plate, another plate near the lower border of the mandible is necessary to neutralize torsional forces.[25]

PEARLS: BASIC MANDIBLE FRACTURE PRINCIPLES

- To avoid damage to the inferior alveolar nerve, surgeons should be familiar with its three-dimensional anatomy.
- Initial biomechanical studies of the mandible modeled this bone as a straight cantilever beam, with the alveolar border under tension and the inferior border under compression. More recent studies have shown that the stress distribution of the mandible depends on the magnitude and position of the biting forces.
- The two basic steps of fracture treatment are reduction followed by stabilization.
- Fracture reduction can be accomplished indirectly (closed reduction) or directly (open reduction).
- Maxillomandibular fixation is the standard method for both reduction as well as stabilization.

- External fixation plays a small but important role in the treatment of mandibular fractures; it can be considered in the atrophic edentulous mandible, extensive soft tissue injuries, severe comminution, and an infected fracture.
- Techniques used for internal fixation can be classified as techniques of absolute stability and techniques of relative stability. Rigid internal fixation is the technique of absolute stability. Bridging, biologic (flexible) fixation, and the Champy technique are techniques of relative stability.
- Rigid internal fixation is accomplished by the use of compression plates, lag screws, and the tension band principle.
- Biologic fixation represents a new paradigm in fracture treatment. Absolute stability is no longer considered an essential precondition for success. Relative stability and callus formation are considered beneficial.
- Not pressing the plate against the bone improves the blood supply to the cortical bone and prevents the formation of early temporary porosity.

REFERENCES

1. Goss C, ed. *Gray's Anatomy*. Philadelphia: Lea & Febiger, 1973:152
2. Rajche J, Ellis E III, Fonseca RJ. The anatomical location of the mandibular canal: its relationship to the sagittal ramus osteotomy. Int J Adult Orthodon Orthognath Surg 1986;1:37–47
3. Rudderman RH, Mullen RL. Biomechanics of the facial skeleton. Clin Plast Surg 1992;19:11–29
4. van Eijden TM. Biomechanics of the mandible. Crit Rev Oral Biol Med 2000;11:123–136
5. *Stedman's Medical Dictionary*, 25th ed. Baltimore: Williams and Wilkins, 1990
6. McCabe J. *Anderson's Applied Dental Materials*, 6th ed. London: Blackwell Scientific Publications, 1985:7
7. Barbenel JC. The mechanics of the temporomandibular joint—a theoretical and electromyographical study. J Oral Rehabil 1974;1:19–27
8. Tams J, van Loon JP, Otten E, et al. A three-dimensional study of bending and torsion moments for different fracture sites in the mandible: an in vitro study. Int J Oral Maxillofac Surg 1997;26:383–388
9. Tams J, van Loon JP, Rozema FR, Otten E, Bos RR. A three-dimensional study of loads across the fracture for different fracture sites of the mandible. Br J Oral Maxillofac Surg 1996;34:400–405
10. Bramley P. Basic principles of treatment. In: Rowe N, Williams J, eds. *Maxillofacial Injuries*. Edinburgh: Churchill Livingstone, 1985:52–53
11. Nepola J. External fixation. In: Rockwood CA, Green DP, eds. *Rockwood and Green's Fractures in Adults*, 4th ed. Philadelphia: Lippincott-Raven, 1996: 229–242

12. Burgess A, Poka A, Browner BD, et al. Principles of external fixation. In: Browner BD, Jupiter JB, Levine AM, et al., eds. *Skeletal Trauma*. Philadelphia: WB Saunders, 1992:231–241

13. Perren SM, Rahn BA, Cordey J. Mechanik und Biologie der Frakturheilung. *Fortschr Kiefer Gesichtschir* 1975;19(33)

14. Spiessl B. *Internal Fixation of the Mandible*, 1st ed. Berlin: Springer-Verlag, 1989

15. Prein J, Rahn BA. Scientific and technical background. In: Prein J, ed. *Manual of Internal Fixation in the Craniofacial Skeleton*. Berlin: Springer-Verlag, 1998;5–8

16. Tencer A, Johnson K. *Biomechanics in Orthopaedic Trauma*. London: Martin Dunitz, 1994:142–157

17. Muller M, Allgower M, Schneider R, et al. *Manual of Internal Fixation*, 3rd ed. Berlin: Springer-Verlag, 1990:12–81

18. Danis R. *Theorie et Practique de L'osteosynthese*. Paris: Masson, 1949

19. Schatzker J. Principles of stable internal fixation. In: Uhthoff HK, ed. *Current Concepts of Internal Fixation of Fractures*. Berlin: Springer-Verlag, 1979:180–181

20. Schatzker J. The eccentric loading of bones. In: Muller M, ed. *Manual of Internal Fixation: Techniques Recommended by the AO-ASIF Group*. Berlin: AO-ASIF, 1991:227

21. Perren S. Evolution of the internal fixation: choosing a new balance between stability and biology. J Bone Joint Surg Br 2002;84:1093–1110

22. Perren SM. Minimally invasive internal fixation history, essence and potential of a new approach. Injury 2001;32(suppl 1):SA1–SA3

23. Perren SM. Evolution and rationale of locked internal fixator technology. Introductory remarks. Injury 2001;32(suppl 2):B3–B9

24. Hofer HP, Wildburger R, Szyszkowitz R. Observations concerning different patterns of bone healing using the Point Contact Fixator (PC-Fix) as a new technique for fracture fixation. Injury 2001;32(suppl 2):B15–B25

25. Champy M, Pape HD, Gerlach KL, et al. The Strasbourg miniplate osteosynthesis. In: Kruger E, Schilli W, eds. *Oral and Maxillofacial Traumatology*. Chicago: Quintessence Books, 1986:19–43

Chapter 11

CONDYLAR AND SUBCONDYLAR FRACTURES

Jose M. Marchena and Zahid S. Lalani

Despite numerous advances in instrumentation and surgical fixation techniques, the management of mandibular condylar fractures remains a controversial topic and has generated a variety of opinions and proposed treatment modalities.[1-5] The controversy relates to indications for operative versus nonoperative management. As with any traumatized joint, the surgeon must choose strategies that carry the least surgical morbidity and risk for long-term degenerative joint disease. This chapter reviews pertinent surgical anatomy of the temporomandibular joint (TMJ), characteristics and classification of mandibular condylar and subcondylar fractures, clinical and radiographic evaluation, and sensible management strategies.

ANATOMIC CONSIDERATIONS

The TMJ is a ginglymoarthrodial joint allowing the condyle to undergo rotational and translational movements with respect to the glenoid fossa. The joint contains superior and inferior joint spaces, which are lined by synovial tissue and are separated by a disk (Fig. 11–1). The disk is attached to the articular eminence and superior belly of the lateral pterygoid muscle anterosuperiorly, to the tympanic plate of the temporal bone posteriorly, and to the medial and lateral poles of the condyle immediately above the capsular attachment. A tight attachment of the disk to the condyle results in displacement of the disk with the condyle in fracture dislocations. The articulating surfaces of the condyle and glenoid fossa are lined by fibrocartilage. The entire joint is surrounded by a capsule, which is attached superiorly to the outer rim of the glenoid fossa and inferiorly to the condylar neck (Fig. 11–1). The lateral

portion of the capsule (also called the temporomandibular ligament) is thicker than the medial portion, which explains the preponderance for medial fracture dislocations of the condyle (Fig. 11–1). The lateral pterygoid muscle attaches to the anterior disk and medial aspect of the condyle (Fig. 11–1), also explaining the preponderance for anteromedial displacement and dislocations.

The condylar process is composed of a body and head separated by the condylar neck. The condylar head is the only intracapsular portion. Fractures occurring below the condylar neck are extracapsular and should be referred to as subcondylar fractures. The blood supply to the condyle is circumferential and derived from branches of the internal maxillary, transverse facial, and superficial temporal vessels (Fig. 11–1). These vessels may be encountered during an open joint approach and can cause significant bleeding. The medially located internal maxillary artery and its branches, in particular, may be injured during manipulation of medially displaced segments causing significant bleeding, which may be difficult to control because of poor access. Meticulous surgical technique must be followed in the medial aspects of the joint because aggressive vascular ligation and muscle stripping can result in aseptic necrosis of the condyle.[6]

The auriculotemporal nerve provides most of the sensory innervation to the joint and is often injured during preauricular approaches to the TMJ. The facial nerve and its branches lie in close proximity to the TMJ and are also prone to injury during an open joint approach. The temporal and zygomatic branches are at risk with preauricular or hemicoronal approaches and the marginal mandibular branch with neck approaches.

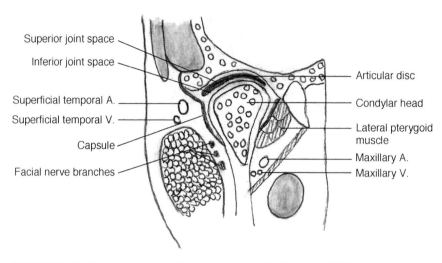

FIGURE 11–1 Anatomy of the temporomandibular joint (TMJ).

CLASSIFICATION AND DESCRIPTION OF CONDYLAR AND SUBCONDYLAR FRACTURES

There are several classifications of condylar fractures. These classifications are based on anatomic location of the fracture, direction of displacement of the condylar segment, or the relationship of the fractured condylar segment to the mandible and the articulating surface of the glenoid fossa.[7] Strict adherence to such classification schemes may be impractical, especially when meaningless roman numbers are assigned. Describing fractures in a way that enables the surgeon to build a mental image of the injured TMJ and the appropriate method of treatment is more practical.

Condylar fractures can be simplistically divided into intra- and extracapsular. Intracapsular fractures are those that involve only the condylar head and result in a short proximal segment (Fig. 11–2A). These usually stay within the confines of the capsule. Fractures below the condylar head, therefore, are extracapsular. This distinction has important surgical implications because most intracapsular fractures are treated nonsurgically for reasons discussed later. In the event that surgery is performed, this designation (intracapsular) would necessitate a preauricular approach for efficient and adequate reduction and fixation.

Extracapsular fractures involve the condylar neck and process. These fractures are also referred to as subcondylar fractures (Fig. 11–2A). The level of fracture has important surgical implications.

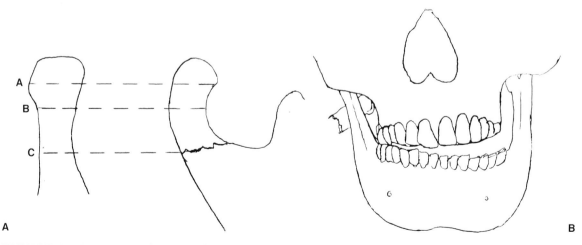

FIGURE 11–2 A: Level of condylar fractures (a, intracapsular fracture, i.e., condylar head; b, condylar neck fracture; c, subcondylar fracture). B: Shortening of ramus secondary to fracture dislocation of condyle causing an anterior open bite on the contralateral side.

Distinguishing between condylar neck and head fractures, for example, can be difficult, and both fractures are often treated with closed reduction. Displaced subcondylar fractures at the level of the sigmoid notch, in contrast, are readily accessible and often treated surgically because they may cause a significant loss of ramus height and alteration in the occlusion.

A description that includes the presence and direction of displacement of the fracture segment and the relationship of the condyle to its articulating surface is also important. Fracture dislocations wherein the condylar segment is out of the confines of the glenoid fossa correspond with capsular rupture and enough angulation of the proximal segment to cause a significant loss of ramus height (Fig. **11–2B**). Open treatment of such fractures is likely indicated to restore ramal height and the occlusion.

CLINICAL ASSESSMENT

Patients with facial injuries should be evaluated according to the Advanced Trauma Life Support (ATLS) guidelines. Those with isolated facial injuries should also undergo evaluation of the cervical spine prior to a detailed maxillofacial examination. Assessment begins with a detailed history about the mechanism of injury because certain patterns of condylar and subcondylar fractures are consistent with specific mechanisms.

COMMON FRACTURE PATTERNS

- A unilateral fracture along with a contralateral mandibular body fracture as a result of blunt trauma to the body of the mandible.
- A unilateral fracture along with an ipsilateral parasymphysis fracture from trauma to the parasymphysis.
- Bilateral condylar fractures with or without a symphyseal area fracture as result of direct trauma to the symphyseal area.

A unilateral fracture of the condylar area along with a second contralateral fracture is usually seen in patients involved in an altercation and sustaining a blow to the side of the face. Bilateral condylar fractures are often found in patients who lose consciousness and fall forward, striking the floor with their chin, which leads to translation of forces to both joints. A similar pattern may be observed in motor vehicle accident victims who strike the steering wheel with their chin. After obtaining a history

on the mechanism of injury, a detailed examination is performed to elicit common findings associated with condylar and subcondylar fractures.

CLINICAL FINDINGS IN CONDYLAR AND SUBCONDYLAR FRACTURES

- Laceration or abrasion over the chin, mandibular body, or preauricular area.
- Pain or tenderness over the affected TMJ.
- Laceration of the external ear canal with or without blood behind the tympanic membrane (may indicate fracture of the glenoid fossa).
- Facial asymmetry with deviation of the chin point at rest.
- Mandibular occlusal cant with an open bite on the nonaffected side along with an occlusal prematurity on the injured side (asymmetric open bite).
- Symmetric anterior open bite (in bilateral fractures).
- Presence of a fracture at another site in the mandible.
- Pain, joint crepitation, jaw deviation, and hypomobility during opening or lateral excursive movements.

Any of these findings may indicate the presence of a fracture. There are two conditions, however, that do not involve a fracture but present with similar findings. Unilateral joint dislocations or intracapsular hematomas show jaw deviation, pain, and occlusal abnormalities similar to those seen in unilateral condylar fractures. Bilateral joint dislocations show a symmetric anterior open bite similar to that seen in displaced bilateral fractures. In the majority of cases appropriate imaging establishes the presence of a fracture.

IMAGING

At least two radiographic views at right angles to each other should be obtained for evaluating condylar fractures. A mandibular series consisting of a posterior anterior skull view, left and right lateral oblique views, and a Towne's view will detect most condylar fractures and also provide information on the direction of displacement. The Towne's view in particular provides an excellent view of the condylar area (Fig. **11–3**). The panoramic radiograph is excellent at detecting condylar and subcondylar fractures, but by itself fails to reveal whether the fractured segment is medially or laterally displaced.

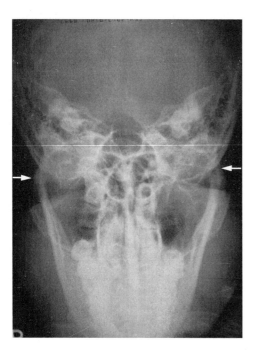

FIGURE 11–3 Towne's view showing bilateral subcondylar fractures.

Computed tomography (CT) has become the gold standard imaging modality for facial trauma. It provides excellent three-dimensional assessment of facial fractures, including the temporomandibular joint, and can be undertaken on most patients regardless of the mental or physical status.[8] Many centers are now including a facial survey CT as part of the head CT protocol in head trauma victims with suspected maxillofacial fractures. Magnetic resonance imaging (MRI) provides excellent soft tissue detail of the TMJ and certainly has a role in the evaluation of internal joint derangement, disk pathology, or joint effusions. For fractures, however, MRI offers no advantage over plain radiography or CT and rarely has a place in maxillofacial trauma.

NONSURGICAL MANAGEMENT

The management of condylar and subcondylar fractures remains one of the most controversial topics in maxillofacial trauma. Experienced surgeons would agree, however, that despite the advances in instrumentation and minimally invasive techniques, most condylar fractures can be treated closed. This is particularly true in children and adolescents, whose fracture dislocations of the condyle can heal perfectly by remodeling or regeneration of a neocondyle with full restoration of joint function.[9]

ACCEPTED INDICATIONS FOR NONSURGICAL MANAGEMENT

- Intracapsular fractures.
- Most fractures in children and adolescents.
- Nondislocated fractures in edentulous patients with preserved jaw symmetry.
- Minimally displaced unilateral or bilateral fractures with minimal alteration of vertical ramus height and the occlusion.
- Absence of mechanical interference with jaw motion.
- Ability to achieve a normal occlusion with simple manipulation.

Patients with nondisplaced unilateral or bilateral condylar fractures and an unchanged occlusion can be managed with a liquid diet for 6 weeks and weekly examination of jaw function and occlusion. This approach is reserved for children and cooperative adults. If any change in the occlusion is noted, intermaxillary fixation is applied with the teeth in the correct occlusal relationship for 1 to 3 weeks. The time period of immobilization depends on the patient's age and nature of the fracture, but should not exceed 3 weeks. Children should not be immobilized for more than 10 days because of the risk for an intraarticular bony ankylosis.[9] Early mobilization decreases the risk of developing extraarticular causes of joint hypomobility, such as muscle atrophy and soft tissue fibrosis, as well as intraarticular causes such as adhesions or ankylosis formation.

After a trial period of 1 to 3 weeks, immobilization is discontinued and the occlusion assessed. If the correct occlusion is reproducible with repetitive jaw function, a trial of daytime functioning without immobilization is attempted. Nighttime immobilization during this trial period is recommended to assure healing and remodeling with the teeth in occlusion at night. Nighttime immobilization also prevents motion at the fracture site from parafunctional activity during sleep like clenching and grinding of teeth. The application of arch bars, therefore, is recommended for patients with condylar fractures because they can be used for immobilization or guidance using elastics at any time. Ivy loops should be reserved for nondisplaced fractures with a normal occlusion and when guidance with elastics is not anticipated.

Many patients experience jaw deviation toward the injured side and decreased mouth opening after release of intermaxillary fixation. Jaw deviation is most likely due to weakness of the lateral pterygoid muscle and stiffness of the other muscles of mastication. Training elastics are used to guide jaw opening until function is symmetric. Hypomobility should be treated aggressively with physical therapy. Physical therapy should be started early with passive mouth opening exercises, followed by active opening and stretching exercises after 4 weeks with continuous evaluation of the occlusion.

SURGICAL INDICATIONS

The indications for an open reduction have been divided into absolute and relative.[10,11] This distinction is not widely accepted due to different training philosophies and experiences. Despite the controversy, however, there are certain conditions that are best managed with an open approach. In many such conditions there is an acute mechanical interference with joint function or with the ability to restore the occlusion with simple jaw manipulation. In others it may be less obvious.

INDICATIONS FOR AN OPEN APPROACH

- Condylar displacement into the middle cranial fossa
- Lateral and medial fracture dislocations
- Presence of an intraarticular foreign body interfering with joint motion
- Inability to manipulate the jaw into occlusion
- Bilateral fractures with an intracapsular fracture on one side
- Bilateral subcondylar fractures with concurrent impacted and comminuted midface fractures
- Medical conditions precluding the use of intermaxillary fixation such as seizure disorders and mental health disturbances

Condylar displacement into the middle cranial fossa may cause a significant loss of vertical dimension, jaw hypomobility, and an alteration of occlusion. Further displacement of the condylar segment with function may also result in intracranial injury. In lateral fracture dislocations, the zygomatic arch interferes with the proximal segment causing jaw hypomobility. An intraarticular foreign body such as a bullet fragment may interfere with condylar movement along the articulating surfaces, causing pain and hypomobility.

In severely displaced fractures or fracture dislocations with significant loss of vertical height and bony contact between segments, it may be impossible to achieve satisfactory occlusion and adequate reduction of the fragments necessary for healing. When there is an intracapsular fracture along with other mandibular fractures, including a contralateral subcondylar fracture, the other fractures must be rigidly fixed, so that the intracapsular fracture can be managed with early physiotherapy. Presence of bilateral subcondylar fractures with comminuted midface fractures may make it impossible to reestablish vertical dimension of the face unless the posterior mandibular height is restored. At least one ramus–condyle unit should be reconstructed prior to addressing the midface. Bilateral intracapsular fractures in the presence of midfacial fractures should be treated closed with aggressive physiotherapy. An open reduction may also be indicated in mentally handicapped patients or those with neurologic movement disorders such as Huntington's chorea, where even a short period of intermaxillary fixation would cause a significant problem.

Each case must be assessed individually, but in some instances, such as an acute mechanical interference with joint function, the need for surgical intervention is obvious. Patients treated with an open reduction should undergo early physiotherapy with occlusal guidance similar to those treated with a closed reduction. Those who have undergone extensive stripping of the lateral pterygoid muscle to facilitate reduction of the proximal segment may never achieve normal lateral pterygoid function. Such patients will have a persistent deviation to the operated side during jaw opening secondary to an inability of the condyle to translate normally.

SURGICAL APPROACHES AND TECHNIQUES

Surgical approaches described for open reduction of condylar and subcondylar fractures include (1) preauricular approaches with or without coronal or rhytidectomy type extensions; (2) submandibular approaches such as the classic Risdon incision or the retromandibular incision; and (3) the intraoral approach. Preauricular approaches and their modifications carry the highest risk for morbidity such as facial scarring, facial nerve injuries, Frey's syndrome, and bleeding.[12] They should be reserved for cases where an arthrotomy is needed for the removal of foreign bodies or for the retrieval of dislocated fragments from the middle cranial fossa or medial aspect of the joint. The intraoral approach is useful for low subcondylar fractures but presents difficulty with orientation and instrumentation, especially with medially displaced fractures. The classic submandibular or Risdon incision is useful for low subcondylar and ramus fractures but can rarely be used alone for high subcondylar fractures. The retromandibular approach described by Hinds and Girotti[13] is most useful for subcondylar fractures and is described in detail. In the presence of a subcondylar fracture along with ipsilateral posterior body fractures, a modification combining the retromandibular and submandibular incision is preferred for simultaneous reduction and plating of the body and subcondylar fractures.

RETROMANDIBULAR APPROACH

The skin incision is ~2.5 cm long and runs from a point ~1.5 cm below the earlobe to the posterior angle, parallel to the inferior aspect of the posterior border of the ramus. It is nearly vertical, ~2 cm behind the posterior border of the mandible (Fig. **11–4A**). The incision is made through skin and subcutaneous tissue to the platysma. The platysma is incised and the underlying tissue bluntly dissected to the mandible by spreading in the direction of the facial nerve. The pterygomasseteric sling is incised, and a subperisoteal dissection is performed superiorly toward the condylar area. Retractors can be placed in the sigmoid notch or on the anterior or posterior borders of the ramus (Fig. **11–4B**). Laterally displaced fragments are usually encountered during the superior dissection. Medially displaced segments can be retrieved by

distraction of the distal segment. The use of muscle relaxants at this point often facilitates manipulation and reduction of the segments. After the fracture is reduced, intermaxillary fixation is applied and the fracture is plated. Placement into intermaxillary fixation prior to fracture reduction may impede with distraction of the distal segment and retrieval of a medially displaced segment.

ARTHROTOMY

An arthrotomy is indicated for the removal of a foreign body and retrieval of medially dislocated fracture segments. A preauricular incision is made, and dissection is performed through skin and subcutaneous tissue to the perichondrium of the tragus. Dissection is then carried deep and anterior in this plane to the capsule of the TMJ. The superior joint space is injected with a vasoconstrictor containing solution and then entered by incising the capsule right below its attachment to the outer rim of the glenoid fossa. The inferior joint space is entered through an incision right below the disk avoiding injury to the fibrocartilage of the condyle. Once manipulation and instrumentation is complete, the integrity and position of the disk are assessed while manipulating the jaw. A torn and malpositioned disk that interferes with condylar movement is repaired and repositioned. Failure to do so may lead to joint

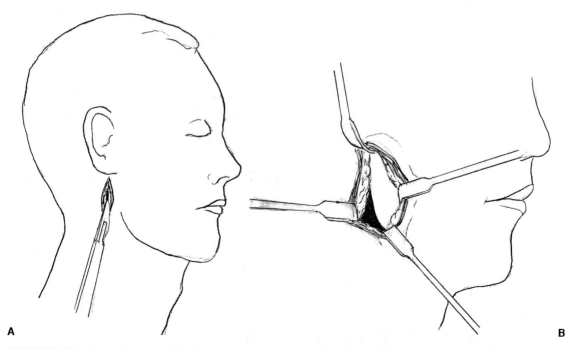

A

B

FIGURE 11–4 A: Retromandibular incision. B: Retromandibular dissection to gain access to mandibular condyle.

hypomobility or internal derangement with pathologic clicking, popping, or crepitus. The capsule is repaired whenever possible.

INTRAORAL APPROACH

The intraoral approach is identical to that for an intraoral ramus osteotomy procedure. An incision is made over the external oblique ridge and carried superiorly along the anterior border of the ramus. The periosteum and the temporalis insertion are stripped superiorly to the level of the sigmoid notch. Subperiosteal dissection is performed posteriorly to the condylar area, posterior border of the ramus, and angle (Fig. **11–5**). The distal segment is then distracted inferiorly to create room to manipulate and reduce the proximal condylar fragment. Medially displaced segments can be pushed laterally by sliding an instrument medial to ramus above the lingula. Fixation is performed with a percutaneous technique after fracture reduction and placement into intermaxillary fixation.

REDUCTION AND FIXATION

The preferred method of fixation is a 2.0-mm plate with at least two screws in the proximal segment and two to three screws in the distal segment (Fig. **11–6**).[14] The operation is started with the application of arch bars. Once the fracture site is

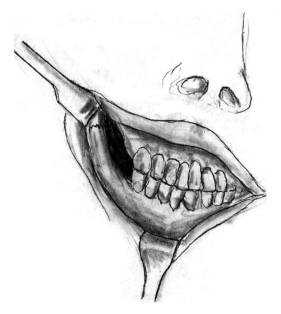

FIGURE 11–5 Intraoral approach to mandibular condyle.

adequately exposed and meticulous hemostasis is achieved, the patient is paralyzed to facilitate distraction of the distal segment and manipulation and reduction of the proximal segment. Once the fracture is reduced and the vertical height of the ramus reestablished, the occlusion is secured by intermaxillary fixation. A 2.0-mm plate is then placed on the posterolateral border allowing for at least two screws on each side of the fracture (Fig. **11–6**). It is advantageous to place the initial screw on the proximal segment, because this will allow the plate to be used as a handle to manipulate and hold the proximal segment in place. Screw placement is facilitated using a trocar with percutaneous technique. A screw is then placed in the distal segment followed by the remainder of the screws. Intermaxillary fixation is released and the occlusion checked with passive mandibular movements. When other mandibular fractures are present, these must be fixated first with the patient in intermaxillary fixation. Intermaxillary fixation is released prior to reduction of the subcondylar fracture. In edentulous patients, a close to anatomic reduction with reestablishment of ramal height is sufficient. Drains are rarely necessary but because the parotid gland is penetrated by the percutaneous instrumentation, a pressure dressing is recommended for 48 hours to help prevent the formation of a sialocele. Minimally invasive endoscopic techniques have been recently developed but have not yet gained widespread acceptance.[15]

COMPLICATIONS

Mandibular trauma may produce a variety of TMJ injuries, such as sprains, disk damage, and condyle fractures. These injuries alone or in combination produce disorders encompassing pain, dysfunction, degeneration, and limitation. Pain may be associated with scarring or impingement of soft tissues. Dysfunction involves alteration of condylar movement and is caused by irregular surfaces and changes in relationships between the disk and condyle. Condylar fractures produce shredding of the disk and joint surfaces 50 to 60% of the time, and these are often greatest with dislocations.[16] The disk tends to follow the proximal segment at the time of fracture displacement and repositioning, but with tearing of the ligaments and capsule, the disk and condyle may assume a new relationship and cause dysfunction.[17] Adhesions are also noted in fractured TMJs and may cause alteration in joint motion.[18]

The complications of open treatment of condylar fractures are associated with surgical access, reduction and fixation of the fractured fragments, and

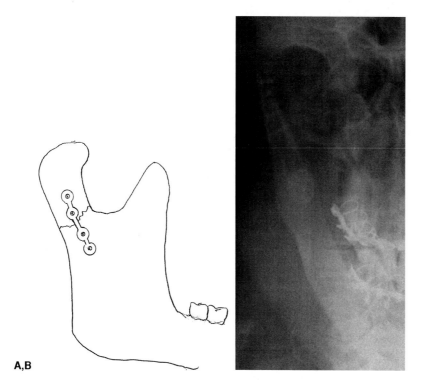

A,B

FIGURE 11–6 A: Diagrammatic representation of application of 2.0-mm plate for condylar fracture. B: Postoperative radiograph of condylar fracture fixed using a 2.0-mm miniplate, with two screws on each side of the fracture.

arthrotomy. Transcutaneous approaches may cause injury to branches of the facial nerve as a result of retraction or direct injury. Stripping of muscles and ligaments off the condyle can result in long-term deviation of the jaw to the affected side. Overseating of the condyle against the glenoid fossa may result in pain and progressive degenerative joint disease or condylar resorption. Popping and clicking has been noted in 4 to 32% of individuals who sustained condylar fractures in childhood in long-term follow-up studies.[19] Despite a perfect anatomic reduction, failure to appropriately seat the condyle (underseating) will lead to an asymmetric open bite upon release from intermaxillary fixation as a result of physiologic superior repositioning of the condyle. This problem is usually caused by inadequate and loosened intermaxillary fixation or malreduction (overlapping) at a coexisting mandibular fracture site. This should be assessed in the operating room by releasing the intermaxillary fixation and evaluating the occlusion prior to extubation.

Open treatment of condylar fractures may also lead to growth disturbances and ankylosis in children.[20–22] The reported rate of ankylosis following condylar fractures in the pediatric population has varied from 0 to 7%.[20–22] The risk of ankylosis following condylar fractures appears to be higher in children less than 6 months of age.[21] It has also

been shown that even though condylar anatomy following remodeling may return to premorbid states, late appearance of facial asymmetry as the child enters the teenage years is not uncommon.[21] Complications associated with closed reduction are related to failure in appropriately correcting vertical ramus height and mechanical interference resulting in malocclusion and internal joint derangement, respectively. Prolonged immobilization used for closed reduction or following open treatment may also lead to joint hypomobility. Postoperative limitation of mouth opening and jaw deviation are very common and often secondary to soft tissue problems. Persistent limitation of mouth opening and jaw deviation is common regardless of the method of treatment.

Causes of Posttraumatic/ Surgical Joint Hypomobility and Jaw Deviation

- Lateral pterygoid muscle detachment, shortening, or atrophy.
- Prolonged intermaxillary fixation.
- Scarring and fibrosis of capsular and ligamentous tissues.

- Intraarticular adhesions.
- Internal derangement secondary to a torn or displaced disk.
- Ankylosis.

PEARLS: CONDYLAR AND SUBCONDYLAR FRACTURES

- Intracapsular fractures where the proximal fragment is short should be treated with closed reduction.
- Most fractures in children and edentulous adults can be treated closed.
- Intermaxillary fixation in children should be kept for a maximum of 10 days.
- Operative management is indicated in patients with low displaced or dislocated subcondylar fractures causing an acute mechanical interference with joint function, loss of vertical dimension, and unstable occlusion.
- A 2.0-mm system with at least two screws on each side of the fracture is recommended.
- All patients treated with a closed or an open reduction should undergo postoperative physiotherapy with occlusal guidance using elastics.
- Persistent joint hypomobility and jaw deviation with function are common sequelae of TMJ injuries.

REFERENCES

1. Ellis E III. Condylar process fractures of the mandible. Facial Plast Surg 2000;16:193–205
2. Krenkel C. Treatment of mandibular-condylar fractures. Atlas Oral Maxillofac Surg Clin North Am 1997;5:127–155
3. Baker AW, McMahon J, Moos KF. Current consensus on the management of fractures of the mandibular condyle. A method by questionnaire. Int J Oral Maxillofac Surg 1998;27:258–266
4. MacArthur CJ, Donald PJ, Knowles J, Moore HC. Open reduction-fixation of mandibular subcondylar fractures. A review. Arch Otolaryngol Head Neck Surg 1993;119:403–406
5. Raveh J, Vuillemin T, Ladrach K. Open reduction of the dislocated, fractured condylar process: indications and surgical procedures. J Oral Maxillofac Surg 1989;47:120–127
6. Iizuka T, Lindqvist C, Hallikainen D, Mikkonen P, Paukku P. Severe bone resorption and osteoarthrosis after miniplate fixation of high condylar fractures. A clinical and radiologic study of thirteen patients. Oral Surg Oral Med Oral Pathol 1991;72:400–407
7. Lindahl L. Condylar fractures of the mandible. I. Classification and relation to age, occlusion, and concomitant injuries of teeth and teeth-supporting structures, and fractures of the mandibular body. Int J Oral Surg 1977;6:12–21
8. Yamaoka M, Furusawa K, Iguchi K, Tanaka M, Okuda D. The assessment of fracture of the mandibular condyle by use of computerized tomography. Incidence of sagittal split fracture. Br J Oral Maxillofac Surg 1994;32:77–79
9. Norholt SE, Krishnan V, Sindet-Pedersen S, Jensen I. Pediatric condylar fractures: a long-term follow-up study of 55 patients. J Oral Maxillofac Surg 1993;51:1302–1310
10. Kleinheinz J, Anastassov GE, Joos U. Indications for treatment of subcondylar mandibular fractures. J Craniomaxillofac Trauma 1999;5:17–23
11. Zide MF, Kent JN. Indications for open reduction of mandibular condyle fractures. J Oral Maxillofac Surg 1983;41:89–98
12. Bernstein L, Nelson RH. Surgical anatomy of the extraparotid distribution of the facial nerve. Arch Otolaryngol 1984;110:177–183
13. Hinds EC, Girotti WJ. Vertical subcondylar osteotomy: a reappraisal. Oral Surg Oral Med Oral Pathol 1967;24:164–170
14. Sugiura T, Yamamoto K, Murakami K, Sugimura M. A comparative evaluation of osteosynthesis with lag screws, miniplates, or Kirschner wires for mandibular condylar process fractures. J Oral Maxillofac Surg 2001;59:1161–1168
15. Lee C, Mueller RV, Lee K, Mathes SJ. Endoscopic subcondylar fracture repair: functional, aesthetic, and radiographic outcomes. Plast Reconstr Surg 1998;102:1434–1443
16. Goss A, Bosanquet AG. The arthroscopic appearance of acute temporomandibular joint trauma. J Oral Maxillofac Surg 1990;48:780–783
17. Chuong R, Piper MA. Open reduction of condylar fractions of the mandible in conjunction with repair of discal injury: a preliminary report. J Oral Maxillofac Surg 1988;46:257–263
18. Chuong R, Piper MA. Open reduction of condylar fractions of the mandible in conjunction with repair of discal injury: a preliminary report. J Oral Maxillofac Surg 1988;46:262
19. McGuirt W, Salisbury PL. Mandibular fractures—their effect on growth and dentition. Arch Otolaryngol Head Neck Surg 1987;113:257–261
20. Amaratunga N. A study of condylar fractures in Sri Lankan patients with special reference to the recent views on treatment, healing and sequelae. Br J Oral Maxillofac Surg 1987;25:391–397
21. Myall R. Condylar injuries in children—What is different about them? In: Worthington P, Evans JR, eds. *Controversies in Oral and Maxillofacial Surgery,* vol 1. Philadelphia: WB Saunders, 1994:191–200
22. Strobl H, Emshoff R, Rothler G. Conservative treatment of unilateral condylar fractures in children: a long-term clinical and radiologic follow-up of 55 patients. Int J Oral Maxillofac Surg 1999;28:95–98

Chapter 12

MANDIBULAR FRACTURES: SYMPHYSIS, BODY, AND ANGLE

James V. Johnson

The mandible is the largest of the facial bones, it develops embryologically from the membrane covering Meckel's cartilage. The portion of the mandible consisting of the symphysis, body, and ramus make up ~90% of its physical content. The alveolar portion lies above the symphysis and body and is the supporting structure for the dentition. The usual complement of adult teeth is 32, and there are 20 deciduous or baby teeth. Eruption of permanent dentition begins about age 6. The deciduous teeth then begin to exfoliate creating a mixed dentition until approximately age 12. During this period, the dentition is difficult to utilize for intermaxillary fixation due to the bell shape of the deciduous molar crowns and partially erupted permanent teeth. For this reason, arch bars are more difficult to place. Ivy or Stout's loops are more appropriate. Exfoliating deciduous teeth or traumatically avulsed teeth makes for a challenging dilemma for intermaxillary fixation, usually requiring splint fabrication and skeletal fixation. Until full eruption of the permanent teeth, the symphysis and body of the mandible contain "wall to wall" teeth with precious little bone for placement of bone plates or screws; placement of screws can injure the developing buds and result in developmental deformity or loss.

For surgical reference, the symphysis of the mandible is that area between the cuspid teeth. The area between the cuspid and second bicuspid is generally referred to as the parasymphysis. The body extends proximally to the ascending ramus. If the third molars are impacted, they may lie in the ramus. Because the symphysis, parasymphysis, and body are dentate, open fractures create a quandary for management of the teeth in terms of removal.

The angle and condylar neck are more susceptible to fracture due to a smaller area of mass in cross section. The angle is usually fractured by lateral forces and the condylar neck and head by anterior-posterior forces. Angle fractures may be separated anatomically into those that lie between the insertions of the pterygomasseteric sling and those that are distal. In general, those that are within the sling are splinted by the muscle mass and aponeurosis and may be more resistant to displacement. If the fracture is distal to the sling, it may be unstable or unfavorable and can displace. Such fractures bilaterally may produce a flail mandible.

The ramus extends vertically. Anteriorly, the coronoid process provides for the insertion of the temporalis muscle. Impacted third molars weaken the posterior body and ramus area predisposing to fracture through the tooth socket. Reitzik et al[1] demonstrated that 40% less force was required to fracture monkey cadaver mandibles with impacted third molars. Such fractures may also occur during removal of impacted third molar teeth or in the first weeks of the postoperative period.

Mandibular fractures in general are displaced by the following muscle groups: the muscles of mastication (the masseter, temporalis, and lateral and medial pterygoid) in angle fractures, and the suprahyoid muscles (the anterior belly of the digastric, mylohyoid, geniohyoid, and genioglossus) in symphysis and body fractures. Bilateral or multiple fractures affected by muscle pull from different directions can result in a flail mandible (Fig. 12–1). Subsequently, this can create a loss of airway control due to compromise of lingual function, posterior collapse of the tongue, and parapharyngeal tissues. A definitive airway (intubation or surgical airway) may be needed, particularly if the injury is aggravated by edema or bleeding.

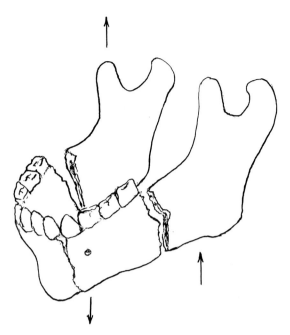

FIGURE 12–1 Flail mandible.

VASCULAR SUPPLY

The vascular supply of the mandible is mainly from the inferior alveolar artery, supplemented by periosteal feeders. The atrophic mandible may have significant loss of alveolar artery diameter, and therefore vascular supply can depend mainly on the periosteal feeders. This can create a problem with postfracture healing. Because of their proximity to the mandible, the facial artery and vein and retromandibular vein may pose problems with bleeding during fracture repair, during an intraoral or extraoral (external) approach. For external surgical approaches, the facial artery and vein or retromandibular vein may require ligation. The internal maxillary artery runs lingual to the ramus and condylar neck at the level of the coronoid, and is usually not encountered at surgery. During open reduction of the ramus, however, it should be avoided. Injudicious penetration through the lingual plate of the condylar neck with a drill places the internal maxillary artery at risk. Also, the maxillary, lingual and facial arteries may be traumatically injured especially from gunshot wounds. In this case, a high suspicion of immediate or impending airway obstruction is imperative and may necessitate a definitive airway. Angiographic studies, embolization, or surgical intervention may be necessary.

NERVE SUPPLY

Sensory innervation of the mandible is from the third division of the fifth cranial nerve. The mandibular nerve enters the medial ramus of the mandible at the lingula and traverses the ramus and body to emerge from the mental foramen in the parasymphysis area. It provides sensory innervation to the teeth, periodontal membranes, gingival and buccal mucosa of the parasymphysis area, and the ipsilateral chin and lip skin. A hallmark of a fracture through the mandibular canal is paresthesia, dysesthesia, or anesthesia of the mental nerve. Sensory innervation of the lingual mucosa, periosteum, and gingiva is from the lingual nerve, whereas that of the lateral perimandibular tissues, buccal mucosa, and gingiva *proximal* to the mental area is from the long buccal nerve. Injury to the lingual nerve is unusual in mandible fractures, except from penetrating trauma.

THE EDENTULOUS MANDIBLE

After tooth loss, the alveolar process may rapidly resorb, resulting in an atrophic jaw. This is particularly problematic in women who have a smaller mandible to begin with. The atrophic mandible is at high risk for fracture even from masticatory force; this risk may be aggravated by postmenopausal osteoporosis. If there is insufficient alveolar bone to support a dental prosthesis, then bone grafts and osteointegrated implants may be necessary to restore dentition.

CLINICAL ASSESSMENT

As part of the clinical assessment of a mandible fracture, the external (extraoral) examination should include the following steps:

- Facial examination to detect swelling, ecchymosis, laceration, puncture wounds, foreign bodies, and facial asymmetry
- Examination of the external auditory canal (EAC) for ecchymosis or bleeding secondary to condylar head dislocation or basilar skull fracture
- Palpation of the EAC to detect pain with condylar motion on mouth opening and lateral mandible excursion, which may indicate condylar fracture. Inability to palpate the condylar head motion along with deviation on opening suggests a fracture dislocation of the condyle head
- Neurologic evaluation of cranial nerves V and VII

The intraoral examination should include the following steps:

- Examination of the lips, tongue, cheeks, palate, tonsillar fossae, perioral mucosa, floor of mouth, and retromolar areas

- Evaluation of the dentition to detect crown fractures, mobility, avulsion, and partially impacted teeth
- Evaluation for malocclusion. An anterior open bite may indicate bilateral subcondylar fractures. Lateral deviation on opening with malocclusion is diagnostic for a unilateral subcondylar fracture
- Evaluation for lingual ecchymosis, which is an indication of fracture

IMAGING

Radiographic studies are covered in detail in Chapter 2; however, several points are important to mention here. The typical plain radiographs performed include the mandible series [posteroanterior (PA), left and right lateral oblique, and Towne's view), and a panoramic view (orthopantomogram, or Panorex). A submental vertex view may also be useful for fracture dislocations of the condylar heads. The computed tomography (CT) scan can be helpful, and in particular the newer three-dimensional reconstruction views can be helpful for more complex fractures, such as comminuted fractures, and fracture dislocations of the mandibular condyle. An example of a three-dimensional reconstruction of a comminuted fracture (from a gunshot wound) is shown in Fig. **12–2**. Finally, stereolithic models generated from CT studies can be helpful in complex fractures; the model may be used to prebend a reconstruction plate for proper fit and contour.

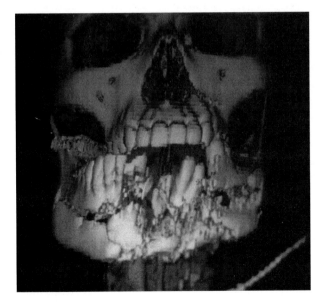

FIGURE 12–2 Three-dimensional computed tomography (CT) of comminuted mandible fracture, from a gunshot wound.

TREATMENT OF MANDIBULAR FRACTURES

The principal objectives in treating mandible fractures are to reestablish the skeletal form of the mandible, the occlusal relationship of teeth (if present), and the function of the jaws, including the temporomandibular joints. Minimal acceptable interincisal distances for opening are ∼ 35 to 40 mm, or "two knuckles." Immediate postoperative opening exercises for patients treated with open reduction and internal fixation (ORIF) are imperative; stacked tongue blades used for progressive stretching are inexpensive and practical. For patients treated with closed reduction, exercises should begin immediately after removal of intermaxillary fixation.

Establishment of form is achieved using closed reduction (along with immobilization), or open reduction. After reduction, the mandible is held rigid to allow osteosynthesis at the fracture site. This is achieved by placement of internal rigid plates; this is a combination of open reduction and internal fixation (ORIF). Although ORIF is not needed for every mandible fracture, some form of ORIF is typically required to achieve adequate immobilization and bone healing for displaced fractures.

THE SEQUENCE OF FRACTURE TREATMENT

ESTABLISH DENTAL OCCLUSION

The most important step in mandible fracture repair is to reestablish dental occlusion. *Remember: if the occlusion is not right, then nothing is right.* After establishment of dental occlusion, the proper mandibular arch form is established next. If a patient has severe malocclusion after fracture repair, that is best re-treated immediately. Unless this can be achieved within the first eight weeks, orthognathic procedures will be needed. Minor occlusal problems, on the other hand, can be managed with occlusal adjustment or orthodontic treatment.

For multiple fractures through the dentition that are unstable, the surgeon can consider utilization of a lingual splint, as shown in Fig. **12–3**. After placement of the splint, the patient is placed into intermaxillary fixation. After proper occlusion is established, the basal bone of the dentate portion of the fractures may be reduced and fixated, and the fractures proximal to the dentate portion are reduced last. If rigid fixation is utilized, the occlusion should be checked immediately after reduction to

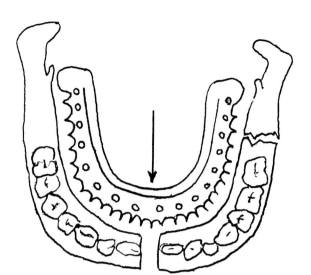

FIGURE 12–3 Lingual splint.

ensure that plating has not displaced a segment causing some malocclusion. For extensive procedures, a short period of intermaxillary fixation postoperatively (less than 1 week) allows edema to subside. The patient may otherwise be biting the tongue or buccal mucosa.

CLOSED REDUCTION

Closed reduction is indicated for nondisplaced or minimally displaced fractures in dentate patients. The jaws are immobilized with intermaxillary fixation for a period of time depending on the type of fracture and the age of the patient. This may vary from approximately 10 days in a 5-year-old child, to 4 to 6 weeks for adults. Intermaxillary fixation is generally contraindicated under the following circumstances: very young children, seizure disorder, severe head injury, the noncompliant patient, sociopathic personality, psychiatric or neurologic disease, dementia, alcoholism, and drug addiction.

Undisplaced or "hairline" fractures through dentate areas of the mandible with repeatable occlusion may tempt the surgeon not to utilize intermaxillary fixation. Although this is an alternative, the judicious surgeon should still consider a short term of intermaxillary fixation. An edentulous patient with a similar nondisplaced fracture, however, may be observed without intermaxillary fixation. This is because in dentate patients, there is constant occlusal loading, which is not true in the edentulous patient. Finally, isolated fractures of the coronoid process are splinted by the temporalis tendons and usually require no treatment.

INTERMAXILLARY FIXATION

Intermaxillary fixation (IMF) includes any method of immobilizing fractures of the jaws. Although historically there are numerous methods, contemporary use includes the following:

- Arch bars and stainless steel wire using either wire or elastics for fixation in adult, dentate patients. This technique may be utilized in conjunction with lingual or palatal splints
- Stout's or Ivy loops in children
- Acrylic splints for partially edentulous, and Gunning splints (including the patients' dentures) for edentulous patients
- Occlusal mandibular splints with circumferential wiring, usually in children
- Four-point screw fixation has become popular in the past few years, particularly to facilitate IMF for patients with HIV or hepatitis (to decrease skin puncture risk for the surgeon). This technique is valuable for that reason; however, it cannot be utilized when postoperative elastic therapy is necessary (for example, for subcondylar fractures). Also, the technique cannot usually be used in patients with limited occlusal contact

SURGICAL APPROACHES

Mandible fractures can be repaired using a transoral approach or an external approach. There are advantages and disadvantages to each. The advantages of an intraoral approach are the lack of facial or neck incision, minimal risk for bleeding or facial nerve branch injury, and, in experienced hands, faster operating time. Parasymphyseal fractures are particularly amenable to an intraoral approach. Disadvantages include the fact that special instruments and meticulous technique are required to achieve adequate bony reduction and plate positioning. There is also increased risk for mental nerve dysesthesia due to stretching, as well as vermilion or commissure abrasion or laceration. Finally, the intraoral approach is impractical for comminuted fractures.

An external approach to the mandible can be achieved by making a skin incision in the submental, submandibular, or retromandibular regions of the neck. Direct incision over the mandible is avoided because of injury to the mandibular division of the facial nerve. Advantages of the external approach include improved access to symphysis, body and angle fractures, as well as comminuted fractures. The disadvantages include a visible scar, increased risk for facial nerve branch paresis, and perhaps longer operative time. Some would debate, however, the relative duration of intraoral versus external procedures; the difference really depends on the comfort level and preference of the surgeon.

SURGICAL TECHNIQUES

A summary of surgical techniques for fracture repair at different sites is shown in Table **12–1**.

DENTATE PATIENT: ANGLE, BODY, OR SYMPHYSIS FRACTURE

Osteosynthesis of mandibular fractures should strive for reconstruction of the basal bone along the lines of tension and compression. These are discussed in more detail in Chapter 10. The tension zone runs along the alveolus to the condylar neck, and the compression zone runs along the inferior border; this is shown in Fig. **12–4**.

For rigid fixation in the symphysis, body, and angle, a small (2.0 mm or less) plate is placed along the zone of tension (the tension band) with monocortical screws. A larger (2.4 mm or larger) plate is placed along the inferior border along the zone of compression. Here, many authors advocate using at least three bicortical screws on each side of the fracture; this is known as the three-screw rule.[2] This terminology is a modification of Spiessl's original use of the term to mandate three screws in the proximal fragment of posterior body and angle fractures. This is due to the relatively thin buccal-lingual width of the inferior boarder (12 to 10 mm). In dentate areas where an arch bar is used, the bar acts as the tension band and a plate is not necessary.

Another technique is to use a 2.0-mm monocortical plate placed only along the tension area for single fractures of the angle, or perhaps in combination with a 2.0-mm plate at the inferior border.[3–5] For angle fractures, another variation is the use of a

three-dimensional strut plate, which is a single unit with the biomechanical advantage of vertical connecting bars between the superior and inferior plates. Holes are drilled monocortical, obviously avoiding the area of the nerve canal. The strut plate in place on an angle fracture is shown in Fig. **12–5**.[6,7] This plate is usually placed transorally.

EDENTULOUS PATIENT

Edentulous patients are usually treated with ORIF. Reconstruction plates (2.4 or 2.0 mm) are an excellent choice for such injuries. The procedure is usually best performed using a neck incision for maximal access and field sterility, and fractures are repaired using the three-screw rule. In addition, autogenous bone grafting may be indicated for the atrophic mandible, as shown in Fig. **12–6**. External pin fixation is a consideration but may have limited application in the severely atrophic mandible. Closed reduction may utilize the patient's dentures or splints secured with skeletal fixation, if there is sufficient alveolar bone.

PEDIATRIC FRACTURES

Pediatric trauma is discussed in detail in Chapter 16, but a brief discussion of pediatric mandible fractures is provided here. Undisplaced fractures may be managed conservatively with IMF using Stout's loops. In addition, if the fractures in the body and symphysis are displaced, an occlusal splint may be fabricated and secured intraoperatively with three circumferential wires. ORIF of severely displaced fractures may be accomplished with monocortical microplates at the inferior border or oblique ridge. The plates may be removed after 6 weeks along with the circumferential wires and loops under general anesthesia as a day surgery. Pediatric patients are allowed to function immediately, even with a

TABLE 12–1 SUMMARY OF TREATMENT OPTIONS

	Closed reduction (IMF +)	Open reduction wire (IMF +)	ORIF 2.0-mm tension band only (IMF ±)	ORIF 2.0-mm tension and compression (IMF ±)	ORIF lag screw (IMF ±)	ORIF 2.0-mm tension, 2.4-mm compression (IMF −)	EPF (IMF −)	ORIF 3-D Strut (IMF −)
Fracture utilization								
Symphysis	+	+	−	+	+	+	+	−
Body	+	+	−	+	+	+	+	−
Angle	+	+	+	+	+	+	+	+

IMF, intermaxillary fixation; ORIF, open reduction and internal fixation.
+ = use; − = do not use; ± = IMF at the discretion of the surgeon.

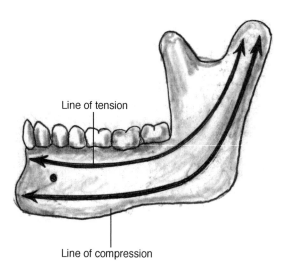

FIGURE 12–4 Tension and compression zones of the mandible.

subcondylar fracture, by placing several large guiding elastics on each side. Elastics are used for a limited time, according to the child's' age: from age 1 to 4 years, for 1 week; age greater than 4 years, for 10 days; age greater than 6 years, for 2 weeks. The treatment goal is repeatable occlusion and increasing range of motion. Potential complications of mandible fractures in children include dysplasia or loss of developing permanent teeth in the line of fracture, malocclusion requiring orthodontic treatment and orthognathic surgery, joint ankylosis and developmental growth problems requiring additional surgery.

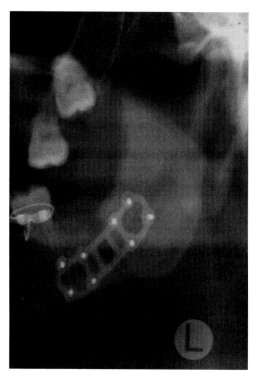

FIGURE 12–5 Mandibular angle strut plate in place.

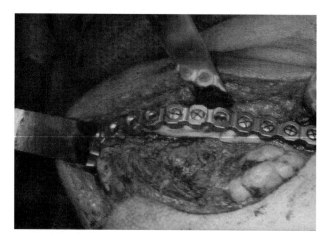

FIGURE 12–6 Fracture of an edentulous mandible, with reconstruction plate.

JOE HALL MORRIS EXTERNAL PIN FIXATION

External pin fixation may be used for most fractures of the symphysis, body, and ramus.[8] Other techniques may be more practical, particularly for the patient who objects to wearing the device, which is shown in Fig. **12–7**. External pin fixation is potentially useful for the infected mandible fracture, continuity defects from trauma or tumor surgery, comminuted fractures including those from gunshot wounds, and fractures in the edentulous patient. The advantages of external fixation include immediate restoration of functional occlusion and jaw mobility, easy correction of occlusion, inexpensive hardware, and it may be left in place for months if needed. Disadvantages include the external appearance of the device, and the need for sufficient bone in proximal and distal fragments. In a condylar fracture with a short proximal fragment or a comminuted

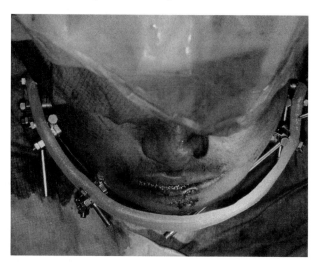

FIGURE 12–7 Joe Hall Morris external pin fixation for gunshot wound of mandible.

ramus, the use of external fixation may require placement of two pins in the zygomatic body for proximal stability, and placement of a hinge between two acrylic bars.

COMMINUTED FRACTURES

Comminuted fractures of the symphysis, body, and angle are a challenging management problem. The basic principle is restoration of occlusion, followed by bony stabilization. This can be achieved using either external pin fixation or a reconstruction plate[9] spanning the bony gap (Fig. **12–8**).

GUNSHOT WOUNDS

For low-velocity injuries with minimal soft tissue loss and comminuted bone, treatment includes debridement and IMF, and ORIF with a reconstruction plate, or external pin fixation. If there is bony loss, delayed bone grafting can be used. For a high-velocity injury with soft tissue and bone loss, treatment includes debridement and IMF, ORIF with a reconstruction plate or external pin fixation, followed by bone grafting or microvascular free tissue transfer (osteocutaneous).

SYMPHYSEAL FRACTURES: SPECIAL CONSIDERATIONS

In a symphyseal fracture with an associated fracture of the contralateral angle, establishment of occlusion can be difficult. The intervening bone is generally unstable and tilted, due to pull of the suprahyoid muscles; this "step" malocclusion may be difficult to reduce. In this case, a lingual splint may be necessary to stabilize the symphyseal area and establish proper occlusion, or the middle fragment can be wire-fixated into place temporarily to

facilitate IMF; then the wires are removed and the fractures plated.

In a symphyseal fracture with a contralateral condylar neck fracture, the condylar neck fracture is often treated closed. Therefore, the patient can have ORIF of the symphysis fracture with closed reduction of the subcondylar fracture, and short-term IMF (i.e., 3 weeks) with functional elastics, followed by function during the day and use of elastics at night for a period of 8 to 12 weeks. The goal is to achieve good healing of the symphysis, and good function of the condylar joint. A lingual splint may be useful to help establish occlusion in these cases as well.

A symphyseal fracture with bilateral subcondylar fractures is particularly difficult. The suprahyoid and mastication muscles create a transverse widening of the distance between the angles of the mandible and a bilateral posterior crossbite malocclusion, as shown in Fig. 12–9. The patient, therefore, has both an occlusal problem as well as a facial aesthetic problem: a widened face. Reduction of this fracture pattern can be difficult. If the patient has an intact maxillary arch and dentition, several methods may be used to aid reduction. A lingual splint, use of a transoral wire between the mandibular first molar teeth with tightening to reduce the molar segments into proper occlusion, use of external manual pressure on the mandibular angles to reduce the transverse distance, and application of a rigid 2.4-mm fracture plate that is overbent to establish the proper symphyseal arch. If there is a concurrent midface fracture with a split palate, there is no stable reference for occlusion. In this circumstance, dental models of both arches are made; the mandibular

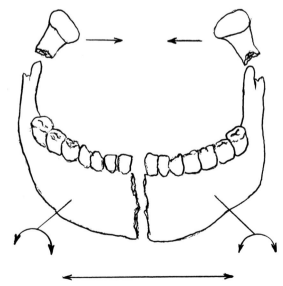

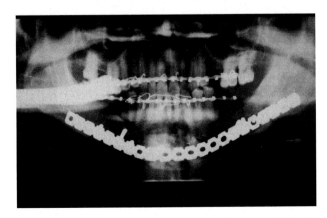

FIGURE 12–8 Comminuted symphysis and body fractures with a reconstruction plate.

FIGURE 12–9 Bilateral subcondylar and symphysis fractures with characteristic displacement of fragments.

model is cut through the fracture site. Determination of the posterior transverse arch width at the first molars may be estimated by using mean arch widths for adults from orthodontic studies, which is 56 mm ± 2 mm from the buccal of the mandibular first molars.[10] The model is glued together at the proper width, and a lingual splint is then fabricated from the repaired model. The maxillary model is sectioned and placed into occlusion with the mandibular model, and a palatal splint can be fabricated.

Angle Fractures: Special Considerations

Fractures through the third molar teeth create a dilemma. Many surgeons fail to recognize the potential complications inherent with teeth in the line of fracture, primarily related to postoperative infection and need for further procedures. In general, teeth in the line for fracture are best removed if they meet removal criteria. Our experience with the mandibular strut plate included routine removal of third molars in the line of fractures.[7] Some recommend leaving third molars during fracture healing with subsequent elective removal as the appropriate management. Therefore, a careful consideration of risks and benefits of removal should be performed. One report recommended that third molars in the line of fracture should be removed under the following circumstances[11]: crown fracture into the pulp, root fracture, partial impaction, severe periodontal bone loss, fracture through the apex, deep caries, dentigerous cyst, and infected fracture. Another study found that third molars had the greatest incident of infection (37.5%), but that postoperative infections were more frequent if the tooth *was* removed.[12,13] The conclusions were that those teeth that do not meet the criteria should not be removed, because there is some benefit to their presence during healing.

Antibiotics

Prophylactic intravenous antibiotics covering skin and oral flora should be administered prior to surgery and discontinued after 24 hours if there was no preoperative infection. In a fracture that is infected before surgery, bone plating may still be used.[14] Prior to fixation, the bone and adjacent soft tissues should be debrided and irrigated to remove foreign bodies and bone sequestra. The author prefers to use a seven- or nine-hole plate, placing the blank middle hole over the fracture to ensure that the other screws are in bicortical bone; at least three screws are used on each side of the fracture. Biomechanical testing indicates that maximum sta-

bility is achieved by no more than four screws in each segment.[15] Therefore, when possible, using the longer plate seems reasonable. Postoperative infections involving unusual organisms such as methicillin-resistant *Staphylococcus* or *Pseudomonas* warrant special consideration. If the plate is stable and appropriate wound care and antibiotic are used, the fracture may go to union as long as there is adequate blood supply and no sequestra; a stable plate buys time for healing, but after healing the plate is typically removed. An unstable plate should be removed and replaced with external pin fixation, or a different (and probably larger) plate.

Absorbable Plates

Absorbable plating for fracture osteosynthesis is a promising technology that will likely play a prominent role in the future. Kallela et al[16] and Suuronen et al[17] report satisfactory use of screw fixation for mandible fractures and orthognathic surgery. Other studies have found good outcomes after use of absorbable plates and screws for mandible fractures in animal studies.[18] Nevertheless, it is premature to advocate resorbable plates and screws for mandibular trauma at this time because of the lack of wide acceptance of the biomechanical stability of plates, the fact that resorbable plates are not inexpensive, and issues concerning foreign-body reactions to biodegradable synthetic polymers.[19]

Summary of Options for Open Reduction of Mandible Fractures (see Table 12–1)

1. Superior border tension zone plate (2 mm) with inferior border compression fracture plate (2.0 or 2.4 mm)
   - Parasymphysis, body, and angle application
   - Utilize three-screw rule on compression band plate
   - Bicortical compression band screws
   - With or without IMF

2. Superior border arch bar (as a tension band) with inferior border compression band plate
   - Symphysis, body, and angle application
   - 2.0-mm monocortical screws
   - With or without IMF

3. Superior border plate only (Champy technique)
   - Angle fracture application
   - 2.0-mm miniplate with monocortical screws
   - Usually without IMF
   - Three screws in each segment

4. Lag screws

- Symphysis and angle application most frequent
- At least two screws placed in symphysis
- One screw placed in angle
- Technique sensitive
- Usually with IMF (angle)

5. Three-dimensional strut plate for angle fractures
   - Angle and body application
   - Uses 2.0-mm monocortical screws
   - Apply plate so that mandibular canal runs between superior and inferior screws
   - Biomechanical stability
   - With or without IMF

PEARLS: SYMPHYSIS, BODY, AND ANGLE FRACTURES

- Establish occlusion first, typically using intermaxillary fixation.
- A lingual splint may be used to establish occlusion in an unstable or comminuted mandible.
- After occlusion is established, perform reduction and fixation of symphysis, body, and angle fractures, typically using the arch bar for a tension band, and an inferior border plate along the compression zone. Plate dentate portion first.
- Whenever possible, the use of three screws on each side of the fracture is ideal for compression plates.
- For missing or comminuted mandibular bone, a reconstruction plate should be used to span the gap; occasionally a bone graft is also placed secondarily. External pin fixation is another option in those cases.
- A lingual splint is useful for bilateral subcondylar fractures combined with a symphysis fracture, to prevent facial widening and malocclusion.
- Consider removal of a third molar in the line of an angle fracture, if criteria for removal are met.

REFERENCES

1. Reitzik M, Lownie JF, Cleaton-Jones P, Austin J. Experimental fractures of monkey mandibles. Int J Oral Surg 1978;7:100–103
2. Spiessl B. *Internal Fixation of Mandible*. Berlin, Heidelberg: Springer-Verlag, 1989:191
3. Champy M, Kahn JL. Fracture line stability as a function of the internal fixation system: an in vitro comparison using a mandibular angle fracture model. J Oral Maxillofac Surg 1995;53:801–802
4. Potter J, Ellis E. Treatment of mandibular angel fractures with a malleable non compression miniplate. J Oral Maxillofac Surg 1999;57:288–292
5. Ellis E, Walker L. Treatment of mandibular angle fracture using two noncompression miniplates. J Oral Maxillofac Surg 1994;52:1032–1036
6. Wittenberg J. Treatment of mandibular angle fractures with 3-D titanium miniplate. J Oral Maxillofac Surg 1994;52(suppl 2):106
7. Guimond C, Marchena JM, Wong MEK, Johnson JV. Fixation of mandibular angle fracture with a multidimensional 2.0-mm strut plate. J Oral Maxillofac Surg 2002;60:49–50
8. Morris JH. Biphase connector, external pin for reduction and fixation of mandible fractures. Oral Surg Oral Med Oral Pathol 1949;2:1382–1398
9. Smith BR, Johnson JV. Rigid fixation of the comminuted mandibular fractures. J Oral Maxillofac Surg 1993;51:1320–1326
10. Ricketts R. Clinical cephalometrics. Angle Orthod 1981;2:130–150
11. Shetty V, Freymiller E. Teeth in the line of fractures: a review. J Oral Maxillofac Surg 1989;47:1303–1306
12. Neal DC, Wagner WF, Alpert B. Morbidity associated with teeth in the line of mandibular fractures. J Oral Surg 1978;36:859–862
13. Lindquist C. Impacted teeth. In: Alling C, Helfrick J, Alling R, eds. *Mandibular and Maxillary Fractures: Impacted Teeth.* Philadelphia: WB Saunders, 1993:333–343
14. Preim J. *Manual of Internal Fixation in the Cranio-Facial Skeleton.* Berlin, Heidelberg, New York: Springer-Verlag, 1998
15. Haug R. What is the ideal number of screws for use in reconstruction plating? J Oral Maxillofac Surg 1992;50(suppl 3):94
16. Kallela I, Iizuka T, Salo A, Lindquist C. Lag screw fixation of anterior mandibular fractures using biodegradable polylactide screws: a preliminary report. J Oral Maxillofac Surg 1999;57:113–117
17. Suuronen R, Laine P, Pohjonen T, Lindqvist C. Sagittal ramus osteotomus fixed with biodegradable screws: a preliminary report. J Oral Maxillofac Surg 1994;52:715–720
18. Quereshy FA, Goldstein JA, Goldberg JS, Beg Z. The efficacy of bioresorbable fixation in the repair of mandibular fractures: an animal study. J Oral Maxillofac Surg 2000;58:1263–1269
19. Bostman O, Hirvensalo E, Makinen J, Rokkanen P. Foreign-body reactions to fracture fixation implants of biodegradable synthetic polymers. J Bone Joint Surg Br 1990;72:592–596

Chapter 13

DENTAL AND DENTOALVEOLAR INJURIES

Mark Eu-Kien Wong, Richard A. Vickers, and Roberta Pileggi

The dentoalveolar complex is composed of the teeth and supporting alveolar processes of the maxilla and mandible. In children, adolescents, and adults, injuries to this area can be attributed to automobile and bicycle accidents, contact sports, missile and projectile injuries, and interpersonal violence, including domestic violence and child abuse. Iatrogenic injury may be the result of dental treatment, endotracheal intubation, or investigative procedures such as laryngoscopy and gastroscopy.

The association between dentoalveolar injuries and facial fractures is considerable as illustrated by a series of 9543 patients with craniomaxillofacial trauma, in which 4763 patients (49.9%) suffered from an associated dentoalveolar injury.[1] In the pediatric population, epidemiologic studies reveal that one out of two children sustains a dental injury, most often between the ages of 8 and 12.[2] The oral cavity is the second most common region injured in preschool children and the fourth most commonly traumatized among 7- to 30-year-olds.[3] In adolescents, contact sports are responsible for dentoalveolar fractures in 36% of the population,[4,5] and the use of mouth guards has been shown to significantly decrease the incidence of such injuries. Crown fracture is the most frequent type of trauma to teeth. Luxation injuries, comprising the incomplete avulsion of a tooth from its socket, usually involve the deciduous dentition, whereas crown fractures are more common in the permanent dentition.[6]

Although appreciation of the gross anatomy is usually sufficient for the diagnosis and treatment of injuries, the extent and eventual outcome is based on the effects of trauma on the microscopic constituents of the dentoalveolar complex. Consequently, this chapter begins with a review of the pertinent anatomy of teeth, the periodontal complex, and the surrounding alveolar bone as a foundation for discussion of the classification and pathophysiology of injury and the ensuing management of these conditions.

APPLIED DENTAL ANATOMY

ANATOMY OF THE TOOTH

In the absence of periodontal disease, which can resorb the supporting alveolar bone, altering the normal relationship between a tooth and its socket, teeth are organized into a suprabony coronal portion, termed the *crown*, and an infrabony radicular component called the *root*. The incisors, cuspids, and mandibular bicuspids are single-root teeth. The maxillary bicuspids occasionally form multiple roots, as do the maxillary and mandibular molars. Maxillary molars usually have three roots, whereas mandibular molars have two roots. The tip of each root(s) is referred to as the *apex (apices)* and contains a small foramen through which passes a neurovascular bundle responsible for the vitality and innervation of the tooth. Both the crown and root of each tooth is composed of two layers of mineralized tissue surrounding a central core of loose, highly vascularized and innervated connective tissue, termed the *dental pulp*. The two layers of mineralized tissue forming the crown of a tooth are enamel and dentine, whereas the radicular portion is composed of cementum and dentine (Fig. **13–1**). Enamel is the hardest tissue in the body and relatively inactive, whereas cementum is histologically and physiologically most like bone, exhibiting constant turnover. Dentine behaves in an intermediary fashion to its mineralized cousins. Although enamel formation is complete at the time of tooth eruption, dentine and cementum, like bone, retain the ability to form and remodel during the life of a tooth. Healing

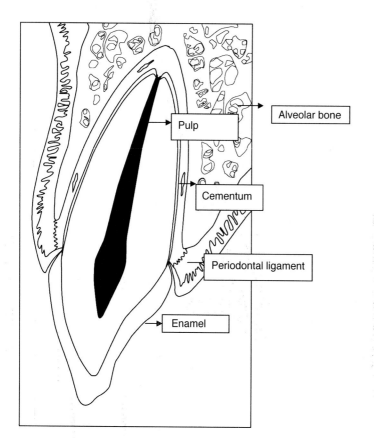

FIGURE 13–1 Diagrammatic representation of dental and periodontal anatomy.

and repair of these tissues, therefore, is possible following injury.

PERIODONTAL LIGAMENT

Teeth are anchored to the surrounding alveolar bone by a network of dense collagen fibers, which attach directly between the cemental surface of the root and the cortex-like inner surface of the alveolar socket (Fig. 13–1). The fibers are interspersed with small neural elements, which transmit sensation when a tooth is displaced or subluxated. Also present within the fibrous network are various populations of cells including undifferentiated osteoprogenitor cells, bone remodeling cells, lymphatics, and a vascular supply. This composite structure is known as the *periodontal ligament* and serves as a suspensory attachment for teeth within their alveolar sockets. The lack of a rigid attachment between teeth and bone and the presence of bone remodeling cells allow for gradual movement of teeth within the alveolar bone. Teeth move physiologically when low forces (e.g., orthodontic traction, habitual tongue thrust) are applied or when positional confinements imposed by adjacent or opposing teeth are removed with tooth loss. The latter effect, which may occur with dentoalveolar injuries, produces a malposed

dentition as teeth drift or overerupt following loss of the adjacent dentition. The dense inner surface of a dental socket is referred to as the *lamina dura* and constitutes an important radiologic landmark in the examination of dental attachments. It is formed by a continuation of the cortical plates of the alveolar bone.

THE DENTAL PULP

The vitality of a tooth is dependent on a dental neurovascular bundle, which enters the pulp through an apical foramen. Radiating from the pulp through the dentine is an array of tubules. These convey nutrients and remove waste from the metabolically active dentine. The principal neurovascular trunk for the maxilla is the superior alveolar artery and nerve, which divides into posterior, middle, and anterior branches. The mandible is supplied by the inferior alveolar artery and nerve posterior to the mental foramen. Anterior to the foramen, the neurovascular supply is provided by the incisive branches of the inferior alveolar vessels and nerve. Tooth vitality is expressed clinically as a function of a tooth's ability to respond normally to electrical stimuli, and thermal changes, as well as crown coloration. These parameters test the presence of an intact neurovascular supply to the tooth. Compromise of the neural supply, as a result of transection or inflammatory compression, produces a hyperesthetic or anesthetic response to electrical and thermal stimulation. Disruption of the vascular supply or vessel network within the pulp causes discoloration of the tooth as products of hemoglobin degradation are released from their intravascular compartment.

PATHOPHYSIOLOGY OF DENTAL INJURY

The response of teeth to injury is largely dependent on the types of tissue involved. When injury is confined to the enamel, alteration in tooth morphology and sensitivity to environmental stimuli, such as pH changes, thermal alterations, and pressure, result. Similar effects are also produced when dentine is traumatized. However, when dentine is injured, exposed dentinal tubules also provide conduits for microbial infection toward the underlying pulp. Pulpal trauma is the most severe form of dental injury because exposure of the pulp to the oral environment often produces a significant inflammatory response, responsible for a compartment syndrome. Edema creates severe pain and ischemia from compression of vascular/neural elements in the pulp, which compromise the vitality of the tooth.

Secondary bacterial contamination serves to aggravate the injury and if sufficient, pulp necrosis ensues, leading to devitalization of the tooth.

Injury to the periodontal complex is capable of producing multiple effects depending on the magnitude and direction of force. Inflammatory reactions of the vascular, lymphatic, and neural network within the periodontal ligament are associated with a concussive state, whereas more severe injuries result in subluxation or avulsion of the tooth, interrupting the neural, lymphatic, and vascular supply. The ability of a tooth to retain its vitality after these types of injury depends on the duration of ischemia and the degree of apical patency, which will either allow or discourage reestablishment of the neurovascular connection. The presence of active osteoprogenitor cells and cementoblasts within the periodontal ligament produces another potential reaction to injury. If these cells are activated, bone deposition within the periodontal space results in ankylosis of the tooth to the surrounding alveolar bone. Ankylosis of the deciduous dentition impedes the eruption of the permanent successors. Inflammatory activation of osteoclastic remodeling cells within the periodontal ligament can produce resorption of the tooth root, termed *external resorption* (Fig. 13–2A). Reduction in anchorage as a result of external resorption leads to tooth mobility or loss. If the pulp undergoes necrosis, the ensuing inflammatory reaction also produces a resorptive response,

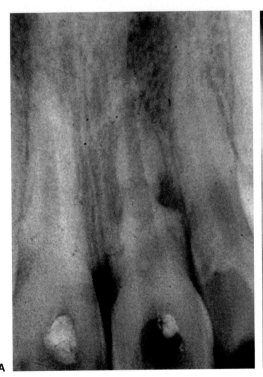
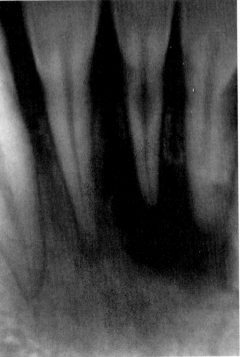

A   B

FIGURE 13–2   A: External resorption of tooth. B: Internal resorption of a tooth.

known as *internal resorption* because it occurs within the pulp chamber (Fig. **13–2B**).

DECIDUOUS AND PERMANENT DENTITION

Humans develop two sets of dentition during their lifetime. The *deciduous* (primary) dentition in each jaw is composed of four deciduous incisors (centrals and laterals), two deciduous cuspids (canines), and four deciduous molars (first and second molars). The appearance of the primary dentition is initiated by the eruption of the deciduous incisors at 6 months, and is completed when the second deciduous molars erupt around $2\frac{1}{2}$ years of age. The permanent tooth buds for the incisors, cuspids, and bicuspids develop in the alveolar bone beneath their deciduous counterparts (the permanent molars do not have a deciduous precursor). Injury to the deciduous teeth can affect development of the underlying permanent teeth, resulting in enamel hypoplasia or dilacerations of the permanent teeth. The *permanent* (adult or secondary) dentition begins to erupt into the mouth at age 6 with the appearance of either the first permanent molars or central incisors. Within each jaw there are four permanent incisors (centrals and laterals), two cuspids (canines), four bicuspids (first and second bicuspids), and four to six molars (first, second, and third molars). The sequence of eruption of the dentition is summarized in Table **13–1**. Between the ages of 6 and 13 years, both deciduous and permanent teeth are present, resulting in a stage of oral development referred to as the *mixed dentition phase*. The eruption of the morphologically larger permanent teeth is responsible for an elongation and widening of the dental arches through enlargement of the alveolar processes. Until this is complete, examination of the dentition during the mixed period often reveals a confusing array of malpositioned, partially erupted teeth, crowded into position by the incompletely developed arches. Recognition of this natural stage of development is important in the management of dentoalveolar injuries.

Development of both primary and permanent teeth is not complete at the time of eruption. Instead, root formation does not begin until the teeth first appear in the mouth. Completion of root formation in the primary dentition takes approximately 1 to $1\frac{1}{2}$ years. Complete root formation of permanent teeth takes twice as long. This developmental progression is important in the management of dental injuries because the presence of an incompletely formed root with open apices offers the best opportunity for reestablishment of a vascular supply to a tooth through a patent root apex.

THE ALVEOLAR PROCESSES

The alveolar processes of the maxilla and mandible constitute the tooth-bearing portions of the jaws. They are continuous with the supporting basal bone and are histologically identical. However, unlike basal bone whose form and structure are maintained by physiologic loads imposed during oral function, the alveolar processes rely on the presence of teeth to provide the functional stimuli necessary for preservation of its morphology. Loss of teeth, therefore, is associated with atrophy of the alveolar bone and a reduction in maxillary or mandibular bone height and width. Concern for the preservation of jaw structure constitutes one of the primary reasons for attempting the replantation of teeth lost or loosened during dentoalveolar trauma. In mandibular tooth-bearing sites, the relative thickness of the cortical plates in the anterior and posterior regions warrants consideration because these dimensions govern the depth that can be safely drilled before tooth roots are encountered. In the anterior mandible, the buccal cortical plate is extremely thin, whereas in the posterior mandible, between 4 and 6 mm of bone thickness overlies the tooth socket.

THE FUNCTIONAL ROLES OF TEETH

For physicians to appreciate the importance of treating dental and dentoalveolar injuries appropriately,

TABLE 13–1 SEQUENCE OF ERUPTION OF THE DENTITION

Teeth	Age of Eruption (range)
Deciduous central/lateral incisors	6–9 months
First deciduous molar	12–14 months
Deciduous canine	16–18 months
Second deciduous molar	24–30 months
First permanent molar, central/ lateral incisors	6–9 years
Permanent canine, first/second premolars, second molar	10–13 years
Permanent third molar	17–21 years

Modified from Scott JM, Symons NBB. The establishment of the deciduous and permanent dentitions. In: Scott JM, Symons NBB, eds. *Introduction to Dental Anatomy.* Edinburgh and London: Churchill Livingstone, 1974:114–127.

the contributions of teeth and their supporting structures to normal function and facial form must be understood. Teeth are important masticatory instruments and their premature loss or malposition compromises an individual's ability to eat. Teeth are also an essential component of facial aesthetics. The loss of anterior teeth, most frequently affected during facial trauma[7] alters appearance, whereas the loss of opposing teeth within the dental arches reduces support to the lower third of the facial skeleton. This produces an overclosed and prematurely aged effect. As described previously, the loss of a single tooth can result in drifting of adjacent teeth or overeruption of an opposing tooth, altering the position of the entire dentition. Speech is yet another activity that relies on the presence of teeth for the production of sounds. Sibilant and fricative sounds involve the placement of the tongue against the palatal surfaces of teeth to prevent anterior air escape. The dentition is also involved in mandibular proprioception and reflexes that coordinate normal muscle activity. The teeth, with their associated periodontal ligaments, provide important sensory input to the muscles of mastication and temporomandibular joints promoting physiologic function of these structures. Finally, the deciduous dentition helps to preserve sufficient space within the dental arches for the subsequent eruption of permanent successors. When primary teeth are lost, crowding of the adult dentition often results as teeth drift into the empty spaces.

DIAGNOSIS OF DENTAL AND DENTOALVEOLAR INJURIES

Several classification systems have been developed to define the various types of injury to teeth and their supporting structures. These systems serve to clarify communication between physicians, facilitate epidemiologic studies, and provide a method for estimating clinical outcomes. The most widely adopted classification, developed by Andreasen,[8] employs categorization of dentoalveolar injuries into those affecting the teeth, periodontal ligament, alveolar bone, and the gingival and mucosal soft tissues. However, for the purpose of management, a simplified set of diagnostic criteria is sufficient. Treating physicians should be able to recognize those conditions that warrant immediate attention, those affecting the management of associated maxillofacial injuries, and injuries requiring referral to an appropriate dental specialist. This process begins with proper diagnosis utilizing appropriate history taking, physical examination, and radiographic investigation.

HISTORY TAKING

Important information contained in the history of patients with dentoalveolar injuries include the age of the patient, conditions that predispose to infection, congenital anomalies of tooth development (e.g., ectodermal dysplasia), and previous dental treatment, especially extractions and orthodontic treatment. It is also essential to define the interval between the traumatic event and presentation for treatment as well as the mechanism of injury. The patient's age is significant, because it establishes the type of dentition present and the expected stage of root development of the teeth. As alluded to previously, teeth with incompletely formed roots and open apices are more likely to survive traumatic avulsion or subluxation, because of their ability to revascularize. A history of anomalies of tooth development and eruption or a history of previous dental extractions helps identify the total number of teeth present prior to the accident. Teeth unaccounted for at the time of initial presentation must be investigated and aspiration must always be considered. Prior orthodontic treatment can change the anatomy of the dental arches and the maxillary and mandibular occlusal relationships. This affects the use of the dentition as an index for the correct reduction of maxillary and mandibular fractures. Knowledge of the mechanism of injury raises suspicion for certain types of injuries. For example, blunt anterior trauma through the lips producing dental fractures may result in the impaction of crown fragments into the soft tissue. Forces applied to the inferior aspect of the mandible can produce subtle vertical fractures of the teeth as they impact against the corresponding maxillary dentition. Questioning care providers on the mechanism of injury can also determine if child abuse or neglect was involved. The interval between injury and treatment is an important variable because it corresponds to the period of potential ischemia of the injured tooth. Permanent teeth that have been avulsed for greater than 2 hours have significantly reduced survival rates and are poor candidates for reimplantation. However, teeth that are subluxated or displaced may retain their vitality and should always be considered for retention unless they are already compromised by significant caries or periodontal disease.

ORAL EXAMINATION

Once the history has been obtained, a careful examination of the facial and oral structures is conducted. Associated fractures of the craniofacial skeleton are noted, especially those involving the maxilla and the mandible, because they have the potential to affect the appropriate identification of dentoalveolar injuries and their subsequent management. Physical examination of the dentoalveolar structures is based primarily on inspection and palpation of the dentoalveolar complex and percussion of the affected teeth. When available, special tests to assess tooth vitality, such as electrical or thermal pulp testing, can also be conducted as part of the physical examination. Inspection of the dentoalveolar structures attempts to identify missing, fractured, or malpositioned teeth through examination of the coronal portions. Injuries to tooth roots contained within alveolar bone require radiographic examination for diagnosis. If the crown of a tooth is missing, the associated alveolar socket is inspected for evidence of retained roots. An empty socket, confirmed with radiographs, suggests tooth avulsion, and efforts are made to locate the missing tooth. Inspection of the crown of a tooth also helps determine the presence and extent of a fracture. If a crown fracture is present, the depth of involvement is significant and a dental consultation is warranted. Teeth displaced as a result of trauma must be investigated further to identify fractures of the roots or supporting alveolar bone. The management of these injuries is discussed in the treatment section of this chapter. Bidigital palpation of teeth suspected of injury can detect mobility, which is suggestive of a fracture, luxation of the tooth, or fracture of the alveolar bone. Percussion of teeth is a method to identify injury to the periodontal complex or fractures of teeth that are not obvious on clinical examination. The blunt handle of a metal dental mirror can be used to tap against the crowns of teeth. Sensitivity upon percussion may indicate a concussive injury to the ligament or a crown fracture. The physical examination of the dentoalveolar complex is completed by an assessment of the gingiva and oral mucosa. Degloving injuries are significant, because of the significant effect on the vascular supply to the dentoalveolar complex and teeth. This supply is especially important in the elderly whose endosteal vascularity is reduced.

Radiographic Examination

In most emergency room settings, the imaging studies available lack sufficient resolution to accurately diagnose dentoalveolar injuries. Even a panoramic radiograph, which is a tomographic study of the maxilla and mandible, is usually obscured in the midline from the curvature of the film. The most suitable studies comprise a combination of dental periapical and occlusal radiographs, readily performed in a dental office with routine equipment.[4,9]

These special films help to confirm the following diagnoses:

1. Root fracture
2. Extrusion or intrusion of the tooth
3. Alveolar and tooth socket fractures
4. Tooth fragments or foreign bodies in the soft tissues

A periapical radiograph can also determine the extent of root development and patency of the apical foramen. Accurate diagnosis of subtle root fractures may be difficult and require multiple views taken at different angulations of the central beam. Foreign bodies in the perioral soft tissue may be localized using radiographs taken at 90 degrees to each other with decreased exposure time (approximately one third). Computed tomography (CT) scans with soft tissue windows can be used to locate displaced teeth or fragments in the deeper tissue planes of the face and neck region.

Management of Injuries to the Dentition

The goal of treatment is to preserve or restore the anatomy, aesthetics, and functional role of the tooth in the dental arch. Crown fractures account for the majority of dental trauma in the permanent dentition (26 to 76%), whereas crown-root fractures are infrequent (0.3 to 5%).[3] The general principles of treatment apply to both the primary and permanent teeth. However, because primary teeth exfoliate during development, efforts to conserve these teeth are not necessarily strenuous. In addition, potential damage to the tooth buds of the developing adult permanent teeth may result from treating traumatic injuries to deciduous teeth. If primary teeth are lost, space-maintaining devices can be constructed by a pediatric dentist to preserve the length of the dental arch for subsequent eruption of the permanent successors.

The principal aim in treating fractures of permanent teeth is to ensure their long-term stability and retention in the dental arch for function and aesthetics. Strategies employed for common dental injuries are based on the extent of damage. This approach is summarized as follows:

Crown Infraction (Incomplete Enamel Fracture with No Loss of Substance)

Immediate treatment is usually not indicated and the status of the dental pulp is evaluated periodically by a dentist for evidence of ischemic injury.

UNCOMPLICATED CROWN FRACTURE (NO PULP EXPOSURE)

If dental services are available at initial presentation, treatment of enamel and dentin fractures may be performed to reduce inflammation and hyperemia while providing protection of the dental pulp against thermal stimuli. A sedative calcium hydroxide dressing is used to insulate the pulp, and, if necessary, a temporary acid-etched resin is applied superficially to protect the dressing. After 6 to 8 weeks, secondary dentin forms in the area of injury and serves as a barrier to the external environment. At this time, a final aesthetic restoration is completed by a dentist. If dental treatment cannot be performed, smoothing rough enamel surfaces with a rotary bur prevents further trauma to the adjacent soft tissue.

COMPLICATED CROWN FRACTURE (ASSOCIATED PULP EXPOSURE)

Treatment for this category of injury depends on the extent of dental pulp exposure, the stage of root development of the tooth and the period of exposure. In general, pulp recovery is more successful when treatment is instituted within 2 hours of injury. After 24 hours, removal of the pulp and endodontic therapy is indicated. The size of the pulpal exposure is an indication of both the extent of injury as well as the potential contamination of the pulp with microbials. Small, pinpoint areas of exposed pulp can be covered with a sedative calcium hydroxide dressing and temporary filling. Larger exposures, however, require partial or complete removal of the dental pulp *(pulpotomy)* and a more extensive assessment of tooth vitality. Treatment also depends on the maturity of the tooth. For partially developed teeth with immature root formation, treatment is directed at maintaining vitality while root formation is completed, a process known as *apexogenesis*. When an injured tooth presents with a mature, closed apex, a grossly contaminated pulp (e.g., exposure for greater than 24 hours), or an obviously necrotic pulp, root canal therapy is indicated and this should be done as soon as possible. If the patient's condition does not permit early intervention, the potential for odontogenic infection must be weighed against the advantages of preserving the fractured tooth, and extraction may be the treatment of choice. When pulpal exposure occurs in permanent teeth with immature apices, a special procedure called *apexification* may be performed as a prelude to formal endodontic therapy. This involves the insertion of calcium hydroxide paste into the pulp canal to promote the closure of the apex through the formation of a calcific bridge, which may take up to 18 months. Final aesthetic restorations of complicated crown fractures are performed at a later date when either the vitality of the tooth has been established or when successful endodontic therapy has completely devitalized the tooth and produced a sterile environment.

CROWN-ROOT FRACTURES

At the initial presentation, emergency treatment of this relatively infrequent injury involves stabilization of the tooth or removal of loose fragments, depending on the location and extent of the fracture. Extended vertical fractures traversing the length of the root or fractures that leave less than two thirds of the root available for tooth retention are indications for removal of the tooth and fractured root. Less extensive injuries are amenable to the use of orthodontic extrusion or crown lengthening procedures for retention and restoration of the tooth in the dental arch.

ROOT FRACTURES

Most root fractures occur in the apical and middle third of the tooth. With this injury, the coronal fragment is immobilized as soon as possible against the root and held with a rigid splint for 12 weeks. Union across the fractured segments can occur through the formation of a calcified bridge, or if mobility persists, a fibrous interphase. Pulp vitality in the fractured root may be preserved through an intact apical neurovascular bundle, while the coronal pulp usually undergoes necrosis. Management of the coronal tissue involves removal of nonvital pulp followed by endodontic treatment at a later stage. If the root is fractured in its cervical third close to the crown, extraction is usually indicated. Preservation of the root may be considered, in which case orthodontic extrusion at a later time may be necessary to produce a functional support for future dental restoration.

INJURIES TO THE PERIODONTIUM

Luxation injuries are the result of a severe impact to a tooth that alters its position in the alveolus. Complete or partial dislocation from the bony socket can also occur. The injury may be isolated to a single tooth or encompass a number of adjacent teeth, involving the surrounding alveolar bone. Andreasen and Andreasen[10] describe five types of luxation injury based on anatomy, therapeutic modalities, and prognosis. The five injuries are concussion, subluxation, extrusive luxation, lateral luxation, and intrusive luxation, and these are managed with a combination of reduction, immobilization, and removal of occlusal interferences. Techniques for the immobilization of teeth or the dentoalveolar complex are discussed in a later section.

CONCUSSION

This is the mildest form of luxation injury, producing neither tooth displacement nor mobility. The patient may experience slight tenderness during mastication, but typically the tooth remains asymptomatic. Pulp nerve testing is unreliable immediately after the injury and should be deferred for 2 weeks.[11] Approximately 2% of concussive injuries progress to pulp necrosis.[12]

SUBLUXATION

Subluxation is characterized by small amounts of bleeding at the epithelial cuff and minor mobility, but the tooth remains in its socket. Sensitivity to mastication and percussion is present. Occlusal adjustment, by the removal of a small amount of enamel from the opposing tooth and stabilization with a splint, may be required for 7 to 10 days to allow inflammation to resolve. The incidence of pulp necrosis and root resorption is less than 5%.[13]

EXTRUSIVE LUXATION

This injury is associated with partial displacement of a tooth along its long axis producing significant mobility and bleeding. The tooth should be repositioned apically as quickly as possible under local anesthesia, and the position maintained with passive, nonrigid splinting of the tooth for 10 to 14 days. The risk of pulpal necrosis after extensive luxation increases with apical closure. A 68% incidence of pulpal necrosis for patients aged 7 to 15 years has been reported for this type of injury.[14]

LATERAL LUXATION

Lateral displacement of a tooth constitutes an even more severe injury, because it involves fracture of the surrounding alveolar socket. There is significant mobility and bleeding at initial presentation and early reduction and alignment of the tooth is necessary. Depending on the severity of trauma, a longer period of immobilization (6 to 8 weeks) may be necessary to promote healing of the bony alveolar complex. Delayed sequelae include pulpal necrosis, external root resorption, and loss of marginal bone or the entire tooth.

INTRUSIVE LUXATION

Teeth with open apices and incompletely formed roots usually reerupt following apical displacement. However, if a tooth is fully developed, intrusion into the alveolar bone represents the most severe form of luxation injury with extensive damage to the pulp, periodontal ligament, and alveolus. The incidence of pulpal necrosis and inflammatory resorption has been reported at 100% and 86%, respectively.[11] Such an injury presents with the tooth impacted and submerged in the alveolus, leaving only a portion of the crown visible. Treatment includes surgical repositioning and alignment of the tooth into the dental arch followed by splinting for 10 to 14 days or longer depending on the severity of associated alveolar fractures. Reduction of the tooth into its proper position may require manipulation with dental forceps if this maneuver cannot be achieved digitally. Other options include the use of orthodontic brackets and wires to extrude the tooth into alignment over a 3- to 4-week period.

AVULSION TOOTH INJURIES

This most catastrophic of all dentoalveolar injuries involves complete disarticulation of the tooth from its alveolar socket. Tooth avulsion occurs in 1 to 16% of all traumatic injuries to the permanent teeth and slightly more frequently in the primary dentition, because of shorter roots. Contact sports and automobile accidents are the most common causes of tooth avulsion with the maxillary central incisors most often affected.[12] The effect of tooth loss is not only physical but also psychological when aesthetics are compromised by this injury.

ISCHEMIA TIME

The avulsed tooth is severely damaged with loss of its blood and nerve supply, laceration of the supporting periodontal ligament, and localized damage to the cemental covering of the root. The goal of treatment is to minimize additional damage to the tooth and provide a favorable environment for reimplantation. The avulsed tooth should be handled gently by the crown, avoiding contact with the delicate cells within the cementum. Gentle irrigation of the root surface with saline helps remove debris and reduce gross contamination. The greatest chance of successful revitalization occurs if the tooth is implanted within the first 15 to 20 minutes of injury into its socket. When a remote consultation is sought concerning an avulsed tooth, information can be provided over the phone to emergency personnel to expedite treatment. If this is not feasible, the clean tooth should be stored in physiologic storage media to preserve viable cells and reconstitute cells and structures that have undergone desiccation following exposure to the environment. These solutions include, in order of preference, Hank's balanced salt solution (commercially available as a Save-A-Tooth system, 3M Healthcare, St. Paul, MN), Viaspan (organ transport medium), milk, and physiologic saline. Saliva may damage the periodontal ligament, and the practice of placing avulsed teeth in the buccal and labial vestibule for transport should be discouraged. Water on the other hand constitutes a hypotonic environment that causes rapid cell lysis.[15]

Preservation of viable periodontal cells attached to the root surface of the tooth is key to successful reimplantation. This process is maximized by bathing the avulsed tooth in a physiologic and biologically conductive fluid, which also serves to minimize exposure to the effects of desiccation. If excessive drying occurs, the damaged periodontal ligament cells elicit a severe inflammatory process over a diffuse area on the root surface.[15] The duration of extraalveolar dry time, the type of storage medium, and maturity of the apex are significant factors that influence the long-term prognosis of reimplanted teeth.[11] A dry time of 60 minutes is considered the juncture where survival of root periodontal ligament cells is compromised. Pulpal necrosis always occurs after an avulsion injury and the combination of bacterial contamination of the pulp and cemental damage results in an inflammatory response. Inflammation triggers both external and internal resorption of a tooth, and these pathologic processes affect its long-term survival.

Teeth that have been avulsed for 2 hours or less and have not been placed in a preservative medium are managed in the following manner. Initially, the tooth is held by the crown and gently rinsed of debris with saline, taking care to avoid contact with the delicate root surface. Reconstitution of the periodontal ligament cells is attempted by immersing the tooth in Hank's solution for 30 minutes. Teeth with open apices should first be soaked in Hank's solution for 30 minutes followed by immersion in an antibiotic solution (doxycycline 1 mg/20 mL), for 5 minutes to reduce pulpal inflammation before reimplantation.

If the extraalveolar dry period is greater than 2 hours, most of the vital periodontal ligament and pulp are assumed to have undergone necrosis. In this case, techniques to remove necrotic tissue, reduce microbial contamination, and strengthen the inorganic structure of the remaining tooth, prior to reimplantation, are employed by suitably trained dental personnel. Removal of the periodontal ligament can be achieved by gently scraping the surface of the root or by soaking the tooth in sodium hypochlorite solution for 30 minutes.[16] The root surface is also treated with citric acid to expose the dentinal tubules, and this is followed by applications of stannous fluoride solution to strengthen the tooth. Placing the tooth in a doxycycline solution helps to reduce the chances of infection. After treating the root surfaces, removal of the pulp and obliteration of the canal is completed using conventional endodontic procedures before the tooth is reimplanted. Teeth that have been avulsed for 24 hours have a very poor prognosis. Between 77 and 96% of teeth exhibit significant resorption as a prelude to failure.

Before a tooth is reimplanted, the alveolar socket is inspected and irrigated with sterile saline to remove coagulum, debris, and loose bone fragments. Deformities of the socket that impair the reimplantation of the tooth can be gently corrected with a blunt instrument to allow passive insertion of the tooth.

PULPAL CONSIDERATIONS

Differing strategies are employed to address the potential of pulp necrosis. A mature tooth with a closed apex can either be replanted or have endodontic treatment performed before implantation and splinting. When the latter approach is adopted, endodontic therapy is commenced after 7 to 10 days using calcium hydroxide intracanal medicament. Teeth with open apices are observed for revascularization of the dental pulp unless the tooth is obviously necrotic. If necrosis ensues, apexification and endodontic therapy is pursued. Radiographs and vitality testing closely monitor all postimplantation stages of avulsed teeth. Pulpal necrosis has been detected radiographically as early as 2 weeks.[17]

MANAGEMENT OF ALVEOLAR FRACTURES

Depending on the magnitude and direction of force, injuries to the mouth may not be confined to the teeth, but may involve the supporting alveolar bone. Fractures limited to a single socket can be reduced with digital pressure and maintained in position by the integrity of the overlying gingiva. However, when larger segments of alveolar process containing multiple teeth are displaced, greater consideration must be given to accurate alignment of the fractures, stabilization of the segments, and reapposition of the overlying soft tissue. The presence of associated maxillary or mandibular injuries should also be considered in the overall treatment plan.

Displaced dentoalveolar fractures should ideally be treated immediately to preserve the viability of the alveolar bone and associated teeth, reduce the incidence of infection, and provide patient comfort. Much can be achieved under local anesthesia in the emergency room setting. After gross debridement of the oral wounds, mucosal or gingival injuries are closed with a resorbable 3-0 suture. A malpositioned segment can usually be reduced with digital pressure using the alignment of the intact arch as a guide. Temporary or permanent stabilization of the segment may be achieved with interdental wires. If a more definitive analysis of the dental arch is required or if an acrylic splint is indicated, dental impressions are taken at this time. Stabilization techniques for dentoalveolar fractures are discussed in the next section. A summary of emergency treatment approaches to the management of dental and dentoalveolar injuries is summarized in Table 13–2.

STABILIZATION TECHNIQUES

Stabilization of reimplanted or mobile teeth is required for healing, comfort, and tooth viability.

Both rigid and nonrigid types of devices are available, and their selection is based ideally on the type of injury present and the intended therapeutic goals. However, technical expertise, availability of the proper armamentarium, and characteristics of the operative site sometimes favor the selection of a particular method of stabilization. Rigid and semi-rigid forms of fixation for dental injuries include interdental wiring, arch bars, and custom-made acrylic splints. These devices are indicated for the treatment of root fractures and fractures of the dentoalveolar complex when absolute stability is necessary to promote either calcific or osseous bridging of the fracture segments. If an adequate clinical crown is present, root fractures are typically treated by the application of a short length of an arch bar secured to the injured tooth (teeth) and at least one to two stable teeth on either side. If an arch bar is used to stabilize a mobile tooth, care must be taken not to extrude the tooth as the circumdental wires are tightened. This can be avoided by adding a second wire that engages the incisal edge of the tooth and ligates it to the bar (Fig. 13–3). The number of teeth incorporated depends on the length of the span and the stability of the anchor teeth. Alternative techniques employ the use of Essig- or Risdon-type wires in place of an arch bar. When the injured teeth

TABLE 13–2 Dental Trauma Algorithm

Crown Fracture		Root Fracture		Tooth Avulsion	
Permanent Tooth	Deciduous Tooth	Permanent Tooth	Deciduous Tooth	Permanent Tooth	Deciduous Tooth
Minor fracture Dental consultation; monitor tooth	Minor fracture Dental consultation; monitor tooth	Assess level of fracture with radiographs	Extraction with fragments	Reimplant as soon as possible	Do not reimplant
Moderate fractures Dental consultation; monitor tooth	Moderate fracture Dental consultation; monitor tooth	Stabilize with rigid splint 4–6 weeks		Stabilize with flexible splint 7–10 days Antibiotics/ tetanus prophylaxis	Early dental consultation for space maintenance
Complex fractures Dental consultation; monitor tooth and extract if infection is a concern	Complex fracture Dental consultation; monitor tooth Extract with early dental consultation for space maintenance	Monitor nerve vitality		Endodontic therapy Dressings ± Apexification Restoration	

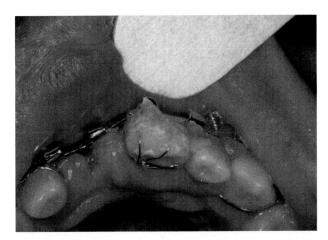

FIGURE 13–3 Rigid arch bar stabilization of subluxated tooth. A stabilizing wire is often placed over the incisal edge of the tooth to prevent extrusion resulting from application of the interdental wire.

possess a short clinical crown, or when a dentoalveolar segment requires stabilization, customized acrylic splints afford the best type of rigid stabilization. The fabrication of these splints involves the production of a plaster or dental stone model of the affected dental arch. If the fractured tooth (teeth) or dentoalveolar segment has not been aligned prior to taking the dental impression, model surgery must be performed before making the splint. This involves cutting the malpositioned structures free of the model and reattaching them with dental wax or glue in their proper position. The acrylic splint is then fabricated as an occlusal overlay, or with coverage of the lingual or palatal surfaces of the fractured alveolus to stabilize the segment (Fig. **13–4**). The acrylic splint is either ligated into position with interdental wires, or if insufficient teeth or short crown heights militate against this, skeletal fixation (e.g., circummandibular, buttress,

pyriform aperture, nasal spine wires) may be employed. A more rapid technique for semirigid stabilization of dentoalveolar injuries involves the application of fast-curing dental resins across the labial surfaces of the teeth (Fig. **13–5**). However, the special materials required for this technique and adequate isolation of the treatment site from blood, saliva, and moisture make this method difficult to execute under normal clinical conditions. Root fractures may need to be stabilized for as long as 3 months, whereas dentoalveolar fractures are usually immobilized for a period of 3 to 4 weeks.[10] Under rare circumstances, fractured alveolar segments cannot be immobilized indirectly through their dental attachments. When this is the case, the segments can be fixated with small bone plates utilizing 1.3- to 2.0-mm-diameter screws drilled to depths no greater than 5 mm. The presence of underlying permanent tooth buds must be taken into account when determining plate placement.

Nonrigid forms of fixation are indicated for the treatment of avulsed or luxated teeth. This form of splinting allows physiologic movement of the tooth and if maintained for the minimal period necessary for periodontal ligament healing, results in a decreased incidence of ankylosis. Current international guidelines recommend that reimplanted teeth should be stabilized for a period of 7 to 10 days. Physiologic stabilization of teeth can be achieved with resilient connectors, such as 24- to 26-gauge stainless steel wire, a straightened paper clip, or 30-lb test monofilament fishing line, attached to the labial surfaces of the teeth with dental resin or orthodontic brackets (Fig. **13–6**). Before the resin or brackets are applied to the teeth, the enamel surface needs to be pretreated with a mild acid (e.g., phosphoric acid). Both acid etching and curing of the resin require a dry environment and this might

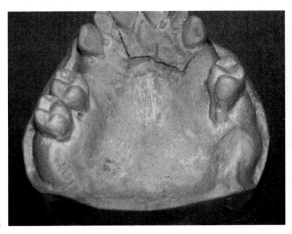
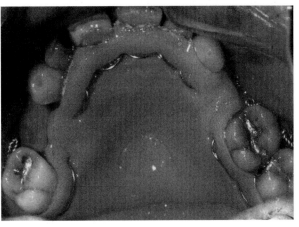

A   B

FIGURE 13–4 A: Sectioning of malpositioned dentoalveolar segment and realignment on dental model. B: Palatal acrylic splint fabricated to support the fractured segment in the correct position. (Courtesy of James V. Johnson, DDS.)

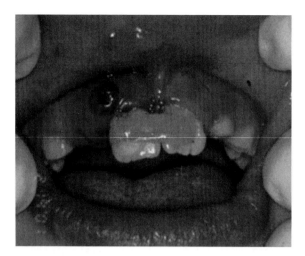

FIGURE 13–5 Rapid-curing dental resins used to provide semirigid stabilization of luxated tooth.

not be available. It is important to note that following the appropriate period of stabilization, removal of the device is performed in stages. The arch wire or nylon connector is removed first and the teeth allowed to further consolidate in their sockets before the resin or brackets are removed.

ADJUNCTIVE TREATMENT MEASURES

Following the reimplantation of teeth or the reduction of a fractured dentoalveolar complex, the occlusion must be adjusted to avoid trauma from the opposing arch. This is achieved by grinding away small amounts of enamel from the opposing teeth. Patients and parents are advised to maintain a soft, nonchewing diet for 2 weeks and to pay special attention to oral hygiene. Gentle brushing with a soft, pediatric toothbrush, supplemented with twice daily chlorhexidine (0.1%) mouth rinses, is part of

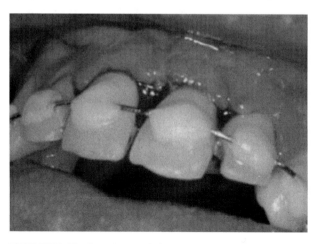

FIGURE 13–6 Nonrigid fixation of mobile tooth with dental resin and flexible orthodontic arch wire.

the postoperative care. Coverage with a systemic antibiotic for 7 days with appropriate dose for age and weight is also recommended. Doxycycline is preferred for mature teeth with closed apices, whereas penicillin is used for immature teeth with incomplete root formation.[2] The need for analgesics is assessed on an individual basis.

For all injuries to the teeth and supporting structures, follow-up evaluations with a dentist should take place as soon as possible and then at regular intervals for up to 5 years. Because pulpal necrosis, inflammatory root resorption, and ankylosis are all potential long-term consequences to trauma, radiographs and dental pulp vitality testing are required for continuous assessment. In addition, occult injury to teeth adjacent to the damaged or avulsed teeth may not develop pathologic changes until long after the initial accident.[15]

PEARLS: DENTAL AND DENTOALVEOLAR INJURIES

- Dental and dentoalveolar injuries may occur separately or in combination. When associated with maxillary or mandibular fractures, failure to recognize and manage appropriately may lead to improper reduction and infection.
- The patient's dental development (i.e., root development), the extent of injury, the duration of ischemia, and conditions of storage affect the prognosis.
- Treatment is aimed at conserving teeth. Relative indications for removal include:
  ○ Fractured or avulsed deciduous teeth
  ○ Permanent teeth with longitudinal root fractures
  ○ Grossly decayed and infected permanent teeth
  ○ Teeth that have been avulsed for 24 hours or more
- Survival of injured teeth depends on the patency of the root apex. Devitalized teeth can still be maintained with endodontic treatment.
- Flexible splinting of luxated and avulsed teeth allows physiologic movement and is more desirable. Rigid stabilization is indicated for alveolar and root fractures.

REFERENCES

1. Gassner R, Bosch R, Tuli T, Emshoff R. Prevalence of dental trauma in 6000 patients with facial injuries: Implications for prevention. Oral Surg Oral Med Oral Pathol Oral Radiol Endod 1999;87:27–33

2. Flores MT, Andreasen JO, Bakland LK, et al. Guidelines for the evaluation and management of traumatic dental injuries. Dent Traumatol 2001;17:193–198

3. Robertson A, Noren JG. Knowledge-based system for structured examination, diagnosis and therapy in traumatized teeth. Dent Traumatol 2001;17:5–9

4. Abubaker AO, Giglio J, Mourino AP. Diagnosis and management of dentoalveolar injuries. In: Fonseca RJ, Marciani RD, Hendler BH, eds. *Oral and Maxillofacial Surgery,* vol 3. Philadelphia: WB Saunders, 2000:45–84

5. Ferrari CH, Medeiros JM. Dental trauma and level of information: mouthguard use in different contact sports. Dent Traumatol 2002;18:144–147

6. Olsburgh S, Jacoby T, Krejci I. Crown fractures in the permanent dentition: pulpal and restorative considerations. Dent Traumatol 2002;18:103–115

7. Luz JGC, Di Mase F. Incidence of dentoalveolar injuries in hospital emergency room patients. Endod Dent Traumatol 1994;10:188–190

8. Andreasen JO. Classification, etiology and epidemiology. In: Andreasen JO, ed. *Traumatic Injuries of the Teeth,* 2nd ed. Copenhagen: Munksgaard, 1981:19

9. Ellis E. Soft tissue and dentoalveolar injuries. In: Peterson LJ, Ellis E, Hupp JR, Tucker MR, eds. *Contemporary Oral and Maxillofacial Surgery,* 4th ed. St Louis: Mosby, 2003:504–526

10. Andreasen JO, Andreasen FM. *Textbook and Colour Atlas of Traumatic Injuries to the Teeth,* vol 3. Copenhagen: Munksgaard, 1994

11. Pileggi R, Dumsha TC. The management of traumatic dental injuries. Texas Dental J 2003;120:270–275

12. McDonald N, Strassler HE. Evaluation for tooth stabilization and treatment of traumatized teeth. Dent Clin North Am 1999;43:135–149

13. Schatz JP, Joho JP, Dietschi D. Treatment of luxation traumatic injuries: definition and classification in the literature. Pract Periodontics Aesthet Dent 2000;12:781–786

14. Eklund G, Stalhane I, Hedegard. A study of traumatized permanent teeth in children aged 7–15 years. Sven Tandlak Tidskr 1976;69:179–189

15. Trope M. Clinical management of the avulsed tooth: present strategies and future directions. Dent Traumatol 2002;18:1–11

16. Krasner P, Rankow HJ. New philosophy for the treatment of avulsed teeth. Oral Surg Oral Med Oral Pathol Oral Radiol Endod 1995;79:616–623

17. Andreasen JO. Periodontal healing after replantation and autotransplantation of incisors in monkeys. Int J Oral Surg 1981;10:54–61

Chapter 14

EXTENDED SURGICAL APPROACHES TO FACIAL INJURIES

Anthony E. Brissett and Peter A. Hilger

Incisions on the face are not as easily camouflaged as on other areas of the body; therefore, thoughtful consideration related to their placement is critical. The goals that should be sought when planning and executing any approach to the facial skeleton are to ensure that adequate exposure is achieved, that anatomy and function are maintained or restored, and that the incisions, once healed, are as inconspicuous as possible. When planning the approaches to expose facial fractures, some general principles should be followed:

PLACE INCISIONS WITHIN RELAXED SKIN TENSION LINES

Relaxed skin tension lines (RSTLs), can best be described as the natural lines of contour that run parallel to the direction of pull of the facial muscles. These lines of contour become more prominent with age as well as with the use or overuse of the muscles of facial expression. Placing incisions within or parallel to the RSTL allows for camouflaging of incisions and creates a less noticeable scar (Fig. 14–1).

USE SITES THAT ARE AS INCONSPICUOUS AS POSSIBLE

The reconstructive surgeon should preferentially choose incisions that lie within the oral cavity, or can be hidden within the hair or within the junction of aesthetic subunits. Although placing incisions in these areas may require more dissection and may make fracture reduction more challenging, the benefits of not having an obvious external incision will greatly enhance cosmetic results. If a laceration is

present in the vicinity that requires exposure, the surgeon should preferentially use it as opposed to creating a new incision.

AVOID DAMAGE TO NEUROVASCULAR STRUCTURES

To minimize damage to anatomic structures, it is critical to consider the path that will be taken during the exposure of facial fractures. Although some sensory neural branches will be damaged regardless of the approach that is taken, the surgeon should make every attempt to preserve as many of these branches as possible. The facial nerve is of the utmost concern when contemplating the placement of incisions as well as the surgical approach. Damage to the facial nerve at any level can result in severe functional and cosmetic abnormalities. A thorough understanding of the anatomic considerations to exposing facial fractures is essential for the head and neck trauma surgeon.

ANATOMY

The supraorbital, infraorbital, and mental nerves are susceptible to injury as they emerge from their bony foramina. The location of the supraorbital nerve can be best identified by palpating the supraorbital foramen at the supraorbital rim. The supratrochlear nerve typically lies in the same plane as the supraorbital nerve, but is approximately 0.5 to 1.5 cm from the midline. Injuries to these nerves result in numbness or dysesthesias of the forehead, scalp, upper lid, and nasal dorsum.

The location of the infraorbital and mental foramina can be approximated by dropping a vertical

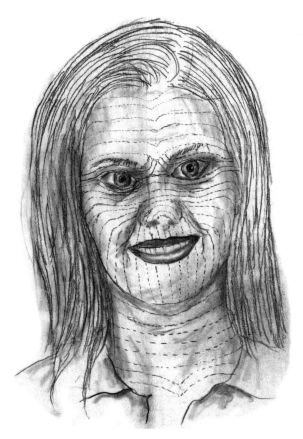

FIGURE 14–1 Relaxed skin tension lines. Placing incisions within the lines of minimal tension create a less noticeable scar.

line from the supraorbital foramen, through the mid-pupil and down to the second mandibular premolar.[1,2] A point on the anterior maxilla 1 cm below the infraorbital rim is palpated along this line to estimate the location of the infraorbital foramen. Injury to the infraorbital nerve creates numbness to the ipsilateral nose, cheek, and upper eyelid. The mental nerve exits its foramen below the second mandibular premolar and provides sensation to the lower third of the face including the lips and buccal mucosa.

There are two common locations where the facial nerve may be damaged when exposing the facial skeleton. The first area is in the upper face where the facial nerve lies deep in the temporal parietal facial layer.[3] At this level, the nerve provides innervation to the frontalis, orbicularis-oculi, and corrugator muscles. Once the facial nerve exits the parotid gland it travels in a plane that is deep in the temporal-parietal fascia over the zygomatic arch and enters the frontalis muscle. The temporal branch of the facial nerve can be found in a triangle, bounded by a line drawn from the bottom of the earlobe to the lateral extent of the eyebrow inferiorly and to the point of the highest forehead rhytid superiorly (Fig. **14–2**).[4,5]

Injury to the temporal branch of the facial nerve typically results in facial asymmetry, brow ptosis, and potential visual field defects.

The second area where the facial nerve is commonly injured is at the junction of the ramus and the inferior aspect of the body of the mandible. The normal course for the ramus mandibularis is to travel in an oblique fashion within the parotid-masseteric or the deep cervical fascia to provide innervation to the mimetic muscles of the perioral region. In general, the ramus mandibularis travels above the inferior aspect of the mandible. However, it has been reported to lie below the inferior border of the body of the mandible in 20% of individuals.[6]

Injury to the marginal branch of the facial nerve results in asymmetry of the mouth. During grimacing, the zygomaticus major and minor muscles are unopposed by the denervated depressor anguli oris muscle, resulting in the inability to show the lower teeth on the affected side. At rest, the tone in zygomaticus major muscle is unopposed by the depressor anguli oris muscle and draws the corner of the mouth up.[1]

SURGICAL APPROACHES

The development of surgical techniques that allow for wide exposure of the facial skeleton while minimizing external incisions have become standards for the management of facial trauma. When using these approaches it is important to adhere to specific technical points to ensure adequate exposure while minimizing the potential for complications.

THE UPPER FACE AND ZYGOMATIC ARCH

The coronal or bitemporal approach is a versatile surgical approach to the upper and middle regions of the facial skeleton, including the zygomatic arch.[7] Three fascial layers are important during this dissection: the temporal parietal fascia, the superficial layer of the temporal fascia and the deep layer of temporal fascia. The temporal parietal fascia is a continuation of the superficial muscular aponeurotic system (SMAS) inferiorly, and the galea and frontalis muscle superiorly. Between the temporal parietal fascia and the temporalis fascia is a plane of loose areolar tissue that is continuous with the loose connective subgaleal tissue of the scalp. The temporalis fascia is a layer of connective tissue that overlies the temporalis muscle. Above the temporal line, the temporal fascia is continuous with the pericranium.

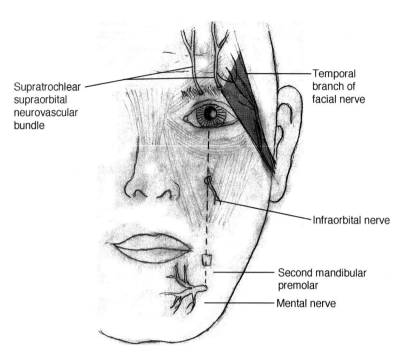

Supratrochlear supraorbital neurovascular bundle

Temporal branch of facial nerve

Infraorbital nerve

Second mandibular premolar

Mental nerve

FIGURE 14–2 The temporal branch of the facial nerve can be approximated by creating a triangle with the boundaries being the earlobe, the lateral brow, and the most superior forehead rhytid.

At the level of the superior orbital rim, it divides into a superficial and deep layer. This area of division is referred to as the temporal line of fusion. The superficial layer of the temporalis fascia continues inferiorly and becomes tightly adherent to the lateral aspect of the zygomatic arch. The deep layer of the temporalis fascia lies on the surface of the temporalis muscle, it continues inferiorly to insert on the medial aspect of the zygomatic arch. The superficial temporal fat pad extends from the temporal line of fusion to the zygomatic arch and separates the superficial and deep layers of the temporalis fascia.

SURGICAL TECHNIQUE

For the majority of females and nonbalding men, the bitemporal incision should extend from the root of the helix bilaterally and should be placed approximately 4 to 5 cm behind the hairline. For men who are balding or have a family history that predisposes them to male pattern baldness, the incision can be placed more posterior. In children, the temporal incision is placed well behind the hairline to allow for the anterior migration of the scar as the child grows.

In general, the head is not shaved. The hair anterior to the incision can be secured within elastic bands, and a sterile drape should be positioned approximately 2 cm behind the planned incision and stapled to the scalp. Injecting 1% lidocaine with 1:100,000 epinephrine into the planned incision line

optimizes hemostasis. The incision should be angled parallel to the hair follicles and should proceed through the galea, leaving the periosteum intact. Initially, the incision should extend from one superior temporal line to the other, to prevent incising through the temporalis fascia and into the temporalis muscle. If the incision needs to be extended inferiorly it should be placed within the preauricular sulcus.

Elevation of the skin flap should proceed in the subgaleal fascia plane to approximately 3 cm above the superior orbital rim. At this point an incision can be made through the periosteum, extending from the anterior aspect of one temporal line to the other. The dissection should then continue in a subperiosteal plane, exposing the forehead and superior orbital rims. To allow for increased exposure of the entire nasal orbital ethmoid region, the supraorbital nerve can be released from its foramen. In addition, the periosteum along the lateral aspect of the orbital rims can be sharply incised to adequately expose the orbital rims as well as the frontal zygomatic sutures.

If exposure of the zygomatic arch is required, an incision should be made through the superficial layer of the deep temporal fascia below the temporal line of fusion. This maneuver exposes the superficial temporal fat pad and establishes a safe plane of dissection to expose the zygomatic arch. Once the arch has been adequately exposed, an incision through the periosteum on the superior aspect of the zygomatic arch should be created. The periosteum is then dissected off of the arch to allow for exposure.

Upon the completion of this dissection, the areas of exposure can include the forehead, frontal sinus and nasal bones, the orbital rims, the zygoma, and the posterior aspect of the malar process (Fig. **14–3**).

CLOSURE

If the periosteum has been divided at the lateral orbital rim, it should be returned to its original position. If a lateral canthotomy and cantholysis has been performed or if the continuity of the lateral canthus has been disrupted as a result of trauma, it will need to be reestablished. Once the bony attachments of the periosteum and muscle have been reconstituted, layered closure of the temporalis fascia and temporal parietal fascia should be performed. A flat suction drain can be placed into the posterior gutter of the scalp incision and brought out through the hair-bearing area, behind the root of the helix. If a suction drain is not utilized we recommend the use of a pressure dressing for 24 to 48 hours. The galeal layer can be closed with slow-dissolving sutures and the skin can be closed with staples. In children, resorbable sutures can be used to close the skin layer. If a preauricular incision was required to increase exposure, the SMAS layer should be reestablished and a suture should be placed in front of the tragus to re-create the pretragal hollow. The skin in this area can be closed with either rapid-absorbing or permanent sutures. Adequate eversion of the scalp incision, as well as the preauricular incision, should be performed to prevent widening of the scar during wound contraction.

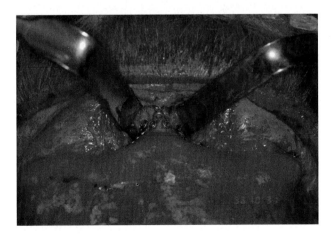

FIGURE 14–3 Exposure following a bicoronal approach with release of the supraorbital nerve and the periosteum of the lateral orbit.

COMPLICATIONS

The most likely postoperative complications that occur following a bicoronal approach to the upper face and zygoma include motor nerve deficits, sensory nerve deficits, hair loss, contour irregularities, and scars.

The primary concern of most surgeons performing this procedure is damage to the temporal branch of the facial nerve. Temporary paralysis is usually the result of neuropraxia, resulting from trauma during the dissection or from excessive traction on the facial nerve, and can persist for up to 6 months. Complete transection results in permanent motor loss. The use of broad retractors, liberal inferior extension, and a thorough understanding of the regional anatomy can prevent this complication.[8]

Some degree of anesthesia is experienced by all patients undergoing this procedure. During recovery, patients commonly complain of shooting pains and pruritus. The areas of hypesthesia or anesthesia typically get smaller with time. Comfort care and support should be provided.

Hair loss at the incision sight is not uncommon. In an attempt to minimize hair loss we discourage the use of Raney clips and monopolar cautery. The judicious use of bipolar cautery assists in preserving hair follicles.

Temporal wasting is often unpredictable and always permanent. The specific pathophysiology of this complication is unclear. Avoiding any dissection into the temporal fat pad is the best way to avoid this dilemma. Approaches to improve the hollowing can include the placement of autologous, heterologous or synthetic fillers, such as fat, AlloDerm, or Gore-Tex.

Meticulous surgical technique is the best way to maximize the appearance of the incision. Standard wound care should include regular cleanings and the application of moisturizing ointments. If the scar appears to become hypertrophic or keloid like, semiocclusive dressings and steroid injections can be used.[9]

A hemicoronal approach should be considered when unilateral exposure of the forehead or zygomatic complex is required. The principles and surgical techniques for the hemicoronal approach are identical to the bicoronal approach, except that the incision extends only slightly across the midline and is then curved anteriorly toward the hairline.

External elevation of the zygoma through a limited hairline incision can, on occasion, successfully reduce isolated fractures of the zygomatic arch. This technique is referred to as the Gilles method[10] and utilizes a 3- to 4-cm incision that is placed above the helical root and extends superior and slightly posterior.[11] Blunt dissection should continue through the temporal parietal fascia and the loose connective tissue to the deep temporalis fascia. The superficial fascia layer of the deep temporalis fascia is incised, establishing the correct plane of dissection to safely expose the zygomatic arch. Blunt dissection should be used to expose the medial aspect of the zygomatic arch. A Boies elevator can then be positioned under the zygoma to lift it back to its normal position. The Gilles method represents a logical starting point when attempting to reduce isolated zygoma fractures. It can dramatically reduce surgical duration and decrease the likelihood of facial nerve damage, and it is not associated with an obvious scar.

THE ORBIT AND PERIORBITAL AREA

ANATOMY

The lower lid consists of four distinct layers: the skin and its subcutaneous tissue, the orbicularis oculi muscle, the tarsus or orbital septum, and the conjunctiva. The orbicularis oculi muscle is oriented in a series of concentric rings that encircle the palpebral fissures and is divided into the pretarsal, preseptal, and orbital segments. The pretarsal portion of the orbicularis oculi muscle overlies the tarsus, the preseptal portion overlies the orbital septum, and the orbital segment extends superiorly over the superior and inferior orbital rims. The orbital septum originates at the orbital rim as the arcus marginalis and is a fascial extension of the periosteum. The tarsal plate is a fibrous layer of tissue that provides support to the eyelid. The conjunctiva that lines the inner surface of the eyelid is called the palpebral conjunctiva; it adheres firmly to the tarsal plate and becomes more loosely bound as it extends inferiorly. The conjunctiva then sweeps onto the globe to become the bulbar conjunctiva.

The medial canthal tendon is a confluence of the upper and lower tarsus as well as the orbicularis oculi muscle. Prior to its insertion on the lacrimal bone, the medial canthal tendon divides into a superficial and deep segment. The superficial segment attaches to the anterior lacrimal crest, whereas the deep segment attaches to the posterior lacrimal crest. The lateral canthal tendon is a confluence of the tarsal plate as well as fibrous extensions from the orbicularis oculi muscle. The anterior portion of the lateral canthal tendon inserts into the periosteum along the lateral aspect of the orbital rim, whereas the posterior portion of the lateral canthal tendon inserts into the periosteum behind the orbital rim at Whitnall's tubercle.

SURGICAL TECHNIQUES

Fractures involving the inferior orbital rim or floor can generally be exposed by utilizing a transconjunctival or transcutaneous incision. The factors considered when deciding what approach to employ include the extent and severity of the trauma, the patient's age, the cosmetic expectations, and the surgeon's experience. In spite of what approach is utilized, the desire for acceptable cosmetic results, combined with adequate exposure, must be achieved.

TRANSCONJUNCTIVAL APPROACH

Over the past two decades the transconjunctival approach for blepharoplasties, as well as for exposure and repair of fractures involving the inferior orbital rim and orbital floor, has gained wide acceptance and popularity. The main advantages of the transconjunctival approach are that it limits external incisions of the lower lid and minimizes the postoperative complication of lower eyelid retraction. The disadvantages of this approach are that exposure to the medial and lateral boundaries of the orbital rim, as well as the orbital floor, are sometimes limited.

When performing the transconjunctival approach, the surgeon should be familiar with the preseptal and retroseptal techniques as well as the extended approach that allows for a wider exposure by detaching the inferior slip of the lateral canthal tendon (Fig. **14–4**). The surgeon should inject 1% lidocaine with 1:100,000 epinephrine into the subcutaneous and conjunctival tissue of the lower lid and lateral canthal area. We also recommend the use of intraoperative intravenous steroids if there are no contraindications.

We begin exposure of the inferior orbital rim by performing a lateral canthotomy and cantholysis. To perform a lateral canthotomy and cantholysis, a horizontal incision is made through the lateral palpebral fissure and extended into a relaxed skin tension line, along the lateral aspect of the orbit. Fine scissors are then used to cut through the inferior portion of the lateral canthal tendon. Once the canthus is released, a Desmarres retractor is used to lift the lower lid away from the globe. Ophthalmic ointment should be placed on the globe and a corneal shield or a Yaeger plate can be used to protect the eye. A guarded needle tip cautery is used to incise through the palpebral conjunctiva, approximately 1 to 2 mm below the inferior aspect of the tarsus. The incision through the conjunctiva should begin lateral to the punctum and extend into the lateral canthotomy incision. At this point a 4-0 silk

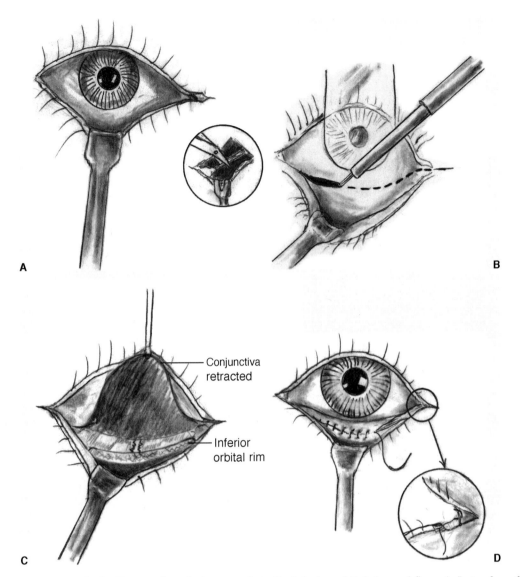

A

B

Conjunctiva
retracted

Inferior
orbital rim

C

D

FIGURE 14–4   Transconjunctival approach to the inferior orbital rim and floor. A: Lateral canthotomy and cantholysis. B: Transconjunctival incision. C: Conjunctiva retracted as a corneal shield, and subperiosteal dissection. D: Conjunctival closure and canthal tendon repair.

suture can be placed through the incised palpebral conjunctiva and pulled superiorly to act as a corneal protector.

If the surgeon is going to approach the orbital rim in a preseptal plane, an incision is made through the conjoined fascia to allow entrance into the preseptal space. Once into the preseptal space, blunt dissection can then be performed that separates the orbital septum from the overlying preseptal layer of the orbicularis oculi muscle. The dissection is then continued toward the orbital rim. If the postseptal approach is to be used, the surgeon should incise through the capsulopalpebral fascia rather than through the conjoined tendon. Once the fascia is incised, the postseptal fat will begin to bulge into the surgical field; visualization of this fat indicates that

the postseptal plane has been entered. Blunt dissection deep to the orbital septum can then proceed to the inferior orbital rim. The periosteum is then incised along the orbital rim. A periosteal elevator can be used to expose the orbital rim, orbital floor, zygoma, and the face of maxilla. During elevation of the periosteum, malleable retractors should be placed to retract the orbital contents. Blunt dissection can then be continued to ensure adequate exposure of the orbital rim and floor. Proponents of the preseptal approach argue that dissecting within the preseptal plane prevents the prolapse of fat into the surgical field and eases dissection and visualization. However, supporters of the postseptal approach argue that increased scarring with accompanying lower lid retraction is more likely to occur when using the preseptal approach. Further investigation to resolve this controversy is indicated.

Closure of the transconjunctival incision should reestablish anatomy and prevent complications that may occur with scarring. Reapproximation of the periosteum should be performed using two to three interrupted sutures. Closure of the conjunctival incision is performed with rapidly absorbing sutures. Particular attention should be placed on reestablishing the position of the lateral canthal tendon and lateral palpebral fissure, if an extended transconjunctival technique has been used. The lateral canthal tendon should be returned to its presurgical position at Whitnall's tubercle. The lateral canthotomy incision is then reapproximated.

Postoperative care should include the use of cold compresses for the first 24 hours, as well as steroid containing eyedrops for 4 days in patients without a history of glaucoma. The use of steroid eyedrops minimizes conjunctivitis during the postoperative period.

Transcutaneous Approach

There are three standard transcutaneous lower lid approaches that provide access to the inferior orbital rim and orbital floor; these are the subciliary, subtarsal/lower lid, and orbital rim approach (Fig. 14–5). The major difference between these three approaches is the location at which the skin is incised as well as the level at which the orbicularis oculi muscle is transected to approach the orbital septum and periosteum. Regardless of which transcutaneous approach is performed, it is recommended that ophthalmic ointment be placed on the globe and in the conjunctival fornix followed by a tarsorrhaphy or a corneal protector. One percent lidocaine with epinephrine 1:100,000 is injected into the subcutaneous tissue of the lower lid as well as the medial and lateral canthal area.

Subciliary Approach

When using this approach a horizontal incision is placed approximately 2 mm below the lash line of the lower lid. The incision begins lateral to the punctum and is carried into one of the periorbital "crow's feet" for approximately 15 mm. Once the skin has been incised there are three approaches that can be used to dissect down to the orbital rim. The first option is to dissect between the subcutaneous tissue and the orbicularis oculi muscle, incising the muscle at the orbital rim to gain access to the periosteum. This technique has been described as a skin only flap. It is associated with several problems, including buttonholing of the thin skin,

flap necrosis, excessive bruising, lower lid edema, and increased likelihood of lower lid retraction. The second option when using a subciliary approach is to incise through the muscle at the same level of the skin incision and dissect down to the orbital rim deep to the orbicularis oculi muscle. This approach results in an increased likelihood of denervating the pretarsal portion of the orbicularis oculi muscle in addition to contributing to contour deformities at the incision line, because of the absence of muscle in this area. In spite of the above disadvantages, a good blood supply to the skin muscle flap is maintained, which minimizes the complications that are associated with the skin only flap. The third option is the stepped skin muscle approach. With this approach, a subcutaneous dissection is performed for a few millimeters and then an incision is made through the orbicularis oculi muscle at a level that is inferior to the skin incision. The preseptal space is then entered, and dissection is continued down to the level of the orbital rim, where the periosteum is incised and elevated to expose the orbital rim and the orbital floor. The major advantage of the stepped approach is that the pretarsal fibers of the orbicularis oculi muscle remain attached to the tarsal plate, which assists with maintaining proper postoperative lid position and minimizes the likelihood of lid retraction.

Lower Lid/Subtarsal Approach

The subtarsal or lower lid approach is a variation of the stepped subciliary technique. With this approach, access to the orbital rim is gained by making a horizontal incision within the subtarsal fold. In the event that significant lower lid edema effaces the fold, the incision should then be placed approximately 5 to 7 mm below the lower lid margin. A small skin-only flap is raised, and the preseptal portion of the orbicularis oculi muscle is divided horizontally to enter the preseptal plane. Dissection then proceeds to the infraorbital rim. Stair stepping prevents contour abnormalities as well as inversion of the scar. In addition, dividing the orbicularis oculi muscle below its pretarsal portion preserves its innervation and assists with maintaining normal lid position. The most obvious disadvantage related to the use of the lower lid approach is a visible scar. However, with meticulous closure this scar is often barely noticeable. Also, because some of the larger lymphatic and vascular channels are disrupted, there is an increased degree of edema that typically resolves over time.

Use of the orbital rim incision represents the most direct approach to the inferior orbital rim. With this approach the incision is placed directly over the

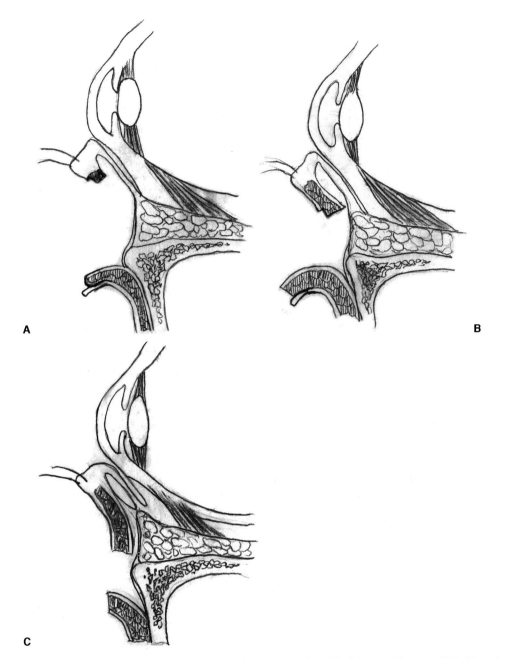

A

B

C

FIGURE 14–5 Transcutaneous approaches to the infraorbital rim and floor. A: Subciliary incision. B: Subtarsal incision. C: Orbital rim incision.

inferior orbital rim and the incision is made through the skin and subcutaneous tissue, the orbicularis oculi muscle, and periosteum to expose the inferior orbital rim. As with the subtarsal technique, the orbital rim approach results in a visible scar as well as prolonged lower lid edema.

CLOSURE

Meticulous closure is necessary to ensure optimal aesthetic results, in addition to the prevention of functional abnormalities. In general, reestablishing

the lateral canthal tendon to the lateral orbital rim, if it has been disrupted, followed by a two-layer closure of the periosteum and skin is satisfactory. If a lateral extension has been performed, the orbicularis oculi muscle adjacent to the lateral orbital rim should be reconstituted. The skin is then closed with a running 6-0 nylon or fast-absorbing gut suture. If there is significant postoperative edema or if the lower lid laxity represents a risk for the development of lid retraction, we recommend supporting the lower lid in some fashion. The most conservative method can be with the use of multiple Steri-Strips that are placed along the lateral aspect of the lower lid. Placement of these strips ensures that the lower lid maintains its position against the globe during healing. This tape can be removed after 1 week. A more direct method of supporting the lid can be accomplished with the use of suspensory sutures, placed through the lower lid and sutured or taped to the brow or forehead. The placements of these suspensory sutures provide upward support to the lower lid and should remain in place for approximately 1 week.

The complications that occur when using the transcutaneous approaches range from prolonged lower lid edema to sclera show and ectropion. Bahr et al[12] compared the complications related to the use of the three transcutaneous approaches in 105 patients. Bahr et al noted a complication rate of 25% for patients with a subciliary incision, 8.8% for patients with a lower lid incision, and 30.4% for patients with an infraorbital incision (Table 14–1).

APPROACHES TO THE SUPERIOR ORBITAL RIM

Exposure of the superior orbital rim and the frontal zygomatic area can be accomplished with a lateral eyebrow or upper lid blepharoplasty incision. These incisions are placed within the lateral aspect of the eyebrow or within the supratarsal crease, respectively. If this incision is made within the lateral eyebrow area, it may result in some hair loss, making the scar more noticeable. If the incision is made within the supratarsal crease, the resulting scar is usually imperceptible. In general, we recommend the use of an incision placed within the supratarsal crease because of its superior aesthetic result.

SURGICAL TECHNIQUE

Prior to anesthesia, the supratarsal crease should be marked. If significant edema blunts the supratarsal

crease, the incision should be placed approximately 10 to 12 mm above the upper lid margin. The planned incision should remain within the supratarsal crease and should generally stop at the lateral orbital rim. If additional access is required, this incision can be carried laterally into one of the relaxed skin tension lines. The incision is made through skin and muscle. Once the muscle is transected, blunt dissection allows for exposure of the lateral aspect of the superior orbital rim. The periosteum is then incised in this area. Periosteal elevators should then be used to expose the lateral aspect of the superior orbital rim, ensuring that the lateral canthus is not disrupted (Fig. 14–6). Layered closure of the periosteum and skin should be completed.

THE MIDFACE

Fractures involving the middle third of the face typically represent a combination of LeFort type fractures. Approaches to this area should facilitate exposure to all fracture sites and fragments within the middle face, in particular, the zygomatic maxillary and nasomaxillary areas.

ANATOMY

The infraorbital nerve is the primary nerve that is at increased risk of injury when exposing the midface; thus careful attention should be maintained during exposure to prevent loss of sensation to the skin and mucous membranes of the midface. During the use of the maxillary vestibular or midfacial degloving approaches, the nasal labial muscles may be detached or disrupted and should be repositioned upon closure to maintain function and aesthetic appearances. The muscles that may be disrupted during this technique include the nasalis muscle, the levator labii superius alaeque nasi, the levator labii superioris, and the levator anguli oris.

TABLE 14–1 DISTRIBUTION OF IMPAIRMENTS IN RELATION TO THE TYPE OF INCISION USED

Impairment	Subciliary incision (n = 16)	Middle to lower eyelid incision (n = 91)	Infraorbital incision (n = 23)
Noticeable scar	0 (0%)	2 (2.2%)	4 (17.4%)
Scleral show	3 (18.8%)	4 (4.4%)	1 (4.3%)
Ectropion	1 (6.3%)	1 (1.1%)	0 (0%)
Edema	0 (0%)	1 (1.1%)	2 (8.7%)
TOTAL	4 (25%)	8 (8.8%)	7 (30.4%)

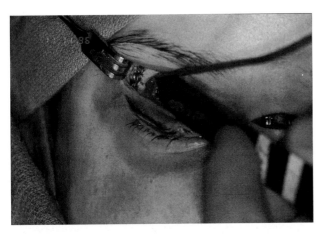

FIGURE 14–6 Exposure of the superior orbital rims through an upper eyelid incision.

SURGICAL TECHNIQUE

Hemostasis should be optimized by injecting 1% lidocaine with 1:100,000 epinephrine into the depth of the upper buccal sulcus (UBS) as well as the canine fossa, anterior nasal spine, and piriform aperture. If a midfacial degloving approach is to be performed, the nasal mucosa should be decongested and injected as with a standard rhinoplasty procedure. Incisions may be unilateral to expose the hemimidface or bilateral to expose the entire midface. In general, if exposure of the entire midface is required, posterior extension of the incision to the first molar is usually adequate. Once the periosteum has been incised, subperiosteal dissection should then proceed in an orderly fashion exposing the canine fossa, infraorbital nerve, inferior orbital rim, medial buttress, piriform aperture, and the zygomatic maxillary buttress. Subperiosteal dissection should then proceed posteriorly along the zygomatic maxillary buttress, exposing the zygomatic arch. Upon completion of this dissection, adequate exposure of the face of the maxilla, the medial and lateral buttresses, as well as the zygomatic arch and the inferior orbital rim should be accomplished (Fig. 14–7). If plating of the inferior orbital rim is necessary, this approach may need to be combined with a transconjunctival approach.

If exposure of the lateral nasal wall, nasal floor and septum, and the inferior aspect of the naso-orbital-ethmoid (NOE) complex is required, rhinoplastic release coupled with the sublabial incision can be performed. The rhinoplastic release requires the addition of a full transfixion incision, as well as intercartilaginous and bilateral piriform aperture incisions that are connected to the upper buccal sulcus incision. The decussating fibers of the nasal septum and anterior nasal spine are sharply incised allowing access to the cartilaginous septum. The

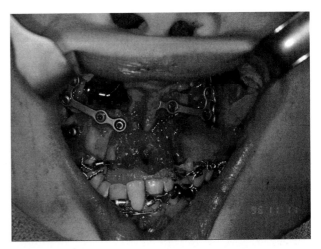

FIGURE 14–7 Open reduction and internal fixation of midface fractures utilizing an upper buccal sulcus approach.

mucosa can then be released off of the septum, nasal floor, and the lateral side wall. Once these areas have been released and exposed, the soft tissue of the midface can be degloved and retracted superiorly.

CLOSURE

Closure following a midfacial degloving approach should reestablish the nasal base as well as the mucosa lining. Reestablishing the alar base width can be accomplished by utilizing an alar cinching technique.[13] Upon completion of this cinching technique the nostril angulation should be reestablished and the nasal base should be symmetric. The intranasal incisions can be closed with chromic sutures, followed by septal splints and nasal packing that should remain in place for 1 week. The UBS incision should be closed with resorbable sutures in a layered manner. The first layer should include periosteum and muscle, and the second layer should contain submucosa and mucosa in a running fashion.

THE MANDIBLE

When approaching the mandible, multiple methods are available depending on the degree of trauma, the areas that require exposure, and the patient's cosmetic expectations. The mandibular vestibular approach or lower buccal sulcus (LBS) approach is the most common technique to expose the mandibular skeleton. The major advantages of this technique are that it does not involve an external incision and it allows the surgeon the ability to continually evaluate the occlusion. In addition, it is rapid and not complicated. Its disadvantages are that exposure of the angle, ramus, and condyle is limited, and the mental nerve is at risk of injury. The transcervical approach allows increased exposure to the inferior aspect of the mandible at the angle and ramus. The major disadvantages are that it involves an external incision, and the marginal mandibular nerve is directly within the surgical field.

ANATOMY

The marginal mandibular branch of the facial nerve takes its origin from the lower division of the facial nerve. As it exits the parotid gland, it travels obliquely to innervate the perioral musculature. For the most part, it courses superior to the inferior aspect of the mandible. However, in 20% of patients it travels below the inferior border of the mandible. The mental nerve exits its foramen at the level of the second premolar and provides sensation to the skin and mucosa of the lower lip and chin. The facial artery and vein can be identified deep to the submandibular gland within the submandibular triangle. As the facial vessels travel superiorly, they course in between the deep and superficial lobes of the submandibular gland and over the inferior border of the mandible at the mandibular notch. As the facial vessels ascend into the face, they are separated from the mandible by periosteum.

TRANSORAL APPROACH

The length of the incision that is used to expose the mandible is dependent on the degree of exposure that is required. The incision may vary from the entire mandible to an isolated area along the body. Hemostasis should be optimized prior to making an incision by injecting 1% lidocaine with 1:100,000 epinephrine into the submucosal tissues.

If necessary, the LBS incision can extend from one retromolar trigone to the other. The surgeon should ensure that an adequate cuff of mucosa remains to facilitate closure and should be cognizant of the location of the mental nerve. The initial incision through the mucosa can be performed with electrocautery. Once the mucosa is incised, the mentalis muscles should be sharply released to uncover the mandible. When the mandible has been exposed along the entire length of the LBS incision, the periosteum should be incised and a subperiosteal dissection should proceed, with careful attention being paid to preserving the integrity of the mental nerve. If necessary, the subperiosteal dissection can continue posteriorly along the ramus, releasing the fibers of the buccinator, masseter, and temporalis muscles. Upon completion, exposure can include the body, angle, ramus, and condyles of the mandible.

Closure should be completed in two layers with resorbable sutures. The first layer should comprise periosteum and muscle, and it is important to reestablish the mentalis muscle anteriorly, to prevent ptosis of the lip and chin.[7] The second layer should include the submucosa and mucosa layers.

TRANSCERVICAL APPROACH

When utilizing the external approach, the surgeon should be sure that the course of the mandibular branch of the facial nerve can be approximated and visualized. In addition, the oral commissure should be exposed to identify if the facial nerve receives stimulation during the dissection. The incision should be placed approximately 2 cm below the inferior border of the mandible and should lie within a relaxed skin tension line. One percent lidocaine with 1:100,000 epinephrine should be injected into the skin and subcutaneous tissue to maximize hemostasis.

The initial incision should be made to incise through skin and the subcutaneous tissue to the depth of the platysma. Sharp dissection can proceed through the 1- to 2-mm-thick layer of platysma muscle once it has been exposed along the entire length of the incision. The marginal mandibular nerve runs within the superficial layer of the deep cervical fascia and can be elevated out of the field. Otherwise, as the surgeon dissects toward the mandible, the facial artery and vein are encountered and can be divided and retracted superiorly. This maneuver allows the ramus mandibularis to retract superiorly. Dissection can then proceed deep to the superficial layer of the deep cervical fascia, exposing the periosteum over the mandible. The fracture sight can be visualized by incising through the periosteum and masseteric muscle. Once completed, exposure should include the body, angle, and ramus of the mandible up to the temporal mandibular joint.

During closure, if the pterygomasseteric sling has been separated, it should be reconstituted. The platysmal layer is closed followed by layered closure of the dermis and skin. A pressure dressing can be applied for 24 hours to close the dead space.

Additional surgical approaches to the mandible include the use of a facelift or rhytidectomy incision, as well as the preauricular approach. The use of a rhytidectomy incision creates a less conspicuous scar; however, the disadvantage is that it requires more extensive dissection and closure, and thus increased surgical time. The preauricular approach facilitates isolated exposure of the condyle and temporal mandibular joint, but places the facial nerve and the superficial temporal artery at risk of injury during dissection. A detailed description of the rhytidectomy and preauricular approaches are beyond the scope of this chapter.

Pearls: Extended Surgical Approaches to Facial Injuries

- Incisions on the face are not as easily camouflaged as those on other areas of the body; therefore, thoughtful consideration about their placement is critical.
- General principles of fracture exposure include placing incisions within relaxed skin tension lines, using sites that are as inconspicuous as possible, and avoiding damage to neurovascular structures.
- The bicoronal, hemicoronal, and Gilles technique can be utilized to approach fractures of the upper face and zygomatic arch.
- The inferior orbital rim and floor can be accessed through the transconjunctival or transcutaneous routes.
- The midface can be easily accessed through an upper buccal sulcus incision.
- Transfacial and intraoral approaches can be utilized to expose mandible fractures.
- Combined approaches may provide the best overall exposure.
- No matter what approach is utilized, the desire for acceptable cosmetic results, combined with adequate exposure, must be achieved.

References

1. Seckel B. *Facial Danger Zones: Avoiding Nerve Injury in Facial Plastic Surgery*. St. Louis: Quality Medical Publishing, 1994

2. Larrabee WF Jr, Makielski KH. *Surgical Anatomy of the Face*. New York: Raven Press, 1993

3. Stuzin JM, Wagstrom L, Kawamoto HK, Wolfe SA. Anatomy of the frontal branch of the facial nerve: the significance of the temporal fat pad. Plast Reconstr Surg 1989;83:265–271

4. Sherris DA, Larrabee WF Jr. Anatomic considerations in rhytidectomy. Facial Plast Surg 1996;12:215–222

5. Correia PdeC, Zani R. Surgical anatomy of the facial nerve, as related to ancillary operations in rhytidoplasty. Plast Reconstr Surg 1973;52:549–552

6. Dingman RO. Surgical anatomy of the mandibular ramus of the facial nerve based on the dissection of 100 facial halves. Plast Reconstr Surg 1962;29:266–272

7. Ellis EI, Zide MF. *Surgical Approaches to the Facial Skeleton*. Philadelphia: Williams & Wilkins, 1995

8. Frodel JL, Marentette LJ. The coronal approach. Anatomic and technical considerations and morbidity. Arch Otolaryngol Head Neck Surg 1993;119:201–207

9. Brissett AE, Sherris DA. Scar contractures, hypertrophic scars, and keloids. Facial Plast Surg 2001;17:263–272

10. Gilles HD, Stone KJ. Fractures of the malar zygomatic compound with a description of a new x-ray position. Br J Surg 1927;14:651

11. Ogden GR. The Gillies method for fractured zygomas: an analysis of 105 cases. J Oral Maxillofac Surg 1991;49:23–25

12. Bahr W, Bagambisa FB, Schlegel G, Schilli W. Comparison of transcutaneous incisions used for exposure of the infraorbital rim and orbital floor: a retrospective study. Plast Reconstr Surg 1992;90:585–591

13. Brissett AE, Sherris DA. Changing the nostril shape. Fac Plast Surg Clin North Am 2000;8:433–445

Chapter 15

Sequencing in Facial Fracture Repair

Becky McGraw-Wall

The sequence with which facial fractures are repaired becomes an issue when there are coexisting fractures of multiple regions of the face. The label "panfacial fractures" is the most common terminology used to describe this clinical situation. Typically, panfacial fractures involve the midface in combination with fractures of the mandible and the frontobasilar region, but the term is often used to describe complex fractures involving the midface and only one of the other anatomic regions. Primarily, this results from the inadequacy of the LeFort classification of midfacial fractures in describing the majority of high impact facial fractures. The complexity of the combination fracture patterns that result from extensive comminution of the midface has led to the use of other, more colorful descriptive terms for these fractures in casual reference (such as "LeFort 4" or "LeFort everything"), but *panfacial fractures* has become the accepted term in medical literature.

The extent of fracture fragmentation makes it difficult to achieve the primary goal of fracture repair, which is to reestablish normal form and function by (1) restoring functional occlusion, (2) reconstructing the facial skeletal supports, and (3) restoring facial architecture to its preinjury three-dimensional contours. Efforts at secondary reconstruction of poor clinical results have been dismal overall, enforcing the need to get things right the first time. Fortunately, there have been advances in fracture management over the past 20 years that have given guidance to surgeons faced with putting the pieces back together, and have given patients better reconstructive outcomes.

SEQUENCING ALTERNATIVES

Improved surgical approaches for craniofacial fracture exposure, as well as the development of rigid internal fixation techniques, have allowed the surgical management of facial fractures to progress from early methods of closed fracture manipulation to external fixation methods, and finally to internal stabilization and immediate bone grafting for reconstruction of facial buttresses. As surgical intervention has gotten more aggressive, various sequencing algorithms have been suggested for successful reconstruction of panfacial fractures. Previously, there have been individual advocates for either a bottom-up versus top-down approach, or an outside framework (centripetal) versus inside-out (centrifugal) approach to facial reconstruction. There have even been advocates for a less-than-systematic approach, piecing the facial skeleton back together from whichever region is the least disrupted, using it as a guide for reconstruction of the remaining face.[1] Each of these sequences has had its own particular advantages and disadvantages, but the plethora of proposed algorithms can be confusing to the novice facial trauma surgeon.

Oral surgeons, who traditionally were more familiar with mandibular surgery than middle and upper facial surgery, advocated a bottom-up approach for reconstruction of panfacial fractures. Based on experience gained dealing with injuries suffered by soldiers in the Second World War, reconstruction was based on reestablishment of occlusion, followed by mandible fracture repair. The reconstructed mandible was then used as the template for reconstruction of the remainder of the craniofacial skeleton. The basis for this approach is that the mandible is the stronger, more stable bone in comparison to the midface, and it is in contact with the maxilla through the occlusion and the skull base via the temporomandibular joint, giving clues to the appropriate vertical height of the face. Usually, reconstruction was initiated from the central, tooth-bearing region of the mandible toward the more lateral and vertical aspects of the jaw.

Craniofacial surgeons introduced wide exposure of facial fractures for accurate reduction and stable fixation, using techniques developed for craniofacial surgery. Reconstruction was initiated from cranial to caudal, using the stable cranial base to begin realignment of the lower facial fractures. Gruss et al[2-4] advocated initiating reconstruction of the external facial frame for the upper face, including the frontal bar, orbital rims, and zygomatic arches. The central portions of the face were then reconstructed within this framework, working from the outside toward the nasoethmoid region of the face. This technique emphasized the importance of the zygomatic arch in establishing the width of the midface, and its impact on controlling facial projection.

Alternatively, other surgeons began to recognize the importance of the central midface anatomy and put emphasis on the initial reconstruction of the nasoethmoid region following reestablishment of the occlusion.[5] The nasoethmoid area is noted to be the key landmark establishing central midfacial width. Although special care is taken to affirm appropriate lateral facial width through the zygomatic complex, it is also recognized that the arch is relatively thin and weak, and when comminuted offers few clues to its correct alignment. The nasoethmoid complex is one of the most difficult regions in which to achieve adequate reconstruction, because there is a tendency for this region to remain widened following fracture repair. The bones and soft tissues of the region are thin and delicate, making it challenging to restore the premorbid contour. Therefore, small errors made when midfacial reconstruction is initiated laterally can be compounded by the time the central component is addressed, leading to suboptimal results.[6] This region is one of the primary focal points of visual attention during social interactions, and minor deformities and asymmetries can be readily evident. Because the results of secondary reconstruction of the nasoethmoid area are generally less than satisfactory, the most favorable results can be attained when midfacial reconstruction is begun in the central core of the midface, working outward toward the orbital rims and zygomatic arches.

Manson et al[7-9] has put sense into all these alternatives by purporting their approach to sequencing panfacial fractures. In their approach, the midface is recognized as a dependent structure, because its projection and width are contingent upon the projection and width of the frontobasilar region above and the mandible below. For treatment purposes, the midface is mentally separated into the upper midface and the lower midface, about the LeFort I level. The upper midface is reconstructed along with the upper facial components in relationship to the more stable cranial base, and the lower midface is reconstructed through its occlusal relationship to the mandible. Both the upper and lower facial components are reconstructed from the central region to the more lateral regions, rebuilding the horizontal buttresses of the face to establish facial width and projection. The vertical buttresses at the LeFort I level are then reconstructed to establish the vertical height of the midface. This approach encompasses the advantages of both the bottom-up and the top-down approaches in relating the more delicate midface to its more stable neighboring structures.

PREOPERATIVE PLANNING

Adequate preoperative evaluation and planning are necessary, as with all surgery. Physical examination should include inspection of areas and patterns of ecchymosis and edema, facial asymmetry, malocclusion, and trismus. Bony step-offs, crepitance, facial instability, and loss of nasal support can be palpated. Careful examination of the eyes should be performed to detect preoperative telecanthus, diplopia, enophthalmos, orbital dystopia, and extraocular dysmotility. An ophthalmology consult is important if signs of orbital injury are present, and to evaluate visual acuity and assess for ocular injury.

Preoperative radiographic assessment using high-resolution computed tomography (CT) scanning is especially necessary in comminuted panfacial fractures prior to repair, to establish the fracture patterns present and the degree of comminution and bone loss. Axial and coronal reconstructions are essential, and sagittal reconstructions can be particularly helpful in evaluating the orbital walls. Radiographic assessment is important for preoperative planning to evaluate which anatomic regions are involved, as well as to assist in the development of a plan for surgical correction of the injuries. In addition, it is helpful to prepare the patient (and family) for which incisions may be required for exposure. More complex injuries require greater exposure of the anterior facial regions via multiple access incisions, and may also require exposure of the posterior mandibular buttresses and cranial base.

Preoperative CT scanning helps determine the degree of displacement and comminution of the fracture elements. Restoration of the three-dimensional parameters of the face depends on adequate reduction and reconstruction of the facial buttresses. The degree of rigid fixation required for reconstruction is directly related to the degree of comminution and amount of displacement of the fractures. More fixation points are required to stabilize fractures as they become more complex. The more comminuted the fractures are, the less stable they are, which requires greater degrees of rigid fixation. This translates into fixation at a greater number of buttress articulations, as the complexity of the fractures increases. Likewise, the more complex the fracture, the greater the need for exposure of all the adjacent bony articulations. In particular, the articulations with the adjacent nonfractured craniofacial bones need to be exposed in complex fractures, to allow for correct anatomic alignment of the fractured regions in relationship with the more stable non-injured facial regions and cranial base.

OPERATIVE MANAGEMENT

Management of panfacial fractures should begin as soon as other, more life-threatening injuries permit. Ideally, fracture repair should occur within 48 hours. When that is not possible, then fracture management within 7 to 10 days is important for optimal results. Early intervention allows for easier reduction of facial fractures, and reduces the errors introduced by fibrous and bony callous formation around the edges of fracture fragments as interfragmentary healing begins. Delayed repair can also be more difficult due to soft tissue scar formation and contraction that can limit adequate fracture reduction.

For sequencing purposes, the facial skeleton should be figuratively divided about the LeFort I plane. The upper midface and cranial base can then be addressed as one unit, and the midfacial occlusal component and mandible as another, separate unit (Fig. 15–1). The upper midface and frontobasilar region is reconstructed relative to the more stable cranium, and the lower midface to the mandible. Once these subunits are individually reconstructed, then the upper and lower facial units can be realigned and fixated at the vertical buttresses of the midface. The order in which the upper and lower facial units are addressed can be adjusted according to the severity of the fractures or physician preference.

Knowledge of the horizontal and vertical facial buttress systems and their contributions to the three-dimensional architecture of the face is essential for successful reconstruction. The primary components of facial width of the upper face are the nasoethmoid complex centrally and the frontal bar and zygomatic arches laterally. For the lower face, the palate and the arch of the mandible from angle to angle determine facial width. The primary components of facial projection for the upper face are the frontal bar, zygomatic arches, and nasomaxillary buttresses. For the lower face, the projection is determined by the mandible from angle to symphysis. Vertical height of the face is determined by the nasomaxillary and zygomaticomaxillary buttresses of the midface, and the posterior mandibular buttress from angle to condyle.

It is important to recognize that the dimensions of the face are interrelated to one another. Facial width and facial projection, in particular, are inversely related to each other. For example, displacement of the zygoma laterally will widen the face, but will also decrease the amount of anterior projection of the midface and malar eminence (Fig. 15–2). Likewise, displaced fractures of the palate or bilateral fractures of the mandible tend to increase the lower facial width and decrease the projection of the lower face (Fig. 15–3).

Exposure of the various fracture components is essential for adequate reduction and management of panfacial fractures. Depending on the facial regions involved with the injury, a combination of incisions is needed to expose the anterior facial skeleton. The coronal incision is used to access the frontal, nasoethmoid, and lateral orbital fractures. It may be extended as necessary to expose the zygomatic arches for rigid fixation. The transconjunctival incision with lateral canthotomy or the subciliary incision is used to access the inferior orbital rim and orbital floor, and the maxillary and mandibular gingivobuccal sulcus incisions can be used to expose the vertical midfacial buttresses and the anterior mandible from angle to angle. A preauricular/retromandibular incision can be used to expose the mandibular condyle as needed for open repair of the condyle.

LOWER FACIAL RECONSTRUCTION

Reestablishment of the occlusal relationship and stable intermaxillary fixation is a prerequisite in panfacial fractures, and is the first key to adequate reduction of the fractures. Frequently, it is necessary to expose the midface fractures and gain better reduction of an impacted midface or widely

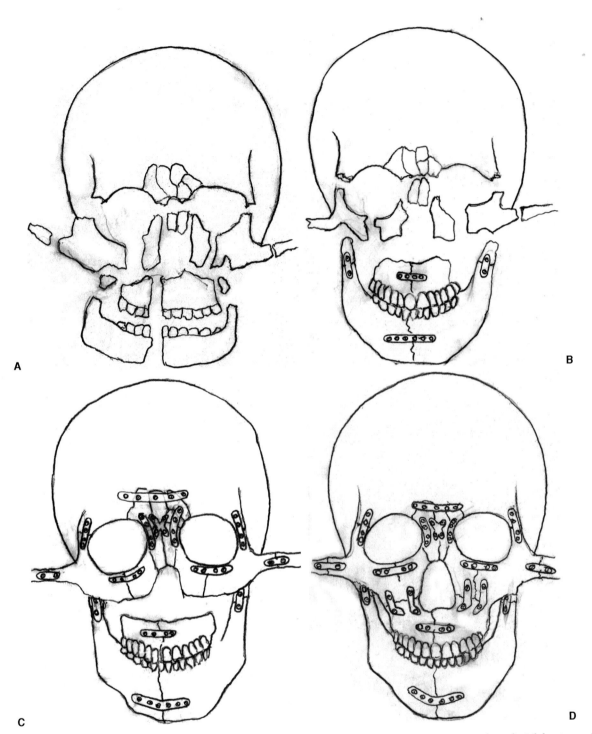

FIGURE 15–1   The order of surgical management of panfacial fractures. A: Depiction of panfacial fractures. B: Palatal fractures are stabilized prior to intermaxillary fixation. If indicated, then rigid fixation of the vertical mandibular component is performed prior to reconstruction of the horizontal mandible. C: The upper midface is reduced and fixated to the skull base and frontal bones. D: After stabilization of the upper and lower midface segments, the two hemiportions of midface are repaired anatomically at the LeFort I level.

displaced fracture fragments prior to placing intermaxillary wires, to accurately reestablish the occlusion. Intermaxillary fixation may need to be left in place for several weeks postoperatively in panfacial fracture repair, depending on the perceived stability

of the repair and the degree of comminution. This is primarily because only the anterior buttresses of the midface are rigidly fixed. The posterior buttresses of the midface are reduced during fracture repair, but are stabilized only through the repaired anterior

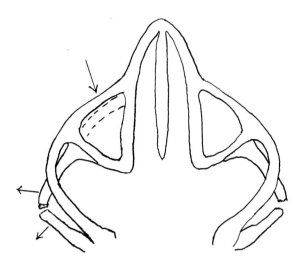

FIGURE 15–2 The zygomatic arch controls both the width and the projection of the midface. Rounding of the normal flat posterolateral aspect of the arch leads to increased width of the midface, but decreased projection.

buttresses of the midface and the occlusal relationship with the mandible. When there is significant comminution of the supporting facial buttresses of the midface, intermaxillary fixation is helpful in preventing postoperative shortening of the posterior buttresses of the midface.

Once intermaxillary fixation is established, and adequate exposure and fracture reduction is achieved, then rigid fixation can begin. The occlusion should be checked both before and after rigid fixation to ensure that the patient has not been pulled out of occlusion. When palatal fractures occur in conjunction with fractures of the mandibular arch, reduction and fixation of the palate need to be addressed following arch bar placement, but before intermaxillary fixation is applied, to reestablish the correct width of the lower central face. Otherwise, the mandibular arch will be set to the widened palatal arch, leading to poor alignment of the facial architecture. Palatal fixation can be achieved through application of a plate on the oral surface of the palate, or the anterior nasal spine and pyriform region. If there is comminution of both the palate and the horizontal mandibular arch, then the occlusion should first be reestablished using fabricated dental splints based on dental impression models.

Mandibular reconstruction proceeds from the central, tooth-bearing regions to the more lateral regions. Comminuted fractures are first pieced together using small miniplates or wires, and then the comminuted segments of the horizontal mandible are joined to the rest of the mandible using a locking reconstruction plate system. Bilateral mandibular fractures have a tendency to flare laterally at the angles, increasing lower facial width,

and to rotate lingually, leading to malocclusion. Applying pressure manually at the angles of the mandible during reduction and fixation can help control facial width and prevent lingual rotation (Fig. **15–3**). Complicated fractures involving the mandibular angles should be exposed through an extraoral incision. Primary bone grafting is used as needed to reestablish the integrity of the mandibular arch.

Open reduction of the vertical component of the mandible is indicated when there are fractures involving both the horizontal and vertical sections of the mandible, and there is loss of vertical mandibular height due to significant displacement or misalignment of the condyle, subcondylar, or ramus region of the mandible. This is particularly true when there are coexisting comminuted fractures of the midface, and when there are fractures

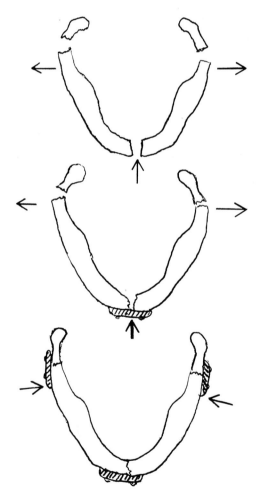

FIGURE 15–3 Bilateral fractures of the mandible can lead to widening of the normal contour of the mandible and decreased projection of the lower face. Manual pressure on the mandibular angles during reduction of bilateral mandibular fractures helps counteract the tendency for these fractures to flare laterally and rotate lingually.

involving the vertical mandibular segments bilaterally. This allows restoration of the vertical height of the lower face, by relating the mandible and the occlusal segment of the maxilla to the more stable cranial base. Once the vertical height of the mandible is set, then the anterior projection of the mandible and lower facial unit can be reestablished (Fig. 15–1). A preauricular incision, extending down into a retromandibular incision can be used to approach the ramus and subcondylar regions of the mandible. The facial nerve should be identified and protected during such an approach.

UPPER FACIAL RECONSTRUCTION

Once occlusal realignment and mandibular reconstruction have been completed, then the upper face can be addressed. Reconstruction should begin with the frontal bone and frontal bar region of the upper face. The frontal sinus should be addressed as indicated by the involvement of the anterior table, posterior table, and nasofrontal drainage regions. The comminuted segments of the anterior table can be removed from the wound and reconstructed on the back table, using microplates or titanium mesh. The frontal bar is then reduced and stabilized using microplates. Orbital roof fractures should be reduced through a subcranial approach,[10] but if unstable, they can be fixated to the frontal bar through an anterior cranial fossa approach. Sinus obliteration or cranialization should then be performed, if indicated. Cranialization should be considered when significant displacement or comminution of the posterior table is present. Obliteration should be considered when frontal sinus drainage is compromised by fracture involvement. Once this is completed, the reconstructed central segment can be rigidly fixed to the nondisplaced lateral regions of the frontal bone. Split calvarial bone grafts are used to reconstruct defects involving the frontal bar or large defects of the anterior table. Hydroxyapatite cement and titanium mesh are also very useful for reconstruction of small contour defects of the anterior cranium and frontal bone.

The reconstructed frontal bone and frontal bar can now provide a stable base for reconstruction of the nasoethmoid fractures. The nasoethmoid complex is the critical determinant of central midfacial width, and is crucial in the reestablishment of the premorbid aesthetics of the central core of the face. Chapter 5 discusses management of these fractures, so only a brief overview is mentioned here. The medial orbital rims and nasomaxillary buttresses are reduced and plated using microplates. This complex is then rigidly fixed to the frontal bar, securing the projection of the central core of the face. The medial orbital walls are then addressed, reducing large fracture fragments, and the bony defects are bone grafted. Positioning of medial orbital bone grafts is facilitated by placement prior to transnasal wiring.

Transnasal reduction of the medial canthal segment is often required in panfacial fractures, depending on the stability and degree of comminution of the nasoethmoid complex. Reduction should be directed posterior and superior to the medial canthal tendon. Attempted "overcorrection" is generally necessary to reestablish the normal intercanthal distance, although it is nearly impossible to actually achieve overcorrection. This is due in part to posttraumatic soft tissue scarring and thickening, but predominantly because of the tendency for these fractures to be displaced laterally and posteriorly, and the general difficulty in reconstructing this delicate region. If the canthal tendons are avulsed off the central segment, then they should be reattached to the transnasal wire using a nonabsorbable suture following stable wiring of the canthal segment.

Upon completion of the nasoethmoid repair, the zygomatic complex fractures are reduced. Restoration of the zygoma and its relationship to the cranial base and nasoethmoid bones is important to correct the three-dimensional architecture of the lateral aspect of the midface. Correct reduction of the zygoma in panfacial fractures can only be achieved by exposure and direct visualization of the fracture sites along the arch, the frontozygomatic suture, and the inferior orbital rim simultaneously. The zygomatic arch determines the width and projection of the midface, and they are inversely proportional to each other. It is important to note that the arch itself is not a true arch, but is flattened posterolaterally, providing anterior projection for the midface. If the arch is reconstructed in a rounded configuration, then the malar eminence will be underprojected and laterally displaced (Fig. 15–2). The key to reduction of the zygomatic arch and the rest of the zygomatic complex lies along the lateral orbit at the junction of the orbital process of the zygoma with the greater wing of the sphenoid. Exploration of the lateral orbital wall should be performed prior to rigid fixation of the zygomatic arch to the zygomatic process of the temporal bone to ensure appropriate reduction.

Once the arch is reduced and stabilized, then the inferior orbital rim can be addressed. Frequently, comminution of the rim makes it difficult to determine proper alignment. The multiple segments tend to be displaced inferiorly and posteriorly. Placing interfragmentary wires and manipulating the fragments anterior-superior prior to plating can be helpful. Also, a nonrigid wire or small microplate along the frontozygomatic suture can be placed to help with determination of the vertical height of the inferior orbital rim prior to rigid fixation, but care must be taken to allow movement in the anterior and medial direction as needed for fracture reduction. Although the frontozygomatic suture area is a good guide to the vertical position of the zygoma, it is a very poor indicator of both projection and horizontal placement of the complex, so it is generally not rigidly plated until after fixation of the inferior orbital rim. Defects of the orbital floors and lateral walls should be reconstructed once the rims have been correctly reduced and stabilized.

RECONSTRUCTION AT THE LEFORT I LEVEL

Following completion of reconstruction of both the upper and lower facial units, the two halves can be realigned and plated along the medial and lateral vertical buttresses of the maxilla at the LeFort I level (Fig. **15–1**). Ideally, midfacial height can be determined using at least one noncomminuted maxillary buttress as a guide. If extensive bone loss or comminution is present at all buttresses, then lip–tooth position may provide information about the correct vertical height of the face. Often, however, there is significant swelling of the lips at this point in the procedure, which makes this a difficult determinant. Bone gaps in the buttress greater than 5 mm should be primarily bone grafted, using calvarial bone or rib graft.

Nasoseptal reduction is performed following reattachment of the upper and lower face. This is facilitated by the stabilization of the anterior nasal spine and maxillary crest, which is achieved with rigid fixation of the maxilla. Cantilevered bone grafting of the nasal dorsum is often necessary to improve the nasal contour due to loss of adequate septal support. Columellar strut grafting for support of the nasal tip may also be required.

Meticulous soft tissue resuspension and repair following wide-access exposure of panfacial fractures is important to prevent postoperative soft tissue ptosis and sagging. A layered closure is essential, including periosteum, fascia, muscle, and skin or mucosa. The periosteum needs to be resuspended at the areas of dissection away from the facial skeleton along the lateral and inferior orbital rims, zygomatic arch, malar eminence, and the mandibular symphysis. Reattachment of the lateral canthal tendon is performed using a permanent suture, and the medial canthal repair should be confirmed to be intact prior to closure of the coronal incision. The fascial layers should be reapproximated, including the deep temporalis fascia and galea. The muscle layers of the gingivobuccal sulcus incision should be repaired; a two-layered intraoral repair helps reduce the incidence of wound dehiscence. The lateral aspect of the orbicularis oculi muscle should also be resuspended. Skin and mucosa closure follow deep layer repair. Nasoseptal splinting is recommended for both septal support and to assist in reduction of hematoma and soft tissue edema in the nasoethmoid region.

SUMMARY

An organized approach to sequencing of panfacial fractures can facilitate successful restoration of the three-dimensional architecture of the face. Facial injuries differ in fracture patterns and extent of comminution, necessitating some degree of flexibility in any surgical management plan. Reconstruction of the facial skeleton should proceed by relating the facial components to their adjacent structures and buttresses in a stepwise fashion. Building from the regions of the face that most impact form and function, and from the regions that offer the most stability and clues to the proper alignment of the surrounding skeleton, to the weaker, more dependent regions of the face affords the most optimal reconstruction results.

PEARLS: SEQUENCING IN FACIAL FRACTURE REPAIR

- There are multiple techniques for sequencing panfacial fractures, including "bottom-up" starting with the mandible, "outside-in" starting with the zygomatic arches, and "inside-out" starting with the naso-orbital region. However, there is no single ideal approach.
- A useful approach is to consider the midface as two subunits, divided at approximately the LeFort I level. The upper midface is reconstructed to the cranium, and the lower midface to the mandibular arch; then the two halves of the midface are realigned at the vertical buttresses.
- Knowledge of the facial buttress system and the three-dimensional relationships of width, height, and projection are essential for successful reconstruction.
- Adequate exposure of fracture sites is necessary before fracture reduction begins.

REFERENCES

1. Manson PN. Some thoughts on the classification and treatment of LeFort fractures. Ann Plast Surg 1986; 17:356–363

2. Gruss JS, Phillips JH. Complex facial trauma: the evolving role of rigid fixation and immediate bone graft reconstruction. Clin Plast Surg 1989;16:93–104

3. Gruss JS, Van-Wyck L, Phillips JH, et al. The importance of the zygomatic arch in complex midfacial fracture repair and correction of post-traumatic orbito-zygomatic deformities. Plast Reconstr Surg 1990;85:878–890

4. Gruss JS, Bubak PJ, Egbert M. Craniofacial fractures: an algorithm to optimize results. Clin Plast Surg 1992;19:195–206

5. Markowitz BL, Manson PN. Panfacial fractures: organization of treatment. Clin Plast Surg 1989;16: 105–114

6. Fritz MA, Koltai PJ. Sequencing and organization of the repair of panfacial fractures. Op Tech Otolaryngol Head Neck Surg 2002;13:261–264

7. Kelly KJ, Manson PN, Vander Kolk CA, et al. Sequencing LeFort fracture treatment (organization of treatment for a panfacial fracture). J Craniofac Surg 1990;1:168–178

8. Manson PN, Clark N, Robertson B, et al. Comprehensive management of pan-facial fractures. J Craniomaxillofac Trauma 1995;1:43–55

9. Manson PN, Clark N, Robertson B, et al. Subunit principles in midface fractures: the importance of sagittal buttresses, soft-tissue reductions, and sequencing treatment of segmental fractures. Plast Reconstr Surg 1999;103:1287–1306

10. Raveh J, Vuillemin T. The surgical one-stage management of combined cranio-maxillo-facial and frontobasal fractures. Advantages of the subcranial approach in 374 cases. J Craniomaxillofac Surg 1988;16:160–172

Chapter 16

PEDIATRIC FACIAL TRAUMA

Carla M. Giannoni

Although trauma is a leading cause of pediatric death, children make up only 5 to 15% of facial trauma victims.[1,2] This is believed to be due to a combination of anatomic, developmental, and social factors. Anatomically the prominent skull and relatively small maxilla and mandible of children make their facial skeleton less exposed to traumatic forces (Fig. 16–1). The normal craniofacial ratio, that is, the ratio of the skull relative to the facial skeleton as viewed in the lateral plane, in a full-term newborn is 8:1 and in an adult is 2.5:1.[3] Children are less susceptible to traumatic facial injury because the skulls of children have a large cancellous proportion and a thin cortex making the facial skeleton more stable. Also, the relative lack of sinus pneumatization in the facial skeleton and the presence of unerupted teeth strengthen the skull and make it more stable and more resistant to trauma. As a child grows there is forward and vertical growth, making the facial skeleton more prominent. Along with facial maturation is dental maturation. Children are born with primary dentition consisting of 20 teeth and secondary dentition of 32 teeth. The primary teeth erupt between infancy and the second year of life. Most children have a complement of secondary dentition by 16 years of age. Additionally, the more protected environment of children with close parental observation of activities and the use of car seats makes children less prone to injury.

The etiology of pediatric facial trauma varies by age and by literature review. The incidence of facial trauma increases with age. Motor vehicle accidents, involving drivers, passengers, and pedestrians, are the number one cause of facial trauma in most series in all age groups (Fig. 16–2). In older children, as in adults, injuries due to falls, equestrian accidents, bicycle riding, altercations, and sports are major causes of facial injury. The higher male-to-female ratio seen in adolescents equalizes in younger pediatric patients, likely secondary to the relatively higher percentage of motor vehicle-related injuries in these younger children and a lower percentage of sports and other injuries related to the recklessness of youth. A useful way to explore the issue of pediatric facial trauma is to divide the pediatric population into three groups based on skull proportions and dentition: infants and toddlers with only primary dentition (ages 0 to 5 years of age), school-age children with mixed dentition (6 to 12 years of age) and adolescents with secondary dentition (12 to 16 years of age). This division is useful in reviewing not only the etiologies of trauma but also the treatments to be discussed below.

EVALUATION OF THE PEDIATRIC TRAUMA PATIENT

As with adults, emergency management follows the axiom of ABC: airway, breathing, and circulation. Airway management of children is similar to that of adults and the need for intubation or tracheotomy is comparable to that of adults. On average, 20% of patients require airway intervention.[1]

In particular, the history should include the mechanism of injury and the estimated energy of impact (low, medium, or high). Lower force injuries are more likely to result in nondisplaced greenstick fractures, whereas higher force injuries are more likely to lead to displaced and comminuted fractures.[4] Physical inspection should be thorough, especially evaluating cosmetic defect, facial asymmetry, malocclusion, hemotympanum, palpable bony step-off, ptosis, bruising, nasal deviation, nasal obstruction, epistaxis, and vertigo (Table 16–1). Asymmetry and tenderness are important signs of

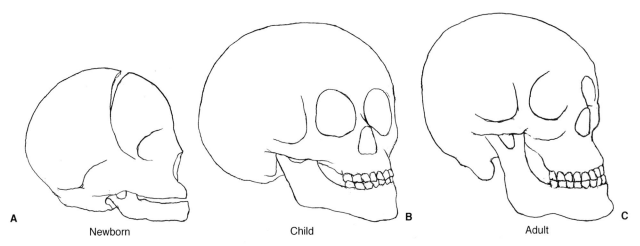

FIGURE 16-1   Skulls of a typical newborn (A), child (B), and adult (C). Note the change in craniofacial relationships that occur during growth and development.

underlying injury. The facial skeleton should be completely palpated, including testing the stability of the palate and bimanual palpation of the mandible at the temporomandibular joint, ramus, body and symphysis. A cranial nerve examination should be performed.

Computed tomography (CT) scanning is used in the majority of pediatric trauma patients, especially to assess the maxillary and orbital bones, and mandibular Panorex is utilized when mandibular fractures are suspected.[3] Plain facial films are rarely

diagnostic. The presence of developing teeth that can obscure a fracture and the high incidence of greenstick fractures in children make the diagnosis of pediatric fracture more challenging. CT scan provides the best detail for a complete assessment of fracture location and pattern of comminution and displacement.[4] CT scanning may be more problematic in children than in adults, as younger children are less likely to be cooperative and may require sedation or even general anesthesia with control of the airway. Often scanning of the facial region

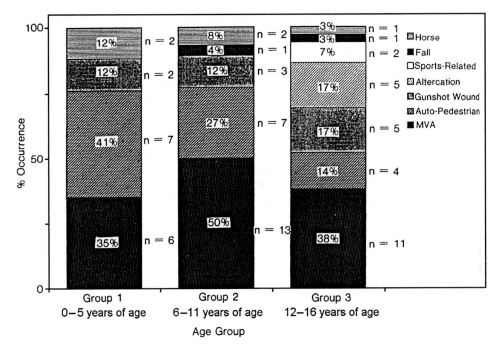

FIGURE 16-2   Mechanisms of facial trauma injury by age group. MVA, motor vehicle accident. (Adapted from McGraw B, Cole R. Pediatric maxillofacial trauma. *Arch Otolaryngol Head Neck Surg* 1990;116:42. Copyright © 1990, American Medical Association. All rights reserved.)

TABLE 16–1 FACIAL INSPECTION OF THE CHILD WITH FACIAL TRAUMA

Site	Sign	Suspected injury or special concern
Nose	Swelling of the septum	Septal hematoma
	Clear rhinorrhea	Skull base fracture (CSF rhinorrhea)
	Nasal obstruction	Nasal fracture
	Epistaxis	Nasal fracture
	Nasal deviation	Nasal fracture
	Cosmetic deformity	Nasal fracture
Orbit	Epiphora /tearing	Lacrimal apparatus injury
	Pseudo-telecanthus	Disruption of medial canthal tendon.
	Palpable step-off	Orbital or zygomatic complex fracture
	Bruising	Orbital or zygomatic complex fracture
Maxilla	Numbness	Injury to V2 nerve
	Malocclusion	Fracture
	Unstable palate	Fracture
Mandible	Asymmetry	Injury to V2 nerve
	Malocclusion	Fracture
	Loose teeth	
Ear	Vertigo	Temporal bone fracture
	Hemotympanum	Temporal bone fracture
Neurologic	Cranial nerve inspection (especially nerves 2, 3, 4, 5, 6, 7, and 8)	Fracture with direct cranial nerve injury or indirect injury by hematoma formation or muscle entrapment

is performed concurrently with CT scanning of the head when assessment of intracranial injury is necessary.

ASSOCIATED INJURIES

Children sustain higher rates of concurrent nonfacial injuries and more often are multiply injured than adults with facial trauma. In a large series of trauma patients, children were much more likely than their adult counterparts to have associated injuries (73% as compared with 58% of adults) and were significantly more likely to have multiple associated injuries (68% of pediatric patients as compared with only 33% of adult patients).[1] These concurrent injuries are most often neurologic and orthopedic, but can also be ocular and soft tissue. The large relative volume of the skull predisposes the child to a higher probability of concurrent skull and central nervous system injury when facial trauma is sustained. Up to 88% of younger patients and 34% of adolescents and adults with facial trauma also sustain head or skull injuries.[3] Additionally, over a third of pediatric patients may have concurrent temporal bone fractures. These findings, though in large part due to cranial volume and prominence, may also be due to the mechanism of injury, which very often includes moving motor vehicles. Thus the pediatric trauma patient requires a comprehensive evaluation for multiple injuries, especially when the mechanism of injury is of moderate or high energy.

FRACTURE PATTERNS

Fracture distribution from three notable pediatric series is summarized in Table 16–2. As may be expected based on anatomic and mechanistic factors, there are age-related differences in fracture incidence (Fig. 16–3). There are relatively more orbital injuries in young children.[3] Maxillary and sinus fractures are rarely seen in children under 12 years of age.[1,2] Severity of injuries also appears to increase with age. Excluding severely injured children who die of head injuries, children under 6 years of age rarely sustain maxillary, orbit, or midface injuries that require treatment except for the occasional closed reduction of nasal fracture.[2] Nasal and mandible fracture incidence increases with age. Happily, favorable mandible fractures are much more common in children than adults with

TABLE 16–2   PEDIATRIC FACIAL FRACTURE PATTERNS{AQ7}

	Gussack, 1987	*McGraw, 1990*	*Koltai, 1995*
Number of children	30	72	62
Mandible	16 (32%)	25 (35%)	18 (32%)
Maxilla (includes zygoma, "panfacial")	4 (8%)	7 (9%)	17 (27%)
Nose	10 (20%)	*	7 (11%)
Orbit	11 (22%)	14 (19%)	11 (18%)
Sinus	9 (18%) (Includes all sinuses)	*	2 (3%) (Frontal sinus only)
Single fracture	21 (70%)	*	*
Multiple fractures	9 (30%)	*	*

*Data not available.

maxillomandibular injuries and are more often able to be managed by observation.[1] Table **16–3** summarizes the management of pediatric facial fractures in one published series.[2] In-depth discussion of the management of each fracture type follows in the text below.

MANAGEMENT

PEDIATRIC NASAL TRAUMA

Nasal injuries are common in both adults and children. Historical information that is particularly important in the assessment of nasal trauma includes the cause of injury, the direction of the blow, and the force of the injury.[5] Though the nose may be injured by trauma directed from the side, below, or the front, it is more susceptible to fracture from lateral trauma. One should inquire about nasal obstruction, the severity of any nasal bleeding, and if there is any clear rhinorrhea suggestive of cerebrospinal fluid (CSF) rhinorrhea. Cheek numbness may indicate a more severe injury of the maxillary complex.

Examination of the nose should be complete including examination of the soft tissues, the

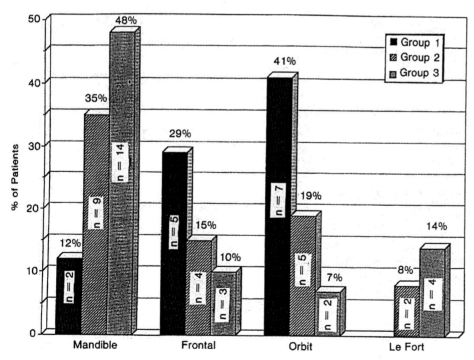

* Group 1: 0 - 5 years of age; Group 2: 6 - 11 years of age; Group 3: 12-16 years of age

FIGURE 16–3   Anatomic distribution of facial fractures by age group. (From McGraw B, Cole R. Pediatric Maxillofacial Trauma; Arch Otolaryngol Head Neck Surg 1990;116:43. Copyright © 1990, American Medical Association. All rights reserved.)

TABLE 16–3 TREATMENT OF PEDIATRIC FACIAL FRACTURES

Number of treated, surviving children	56*
Mandible	18
Observation	7 (39%)
MMF	10[†] (56%)
ORIF	3 (17%)
Maxilla + ZMC + panfacial	16
ORIF	13 (81%)
Nose	7
Closed reduction	7 (100%)
Orbit	11
ORIF	4 (36%)
NOE	2
ORIF	2 (100%)
Sinus	2
ORIF	2 (100%)
All fractures	
Observation	17 (30%)
ORIF	24 (55%)

*Six of 62 children in this series did not survive their other injuries and were not treated.
[†]Estimated; this is a maximal number of children receiving maxillomandibular fixation based on available data.
MMF, mandibular-maxillary fixation; NOE, naso-orbital-ethmoid; ORIF, open reduction and internal fixation; ZMC, zygomatico-maxillary complex.
Adapted from Koltai PJ, Radkin D, Hoehn J. Rigid fixation of facial fractures in children. J Craniomaxillofac Trauma 1995;1:32–42.

septum, the nasal bones, and the nasal vault. Nasal symmetry should be assessed. It is helpful to compare posttraumatic appearance to that of the patient's likeness in a recent photograph to fully assess cosmetic changes. Adequate examination cannot usually be completely performed before swelling has subsided. Practically speaking, this means that the emergency department evaluation should focus on the acute complications of facial trauma that require urgent intervention such as septal hematoma, CSF rhinorrhea, soft tissue injuries requiring closure, and associated injuries to the orbit and maxillary complex. Radiographs are rarely helpful in the assessment of simple nasal fractures, but CT scan may be indicated when more severe injuries are suspected. It is important to allow 3 to 5 days for swelling to regress before making final decisions about surgical intervention. Plans for an interval examination in the office should be made so that the functional and cosmetic appearance of the nose can better evaluated. This examination should be carefully timed such that swelling has regressed but healing has not occurred to a significant degree. Because of the high osteogenic potential in children, there is a narrower window of opportunity to perform closed reduction, usually less than 10 days. Final decisions regarding surgical intervention can be made after this interval examination.

Surgical intervention for pediatric nasal fractures is similar to that of adult nasal fractures with some notable exceptions. The goal of treatment is to restore a bilaterally patent nasal airway, restore the cosmetic appearance of the nose, and prevent complications of untreated injuries. Septal hematomas should be drained urgently (less than 24 hours or so as necrosis can begin in as little as 48 hours). Failure to diagnose and treat a septal hematoma may result in loss of septal cartilage and development of a saddle-nose deformity. With the exception of septal hematoma, there is rarely any harm, and usually there is benefit, in delaying treatment until the majority of the swelling has subsided. Septal deviations and dislocations should be treated as conservatively as possible, as the septum is a primary growth center.[5] In children with symptomatic fractures, closed reduction is the procedure most often indicated. Any significant intervention with pediatric patients, including closed reduction, requires general anesthesia. Often closed reduction is easier to perform in children than in adults. Open reduction is rarely indicated in children but should be performed when necessary for adequate reduction of severe injuries. Chronic nasal obstruction secondary to nasal injury can itself contribute to disorders of facial growth, and injuries causing significant nasal obstruction should be addressed. When deciding to perform open reduction, one must balance the risk of further disturbance of the nasal growth centers with the need to restore nasal function and cosmesis.

NEWBORN NASAL TRAUMA

Newborns presenting with asymmetric flattening of the nasal tip are often believed to have injury secondary to their delivery. This is not always the case; it may also be secondary to intrauterine positioning. Though surgical reduction has occasionally been advocated, it is rarely necessary, because in the vast majority of newborns the deformity resolves without intervention.[6]

MANDIBULAR FRACTURES

Mandibular fractures are the second most common facial fracture in young children and the most common facial fractures in children requiring hospitalization.[6] Mandibular fractures account for 20 to 30% of facial fractures in children. The mechanism, in most cases, is blunt trauma with a blow to the chin.

Management of mandible fractures, more than with other facial fractures, is in large part dependent on age and dentition.[7] Management of children with primary or mixed dentition is complicated by several factors. First is the presence of secondary, unerupted teeth in the mandible body until 6 years of age or longer. Open reduction with internal fixation (ORIF) with a plate in preadolescent children places their secondary dentition at significant risk of injury, and thus only monocortical plating should be performed. Second is the difficulty of maintaining secure mandibular-maxillary fixation (MMF) when the teeth are not present or are not firmly anchored in the mandible. Primary dentition is not completely present until 2 years of age, and fixation cannot rely on arch bars for traditional MMF. After the age of 2 the roots are fairly firm and may theoretically hold arch bars until around 5 years of age. Despite the firm roots, however, the shape of primary teeth with a crown very close to the gingival margin may not permit secure arch bar placement. At age 5 the primary dentition gives way for secondary dentition, and during the process there is resorption of the deciduous roots, making the teeth less firm. Thus, in most preadolescent children, intermaxillary fixation cannot depend on arch bars and requires lingual splints and/or circummandibular wiring. The process of preparing lingual splints is time-consuming and exacting because dental impressions with reconstruction of the prefracture occlusion is required. After 12 or 13 years of age the secondary teeth form stable support for MMF, and the mandible can be treated with open fixation much as in adults. Happily, epidemiologic factors make pediatric mandible fractures in younger children less common and easier to treat.[8] Favorable mandible fractures are much more common in children, 55% versus 15% of adult mandible fractures, and pediatric patients with maxillomandibular injuries are more likely to be managed by observation than are adults.[1,2]

The management of mandible fractures is heavily influenced by the continued facial growth of children, which is impacted by a child's high metabolic rate and enhanced periosteal osteogenetic potential. Generally younger children heal more quickly and have fewer long-term problems than older children, so a particularly conservative approach is advocated in children under the age of 6. For condyle fractures, if there is an open bite deformity, retrusion, or limitation of movement, MMF is recommended.[7] For arch and body fractures, if there is normal occlusion and mobility, then soft diet is recommended; if there is malocclusion and movement limitation, then MMF is recommended, with monocortical miniplate ORIF in children younger than 12 years, and traditional bicortical ORIF for children 12 or older.[7]

The condyle is the most commonly fractured site, accounting for 40 to 70% of pediatric mandible fractures and over 75% of cases in very young children. These fractures may be unilateral or bilateral and may be isolated or seen in combination with other body or angle fractures. Condylar fractures can almost always be treated conservatively.[8] The main question is whether or not MMF is necessary. If the occlusion and mandibular movement are normal, then most children do not require any intervention other than eating a soft diet for a few weeks. In cases where MMF is utilized, a short period of less than 3 weeks is recommended. Ankylosis of the temporomandibular joint is a debilitating complication of mandible fractures and their treatment. This can be best avoided by early mobilization and movement exercises after only 2 to 3 weeks of MMF. Early mobilization is advocated in all children under 12 years of age, whereas teenagers may be treated as adults.

Angle, body, symphyseal, and parasymphyseal fractures are more likely to require immobilization and occasionally ORIF than are condylar fractures. Treatment usually depends on the state of distraction of the segments. Nondisplaced and incomplete fractures require only soft diet. Need for immobilization with MMF depends on the degree of displacement and the loading forces, favorable or unfavorable, on the fractured segments.[9] When ORIF is performed, only monocortical plates should be used to prevent tooth bud injury.

Long-term follow-up is necessary to determine if adequate and symmetrical facial growth and development occurs after mandibular trauma. Though facial growth is self-reported to be good in most mandibular fracture patients, the majority of patients may be found to have mild asymmetry identified by a trained examiner or by cephalometric examinations. Approximately 20% of patients will have clinically significant asymmetry later in life.[10] This asymmetry is almost exclusively deviation to the side of condylar fracture. Routine use of pterygoid muscle exercises and the use of nighttime elastics for 6 to 8 weeks after release of MMF may improve outcome. Children between 4 and 12 may be at greater risk for developing secondary growth disturbance because of the active growth of the mandible during this period. If functional occlusion is not achieved by 14 to 15 years of age then orthodontic or orthognathic surgery can be performed. Interestingly, in the general adolescent population the rate of orthodontic or orthognathic treatment due to mandibular fractures is similar to the rate due to nonfracture mandibular processes.[11]

Dental prognosis is generally good for affected unerupted secondary dentition. Mandibular fractures may involve unerupted teeth one third of the time, but delayed or noneruption occurs in only ~ 20% of affected teeth.[10,12] Though the numbers are small, it appears that ORIF increases the risk of poor outcome for tooth buds in the line of fracture. Nonunion and infection is distinctly uncommon in pediatric mandible patients. Patients may be placed on antibiotics to cover oral flora. Unless completely avulsed, tooth buds in the line of fracture and even those believed injured by treatment are left in place and managed expectantly.

MAXILLARY, ORBITAL, AND NASOETHMOID INJURIES

CT scan is the diagnostic study of choice for the evaluation of nasoethmoid, orbital, and maxillary buttress fractures. CT also often demonstrates the mandibular condyles and temporomandibular joint, which are susceptible to injury when impact occurs in these midface regions. Timely recognition of fractures is important because repair needs to proceed more rapidly than in adults because of children's relatively faster healing. As with nasal fractures, a brief period of observation, 4 days or so, while swelling subsides may be necessary. Waiting more than 8 or 10 days for fracture repair may lead to immobile fractures that cannot be reduced.[13]

The vast majority of these upper face fractures rely on the same surgical management principles that are used for adults. Fortunately, the relatively more resilient pediatric facial skeleton is less likely to sustain higher energy fractures that require repair.[2] Low-energy injuries resulting in nondisplaced fractures are often seen. Generally only fractures that are displaced and causing functional or cosmetic problems need reduction, and those can be treated with closed techniques. Others, typically those that are comminuted and displaced, may require open reduction, and sometimes rigid fixation.

Close examination of the face for symmetry and for telecanthus is important such that medial canthal tendon displacement is recognized when present. When repairing these fractures, the surgeon must take care in these cases not to set the intercanthal distance too wide. Since half of orbital growth is already achieved by 3 years and near mature size is reached at 8 years of age, the orbits may already be near adult configuration in the majority of trauma victims.[13] One should always consider the possibility of concurrent injury of orbital contents and obtain ophthalmologic consultation when indicated.

The surgeon should be sensitive to the continued growth of the pediatric face and utilize techniques that are minimally disruptive when open fracture reduction and fixation are required. Whether intended or accidental, bony disruption and injuries to the overlying soft tissues can alter significantly the growth of the nasomaxillary complex. Good technique consists of anatomic reduction of fractures, minimal periosteal elevation, and careful repair of soft tissues.[13] Cosmetically pleasing surgical approaches, such as the bicoronal and sublabial incisions and the transconjunctival approach to the orbit floor, should be used in children in appropriate situations. An exciting new frontier for the repair of facial fractures in children is the availability of bioresorbable plating systems. Resorbable plates may lessen the impact of the repair on further facial growth.

The vast majority of pediatric patients have satisfactory outcomes from repairs following their facial trauma, despite the liberal use of observation alone in the care of many younger pediatric patients. Favorable fractures, high osteogenic potential with early healing, and overall good health probably play important roles in these good outcomes. Residual deformity, facial growth abnormalities, malunion, infection, and malocclusion affect the occasional pediatric patient.[2] Additionally, children rarely may develop chronic sinusitis or plate exposure and require additional surgical intervention. Because of children's more rapid healing, early primary intervention when required may improve outcome.

BIORESORBABLE FIXATION PLATES

Titanium metal plates have some potential drawbacks when used in the pediatric patient. Risk factors entailed in their use in the pediatric patient include interference with normal craniofacial growth; potential visibility and palpability; tenderness and thermal sensitivity of the plates; interference with diagnostic imaging techniques; and possible intracranial translocation of the plates and screws, with inflammation of the adjacent dura and cerebral tissue.[14] Clinicians have looked for alternatives to metal plate fixations, and thus there has been much interest in biodegradable plate fixation. Animal models using bioresorbable bone fixation have showed promising results, and there is now a modest history of plate use in pediatric patients.[15]

Resorbable plates and screws are usually made of macromolecular chains of repeating polymer subunits of poly-α-hydroxy acids, the same polymers as are used in the manufacture of resorbable sutures. The three most common polymers utilized in the six commercially available resorbable plating systems are polyglycolic acid (PGA), poly-L-lactic acid (PLLA), and poly-DL-lactic acid (PDLLA). PGA has the greatest strength of the three, but also loses that strength and mass more quickly. PDLLA has lower strength and an intermediate length of degradation, and PLLA is intermediate in strength and has the longest degradation time. All three polymers are stable at body temperature, but when heated become soft and flexible. This is important in adjusting the plates for fixation of the convoluted bony surfaces.

The biologic degradation of these plates occurs in two phases. The first phase is hydrolysis, where the strength is lost because the long macromolecule chains are cleaved into shorter polymeric chains, and the second is the metabolic phase, where the plate volume is lost as macrophages phagocytose the polymers, which are eventually metabolized by the liver into CO_2. Following this second phase of biodegradation, there is bony in-growth into the space previously occupied by the plates.

Resorbable plates were first introduced into clinical use in the mid-1990s and have primarily been used since that time for craniofacial procedures of the middle and upper face to repair congenital defects, as well as trauma cases. Existing studies have shown that resorbable plating systems can provide adequate rigidity and immobilization through routine osteosynthesis within the upper and middle facial skeleton. This means that resorbable plating systems are not only viable, but possibly a preferred method for elective pediatric craniofacial reconstruction as well as repair of orbital and maxillary fractures that require open reduction and internal fixation. In a retrospective study, Imola et al[15] found that bony healing, rates of anatomic union, and incidences of complications such as infection, poor healing, and plate extrusion were comparable to those seen with traditional metal plate fixation for all nonmandibular fractures and other craniofacial procedures. An intense inflammatory response, initially reported as a significant

drawback to this technique, has not been seen with the newer bioresorbable plates. These authors noted that palpable and/or protuberant hardware was a common adverse effect after surgery, but this was not considered a complication because it uniformly regressed as the plates were resorbed and was not a persistent problem.

Because of high complication rates, including delayed healing, infection, and plate extrusion, resorbable plate use is not recommended for repair of mandibular fractures. These complications are likely due in large part to the significant muscular forces on plates that occur during mastication. Indeed, for all facial fracture repairs, the necessary tensile strength and reconstructive parameters should be considered individually. Patients who have significant amounts of bone loss or who require repair of areas that have considerable masticatory or other muscular forces may not be candidates for resorbable plate systems. Possibly in the future there will be development of resorbable plates that have greater strength.

One inventive application of resorbable systems in the treatment of mandibular fractures has been reported: a novel technique for maxillomandibular fixation.[16] In this technique the author places a resorbable screw into each zygoma and attaches each screw to a large circummandibular suture. Seven patients with condylar fractures were treated with a total fixation time of 3 weeks in all cases. All these fractures progressed to complete healing and patients had unrestricted oral opening. The author also found that five of these children could have the suture removed in the office; the resorbable screw was allowed to go on to a natural biologic absorption. As additional experience with these plating systems accumulates, it is expected that other unique and original uses for repair of traumatic injuries will be developed.

Most resorbable plating systems have an array of plate and screw sizes and configurations comparable to titanium offerings (Fig. **16–4**). The resorbable mesh, which can be cut and contoured to complex surfaces, can be particularly useful in patients with complex fractures. The use of bioresorbable plates is not without its drawbacks, however. The technique of resorbable plate fixation can require extreme precision, and thus there is a significant learning curve with initial procedures lasting quite a bit longer than conventional metal plate fixation procedures.[17] Resorbable plates and screws are molded and bent to their ideal configuration using heat instead of force. Plates are heated with a heat pack, a hot air heating device, or a hot contour pen, or are placed in a metal bath, depending on the particular

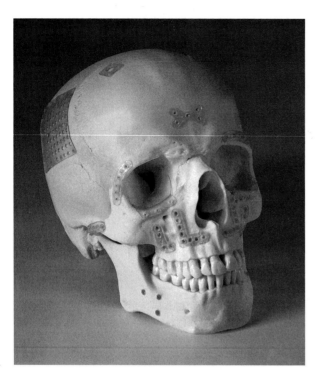

FIGURE 16–4 Example on a model of the variety of bioresorbable plate offerings and their possible anatomic uses. (Product graphic for Lactosorb®. Copyright © 2004 W. Lorenz Surgical. All rights reserved.)

product used. This molding and bending can be somewhat more delicate than bending of conventional titanium plates. Additionally, the plates and screws are bulkier than conventional metal plates and have a more prominent profile when placed. The resorbable plates and screws can be less forgiving than conventional metal plate fixation, and the screws in particular seem to be more susceptible to screw head shearing or thread stripping. Because many of the screws are not self-tapping, it is important that the initial holes be carefully drilled to an adequate depth beyond the screw length and then the hole tapped for its full length so that the screw can completely fix in place. With experience the amount of time to achieve stable fixation using resorbable plates may become only minimally longer than using conventional metal plates. As greater experience is gained and products are modified, these issues are likely to become less of a problem.

Though resorbable plates have been used in pediatric craniofacial surgery for barely a decade, they have enjoyed a successful track record and their use is routine in many centers today. Many of the lessons and principles used in elective craniofacial procedures can be carried over into the realm of the repair of pediatric facial-maxillofacial trauma. The outlook for use of resorbable plates in pediatric facial trauma is bright.

Special Consideration in the Pediatric Patient with Facial Trauma: Child Abuse

Child abuse may occasionally be a factor in pediatric patients with facial trauma. The rate of incidence of child abuse and neglect in the United States ranges from 15 to 42 per 1000 children.[18] Abused children are usually young: 67% are younger than 1 year of age, and 80% are younger than 3 years of age.[19] Children with congenital anomalies, mental retardation or other handicaps, and chronic or recurrent illnesses are at increased risk of incurring abuse. Historical, physical, and parental factors that may raise the suspicion of child abuse as an etiology of facial trauma are summarized in Table **16–4**. The history should begin with open-ended questions about how the injuries were sustained. Interviewing a child alone may be necessary. Evaluation of the general appearance of the child as well as examination of the entire body should be performed. Other head and neck manifestations of child abuse are summarized in Table **16–5**. In some cases laboratory evaluations including clotting studies, chemistry panels, urine chemistries, and toxicology screens may be required to evaluate for other disorders or injuries. It cannot be emphasized too strongly that injuries inconsistent with the proposed mechanism should be further investigated.

Radiographic evaluation for suspected child abuse primarily depends on the suspected injuries and the age of the child. Associated disorders, such as bony dysplasia, and extent of injuries can be evaluated by appropriate radiographic studies. A skeletal survey may be recommended especially if child abuse is suspected and the child is under 2 years of age.[20] The standard skeletal survey includes anteroposterior (AP) and lateral views of the skull and chest; lateral views of the spine; AP views of the pelvis, long bones of the extremities, and feet; and posteroanterior oblique views of the hands. Skull fractures may require both plain radiography and CT scanning for complete evaluation.[21] Skull base and temporal bone fractures are evaluated best with CT, but skull fractures may be detected more reliably by plain radiographs. Central nervous system injuries may occur in children who are shaken violently and those who are injured by high-energy impact forces. Magnetic resonance imaging or CT scanning can be used to detect and follow these injuries. Blunt trauma to the spine, chest, or abdomen may also be seen in the intentionally or unintentionally injured child.

TABLE 16–4   Summary of Common Factors and Findings that May Raise the Suspicion of Child Abuse

History	• History provided is inconsistent with the injuries of the child • History provided is inconsistent with the developmental stage of the child • History provided is not plausible • History changes in repeated versions given by the same caretaker • History is vague • No explanation of injuries is offered
Physical exam	• Injuries are not consistent with the history • Multiple injuries are seen and are in various stages of healing • Coexisting injuries are present (bruises, burns, fractures) • Injuries pathognomonic for child abuse exist (e.g., cigarette burns) • Child behaves inappropriately (child is too compliant with the examiner or is withdrawn, passive, or depressed; or is violent) • Of note: poor caregiving correlates more strongly with neglect and/or poverty than with abuse
Parental behavior	• Arguing, roughness, or violence is observed • Emotional interaction between parents or between parents and children is poor • Response to the severity of the injury is inappropriate • There is a delay in seeking medical care • Parent offers a partial confession

Data obtained from Endom EE. Diagnostic evaluation and management of suspected child abuse. UpToDate Web site. Available at: http://www.uptodate.com.

The goal of the diagnostic evaluation of the child with suspected abuse is to determine whether the level of suspicion is sufficiently high to warrant making a report to Child Protective Services (CPS).[22] All 50 states have laws requiring physicians to report child neglect to CPS, although the specific mechanism varies by state. Complete documentation of factual information should be made. Photographs are useful adjuncts to the medical record. If consultation with a multidisciplinary team (e.g., social worker, nurse, physician with more extensive experience in the management of child abuse) is available, it should be obtained.[18] Most states provide immunity from legal liability for reporters in good faith. Though serious consequences may occur for the family if the report is unsubstantiated, the

TABLE 16–5   Head and Neck Manifestations of Possible Child Abuse

Orofacial injuries	• Fractures of the maxilla, mandible, or other facial bones • Concerning burn or bruising patterns (see below) • Dental fractures or tooth discoloration from repeated trauma • Bruising, lichenification, or scarring at the corners of the mouth from being gagged • Oropharyngeal gonorrhea or syphilis • Black eyes (periorbital ecchymosis) from direct trauma • Basilar skull fractures ("raccoon eyes," Battle sign, or hemotympanum) • Hair loss from being pulled by the hair
Bruising patterns that may be associated with abuse	• Patterns or history not consistent with natural play and/or the developmental stage of the child • Handprints or finger marks • Belt marks (lines or buckle marks) • Loop marks (from trauma with a doubled-up wire, rope, or electric cord) • Linear bruising or petechiae of the apical rim of the pinna • Ligature marks or rope burns may be seen on the neck or at the corners of the mouth (due to strangling or gagging) • Bruises in multiple stages of healing
Burn patterns that may be seen with abuse	• Brands/contact burns • Cigarette burns • Burns from caustic materials or scalding liquids • Immersion burns • Microwave oven burns • Stun gun burns

Data obtained from Endom EE. Epidemiology and clinical manifestations of child abuse. UpToDate Web site. Available at: http://www.uptodate.com.

potential consequences for the child of unreported child abuse are more serious because the consequences may be life-threatening injury or death. An abused child has a 50% chance of incurring further abuse and a 10% chance of dying if abuse is not detected at the initial presentation.[23] The National Clearinghouse on Child Abuse and Neglect provides additional information and resources regarding prevention, management, and statutes regarding reporting of child abuse and neglect (*http://www.calib.com/nccanch/*).

OROPHARYNGEAL TRAUMA

Children (especially toddlers) by their nature, have a tendency to run and play with objects in their mouth. Thus, intraoral trauma is a common occurrence. Although the vast majority of these injuries to the soft palate, tonsil, and posterior pharyngeal regions are minor, there is potential for serious injury. Anatomically, the close proximity of the carotid artery, vagus nerve, sympathetic plexus, glossopharyngeal nerve, hypoglossal nerve, and jugular vein in the lateral aspect of the soft palate and pharynx make them particularly susceptible to penetrating traumatic injury (Fig. **16–5**). Injuries typically occur due to (1) falling on an object carried in the mouth, (2) direct force applied to an object being held in the mouth, or (3) falling or running into a stationary object with the mouth open.[24] The vast majority of children affected with this type of injury are toddlers with a mean age of 3 to 4 years.[24–27] There is generally a male predominance, although this varies widely between studies. The most common offending objects are sticks, pens and pencils, and toothbrushes, but an extremely wide variety of other objects have been known to cause traumatic intraoral injury.

Oropharyngeal trauma is common and usually heals without incident but it may on occasion lead to development of rare, severe neurologic sequelae.[28] It is therefore necessary to have a rational and thoughtful approach to the treatment of children with these traumas. Although the evaluation and management of patients should be individualized, in general the following questions need to be addressed: (1) Are any radiologic studies necessary? (2) Is hospitalization necessary? (3) Is any surgical intervention necessary? (4) Are antibiotics necessary? (5) Is anticoagulation or other medial treatment necessary?

Evaluation of the child with intraoral trauma is aimed at determining the extent of soft tissue injury and determining if there are secondary injuries to any of the underlying neurovascular structures. A thorough head and neck and neurologic examina-

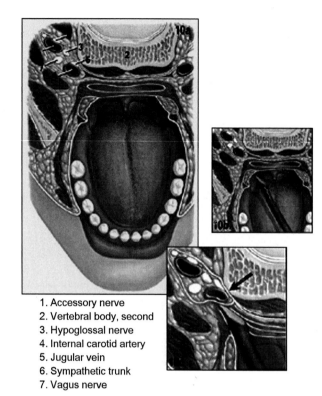

1. Accessory nerve
2. Vertebral body, second
3. Hypoglossal nerve
4. Internal carotid artery
5. Jugular vein
6. Sympathetic trunk
7. Vagus nerve

FIGURE 16–5 The mechanism of carotid injury secondary to impalement from a palatal foreign body. (From Handler S. Soft palate trauma in a child. *Patient of the Month Program*, vol. 28, number 1, 1998. © 1998, American Academy of Otolaryngology. Decker Electronic Publishing, Inc.)

tion should be performed. Interval examination may be required because in patients with carotid artery injuries there may be a lucid, asymptomatic period that may last for hours or even days before the development of neurologic symptoms.[27] Findings commonly associated with blunt internal carotid artery trauma include (1) hematoma in the lateral neck area, (2) ipsilateral Horner's syndrome, (3) transient ischemic attacks, (4) focal neurologic deficits, and (5) hemiparesis in an alert and oriented patient.[26]

Carotid artery injuries range from temporary spasm to intimal tears with development of mural thrombus to compression and even to complete occlusion. In patients who have sustained trauma to the internal carotid artery, the mechanism of the development of neurologic sequelae is theorized to occur as follows: the internal carotid artery becomes trapped against the transverse process of the second or third cervical vertebrae or against the skull base, which results in an intimal tear of the vessel.[24] This tear may further lead to either dissection or formation of a mural thrombus. Although these injuries tend to be focal and not as diffuse as those sustained in less localized blunt trauma such as a motor vehicle accident, nonetheless, they can lead to embolic phenomenon due to an ascending thrombus eventually affecting the middle cerebral artery.

Patients in whom carotid artery injury is suspected because of neurologic symptoms, presence of a cervical hematoma or injury seen on radiographic imaging, should have carotid arteriography. Arteriography is the "gold standard" for evaluating patients for carotid injury; however, the test itself carries some risks, and is not widely available in many emergency centers 24 hours a day. Thus, generally, this test should be reserved for patients in whom there is a high suspicion of carotid artery injury. Although invasive angiography is considered the gold standard for determining the site and extent of carotid artery injury, the radiologic literature does support the use of magnetic resonance angiography (MRA). In some studies MRA has shown an equal sensitivity to detecting carotid artery injury when compared with invasive angiography.

Several authors have promoted the use of CT of the neck with intravenous contrast as a screening examination for patients with lateral or pharyngeal trauma. As well as being readily available in the majority of emergency centers, this test has the advantages of providing additional information about the presence of free air in the neck and potential information about injury to other cervical structures.[25,28] It may also give information about a retained foreign body. Other screening tests that may be used in appropriate situations are soft tissue lateral neck film (to determine if retropharyngeal air is present), chest radiograph (to rule out pneumomediastinum), carotid Doppler, and ocular pneumoculoplethysmography.[26] These tests each have different advantages and disadvantages; it should be remembered that angiography or possibly MRA may be necessary to confirm and delineate any actual carotid artery injuries.

Hospitalization of children with palatal injuries has undergone an evolution ranging from discharge to compulsory hospital admission for observation. A balanced approach to these patients would suggest that child certainly should be hospitalized if there are signs of infection or retropharyngeal or thoracic free air, or if there are signs of carotid injury. The majority of patients, however, can be managed as outpatients if there is reliable adult supervision of the child and appropriate education is given. Table 16–6 provides a sample instruction sheet for the parents of children with a palatal injury. Because generally there is a lucid period between the onset of injury and the onset of neurologic sequelae that may

range from hours to days, this observation should occur for a minimum of 48 to 72 hours. As discussed above, radiologic evaluation of a child with oropharyngeal trauma is somewhat controversial but should be performed when injury is suspected.

Surgical intervention is not commonly required in the treatment of these lesions. Surgical intervention is usually directed at closing large through-and-through defects of the palate and removal of impaled foreign bodies. Other surgical procedures sometimes indicated in specific patients are laryngoscopy and bronchoscopy; needle aspiration of the retropharynx; and incision and drainage of retropharyngeal abscess and neck exploration, particularly for proximal and distal control of the carotid artery before removal of impaled foreign body. Fortunately, in most series, fewer than 10% of patients required surgical intervention for closure of the defects, and fewer than half of the hospitalized patients required any surgical intervention at all. Note that it is generally agreed that a patient with a retained intraoral foreign body should be taken to the operating room for controlled removal of the foreign body, possibly with distal and proximal control of the carotid artery depending on radiographic imaging and whether or not there is obvious carotid artery involvement.

Oral injuries over 1 cm in size benefit from antibiotic coverage to prevent secondary infection. Most authors recommend routine prophylactic antibiotic coverage for patients with oropharyngeal trauma. The risk of infection is small, but in one

TABLE 16–6 Sample Instruction Form for Observation of Pediatric Oropharyngeal Trauma Patients

A child with a palatal injury should be observed for at least 48 to 72 hours after injury. If any of the following symptoms occur, a doctor should be contacted immediately:

- Blurred vision
- Decreased level of consciousness (child is drowsy, does not wake, does not recognize familiar people or objects)
- Convulsions (seizures or fits)
- Vomiting
- Weakness of an arm or leg (child stumbles, falls more than usual)
- Irritability (child is fussy, cannot be calmed)
- Headache
- Bleeding from the mouth

Adapted from Handler S. Soft palate trauma in a child. *Patient of the Month Program*, vol. 28, number 1, 1998. © 1998, American Academy of Otolaryngology. Decker Electronic Publishing, Inc.

series of 48 patients, even with the use of oral prophylactic antibiotics, one patient did require readmission and treatment with intravenous antibiotics for a development of a retropharyngeal abscess.[25]

In a child with a suspected or obvious carotid artery injury, treatment is aimed at the prevention of neurologic sequelae. How this goal is achieved, however, is controversial. Many authors recommend anticoagulation because some research has shown that improved vascular flow to infarcted areas may occur with the use of anticoagulation. On balance, however, there is also concern that its use may convert an ischemic focus to a hemorrhagic infarct, as can be seen in anticoagulation of patients sustaining other cerebral vascular accidents. Once anticoagulation with heparin has been started, it does appear prudent to continue with outpatient anticoagulation with aspirin for a period of several months until complete intimal healing as occurred. Further treatment of patients with thrombosis with thrombolysis of surgical accessible vessels may be cautiously considered.

In summary, intraoral injuries are common, especially in toddler children, and, although usually minor, there is the potential for severe neurologic sequelae. Evaluation and treatment should be aimed at determining if surgical intervention is necessary; determining if carotid injury is likely and if performing angiography is necessary possibly by performing screening CT of the neck; determining if hospitalization is necessary; preventing infection; and providing education of the family as to what signs and symptoms should warrant return to the hospital. Treatment of patients with documented carotid injury may include anticoagulation, but treatment should be individualized for the particular patient and particular injury. Awareness of the lucid interval that may exist between the time of injury and the presentation of neurologic symptoms is imperative.

PEARLS: PEDIATRIC FACIAL TRAUMA

- Pediatric facial dimensions impact the patterns of injury that are sustained.
- Prominence of the skull and orbit, especially in younger children, leads to higher incidence of associated, often cranial, injuries.
- Continued facial growth and rapid osteogenesis affects treatment choices.
- Children require more rapid fracture reduction because of quicker healing.
- Mandibular injuries can often be treated by closed techniques.

- Children should receive short periods of immobilization of the mandible to prevent temporomandibular joint ankylosis.
- Resorbable fixation plates are best used in the repair of nonmandibular facial fractures and may improve long-term facial growth when compared with permanent plates.
- Outcomes for repairs of facial trauma are generally good.
- Patients with penetrating lateral oropharyngeal trauma may require CT scan and possibly arteriogram to identify secondary vascular injuries, but many patients can be safely observed by an educated caregiver.

REFERENCES

1. Gussack GS, Luterman A, Rodgers, Powell RW, Ramenofsky ML. Pediatric maxillofacial trauma: unique features in diagnosis and treatment. Laryngoscope 1987;97:925–930
2. Koltai PJ, Radkin D, Hoehn J. Rigid fixation of facial fractures in children. J Craniomaxillofac Trauma 1995; 1:32–42
3. McGraw B, Cole R. Pediatric maxillofacial trauma Arch Otolaryngol Head Neck Surg 1990;116:41–45
4. Manson PN, Markowitz B, Mirvis S, Dunham M, Yaremchuk M. Toward CT-based facial fracture treatment. Plast Reconstr Surg 1990;85:202–212
5. Colton JJ, Beeknuts GJ. Management of nasal fractures. Otolaryngol Clin North Am 1986;19:73–85
6. Koltai PJ, Rabkin D. Management of facial trauma in children Pediatr North Am 1996;43:1253–1275
7. Koltai PJ. Craniofacial skeletal trauma in childhood: child with facial trauma. In: Cotton RT, Myer III CM, eds. *Practical Pediatric Otolaryngology*. Philadelphia: Lippincott-Raven, 1999:729
8. Thaller SR, Madourakh S. Pediatric mandibular fractures. Ann Plast Surg 1991;26:511–513
9. Chu L, Gussack G, Muller T. A treatment protocol for mandible fractures. J Trauma 1994;36:48–52
10. McGuirt WF, Salisbury PL. Mandibular fractures Arch Otolaryngol Head Neck Surg 1989;113:257–261
11. Demianczuk AN, Verchere C, Phillips JH. The effect on facial growth of pediatric mandibular fractures. J Craniofac Surg 1999;10:323–328
12. Koenig WR, Olsson AB, Pensler JM. The fate of developing teeth in facial trauma: tooth buds in the line of mandibular fractures in children. Ann Plast Surg 1994;32:503–505
13. Crockett DM, Funk GF. Management of complicated fractures involving the orbits and nasoethmoid complex in young children. Otolaryngol Clin North Am 1991;24:119–136
14. Honig JF, Merten HA, Luhr HG. Passive and active intracranial translocation of osteosynthesis plates in adolescent minipigs. J Craniofac Surg 1995;6:292–298

15. Imola MJ, Hamlar DD, Shao W, Chowdhury K, Tatum S. Resorbable plate fixation in pediatric craniofacial surgery: long term outcome. Arch Facial Plast Surg 2001;3:79–90

16. Eppley BL. A resorbable and rapid method for maxillomandibular fixation in pediatric mandible fractures. J Craniofac Surg 2000;11:236–238

17. Imola MJ, Schramm VL. Resorbable internal fixation in pediatric cranial base surgery. Laryngoscope 2002; 112:1897–1901

18. Ludwig S. Child abuse. In: Fleisher, GR, Ludwig S, eds. Textbook *of Pediatric Emergency Medicine*. Philadelphia: Lippincott Williams & Wilkins, 2000:1669

19. Endom EE. Epidemiology and clinical manifestations of child abuse. *UpToDate web site*. Available at *http://www.uptodate.com*

20. Endom EE. Diagnostic evaluation and management of suspected child abuse. *UpToDate web site*. Available at *http://www.uptodate.com*

21. Diagnostic imaging of child abuse. *Pediatrics* 2000;105: 1345

22. American Academy of Pediatrics Committee on Child Abuse and Neglect. Shaken baby syndrome: inflicted cerebral trauma. *Pediatrics* 1993;92:872–875

23. Saade DN, Simon HK, Greenwald M. Abused children. Missed opportunities for recognition in the ED. Acad Emerg Med 2000;9:524

24. Hellmann JR, Shott SR, Gootee MJ. Impalement injuries of the palate in children: review of 131 cases. Int J Pediatr Otorhinolaryngol 1993;26:157–163

25. Ratcliff DJ, Okada PJ, Murray AD. Evaluation of pediatric lateral oropharyngeal trauma. Otolaryngol Head Neck Surg 2003;128:783–787

26. Schoem SR, Choi SS, Zalzal GH, Grundfast KM. Management of oropharyngeal trauma in children. Arch Otolaryngol Head Neck Surg 1997;123: 1267–1270

27. Radkowski D, McGill TJ, Healy GB, Jones DT. Penetrating trauma of the oropharynx in children. Laryngoscope 1993;103:991–994

28. Handler S. Soft palate trauma in a child. *Patient of the Month Program*, vol 28, number 1. American Academy of Otolaryngology, 1998

Chapter 17

Auricular Trauma

C.Y. Joseph Chang

Injuries to the auricle can be categorized as hematoma, laceration, partial avulsion, or complete avulsion. This chapter provides an overview of evaluation and management of these injuries. Table **17–1** summarizes the injuries and treatments.

Anatomy

The pinna is composed entirely of soft tissues. The cartilage forms the structural framework of the pinna and defines the overall shape as well as the intricate folds and contours. The skin is closely adherent to the underlying perichondrium on the anterior surface. On the medial surface, there is a thicker subcutaneous layer separating the skin from the perichondrium. The lobule is the only auricular structure that is not supported underneath by cartilage.

Evaluation

In general, the type and extent of injury can be fully assessed by visual inspection. The examination should include assessment of adjacent structures such as the external auditory canal, facial nerve, and Stensen's duct, which could be injured concurrently. In cases of auricular laceration, the examiner should determine whether the injury involves the skin and subcutaneous tissues only or whether the cartilage and perichondrium are involved. If there is an avulsion, the avulsed piece should be identified for potential use in the repair.

Hematoma

Auricular hematomas most commonly occur as a result of blunt trauma to the auricle. The hematoma is thought to form after the skin and perichondrium are sheared from the underlying cartilage, causing formation of a potential space and hemorrhage. Examination typically shows a bulge under the skin that obliterates the normal cartilaginous contour of the pinna. The area is typically fluctuant and tender. There should be no findings suggestive of infection such as cellulitis, which could indicate the presence of abscess. The main sequela of untreated auricular hematoma is the so-called cauliflower ear, which is a permanent deformity that results from damage to the cartilaginous framework and formation of soft tissue fibrosis and calcification. The auricular hematoma is most easily treated early, within 2 weeks of the injury, at which point the hematoma can be drained through an incision overlying the area. To prevent reaccumulation of blood, a bolster should be applied to provide pressure within the various affected areas. The bolster can be made with various items, but petrolatum gauze rolled into shape works quite well (Fig. **17–1**). The bolster should be applied with through-and-through sutures, and left in place for at least 5 days.

If the hematoma is not treated early, granulation tissue and early fibrosis can occur. In these cases, the wound may need to be debrided prior to placement of the bolster as described previously. If the injury is left untreated for 2 months or more, permanent damage of the cartilage, with calcification and overlying fibrosis, can occur, resulting in permanent deformity of the auricle. Once this permanent deformity occurs, the appearance of the auricle can

TABLE 17–1   SUMMARY OF THE INJURIES AND TREATMENTS OF AURICULAR TRAUMA

Injury	Treatment
Hematoma	Incision and drainage with placement of bolsters
Laceration	Primary repair, including repair of cartilage as needed
Partial avulsion	Primary repair, including repair of cartilage as needed; the wound requires close observation for onset of necrosis
Complete avulsion, small segment < 1 cm	Primary repair and reattachment of avulsed section, including repair of cartilage as needed; the wound requires close observation for onset of vascular compromise
Complete avulsion, total or near total	1. Reattachment with microvascular vessel anastomosis 2. Placement of de-epithelialized cartilage framework in postauricular subcutaneous pocket for later reconstruction 3. Reattachment without vessel repair; probable high chance of failure with loss of cartilage

be improved with reconstructive surgery, but the original appearance of the pinna cannot be restored.

LACERATIONS

As in all repairs, the wound should be cleared of all debris and irrigated prior to prepping and draping. Auricular lacerations are best repaired primarily as with any other open wound due to trauma. If cartilage has been damaged, the lacerated edges should be reapproximated with absorbable suture. Subsequently, the overlying skin can be closed. In general, it is difficult to perform layered closure of the lateral aspect of the pinna because there is inadequate subcutaneous tissue. On the medial aspect, a layered closure can be performed. The cartilage repair can be performed with 5-0 or 6-0 absorbable suture such as chromic gut. The skin repair is usually performed with 5-0 or 6-0 nylon or fast absorbing gut.

Complex and large lacerations are often challenging to close. The various edges of the lacerations should be brought together, and any injured cartilage should be sutured first. It is important to minimize debridement of skin; only completely nonviable or crushed tissues should be removed.

Lacerations that involve the meatus require close attention to the adequacy of skin coverage. If no skin has been lost, primary closure should prevent meatal stenosis. If there has been significant skin loss or separation of the meatus from the external auditory canal, the meatus and canal should be aligned and a meatal pack consisting of material such as polyethylene mesh or Silastic should be used. The packing can be removed in 7 to 14 days. If meatal stenosis or atresia occurs, a meatoplasty with skin graft corrects the problem in most cases.

PARTIAL AND TOTAL AVULSIONS

When there is a segment of tissue partially or completely detached from the remaining pinna, repair should be performed with the goal of restoring as much of the original anatomy as possible.

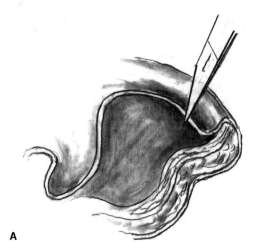

A

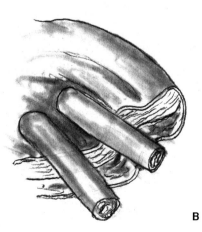

B

FIGURE 17–1   A: Auricular hematoma being incised. B: Bolsters applied to prevent recurrence of hematoma.

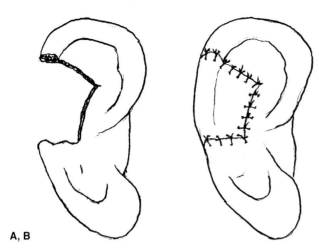

A, B

FIGURE 17–2 A: Avulsion injury of small section of pinna. B: Avulsion section reattached.

Because it is difficult to replace the skin overlying the auricle secondarily, it is important to preserve as much tissue as possible during the initial repair. Regardless of how small a pedicle exists to a partially avulsed portion, the tissues should be replaced and sutured. Due to the robust blood supply to the pinna, a relatively large area of partial avulsion often survives even if the associated pedicle is quite small. Similarly, completely avulsed portions often survive if replaced and sutured, as long as the reattached section is less than 1 cm in size (Fig. 17–2). The cartilage should be secured first with absorbable sutures, followed by repair of the skin and subcutaneous tissues. The reattached area needs to be monitored closely for evidence of vascular compromise and tissue necrosis.

If the avulsed portion is larger, survival of the avulsed segment after primary repair becomes problematic. In these cases, it is more prudent to bury the avulsed cartilage under the skin in an adjacent postauricular pocket after removing all overlying skin. The cartilage may later be used in reconstruction using local skin flaps.

In cases of skin avulsion with intact underlying cartilage, the treatment approach depends on the depth of injury. If the perichondrium is intact, the open area can be allowed to heal by secondary intent for small areas (<3 mm), or skin grafted either primarily or in a delayed fashion after initial cleaning and debridement of the wound. If the perichondrium is not intact, the underlying cartilage is at risk for infection and subsequent resorption. In these cases, the exposed cartilage can be resected if the injury is in a concave area such as the concha, or covered by a rotational flap of tissue from surrounding areas otherwise. The exposed tissues can then be covered by skin graft. A skin graft should not be placed directly over cartilage without perichondrium because there is not adequate blood supply to support the graft.

In cases of avulsed tissues that are not available for replacement during initial repair, the remaining pinna should be repaired primarily. The repair should be aimed at restoring the original shape of the pinna, even if the repair results in a reduction in its size. Deformities such as the "cup ear" should be avoided. After the initial healing period, auricular reconstruction may be possible if needed, depending on the nature of the defect.

Complete avulsions of all or a large part of the auricle are a challenging problem. The avulsed tissue should be kept cool but not frozen prior to reattachment. There has been some success reported with simple reattachment without microvascular repair,[1] but the success rate is thought to be quite low. Another option is to remove the skin from the avulsed cartilage and to implant the cartilage under the postauricular skin for secondary reconstruction. A similar technique involves dermabrasion of the avulsed segment, reattachment and placement in a postauricular pocket. At 2 to 3 weeks, the buried portion is exposed and allowed to reepithelialize.[2,3] If a microvascular team is not available, these options may be considered. However, the current practice is to perform reattachment with microvascular anastomosis.[4,5]

Reattachment of an avulsed pinna using microvascular techniques has been described since 1980. The main technical difficulties include finding blood vessels adequate for anastomosis, especially on the venous side, and then finding appropriately sized donor vessels for anastomosis to these tiny vessels of the pinna. The venous anastomosis is often tenuous, and the repaired pinna typically develops significant venous congestion. Various treatments have been implemented to alleviate this problem, including administration of heparin, aspirin, and low molecular weight dextran, as well as placement of stab wounds in the reattached tissues to allow egress of venous blood. More recently, the use of leeches has garnered interest. The leeches release an anticoagulant into the reattached tissue and remove venous blood from the area.

INFECTION

An infection occurring in the pinna is especially problematic because spread of infection to the cartilage can result in chondritis and subsequent loss of the pinna's structural integrity followed by significant auricular deformity. It is important to prevent infection after trauma, especially after bite wounds. Prior to repair, the wound should be thoroughly cleared of debris and irrigated. In most cases not involving bite injuries or severe contamination of the wound, primary closure with a dose of intravenous antibiotics and oral antibiotics for 5 to 7 days is adequate (Table 17–2).

Based on a review of human bite wounds to the face, Stierman et al[6] identified several factors that predispose patients to wound infection. These include wounds closed primarily, presence of exposed cartilage, avulsion injury to the ear, and less than 48 hours of intravenous antibiotics. Therefore, cases at significant risk of infection should be treated aggressively with intravenous antibiotics and delayed repair as needed. Antibiotic coverage for routine wounds should cover gram-positive organisms such as *Staphylococcus* and *Streptococcus*. For bite injuries, the coverage should be broadened to cover oral organisms such as *Corynebacterium* and anaerobes.

Wound infection requires immediate treatment with systemic antibiotics. Superficial or mild infections can be treated with oral antibiotics, but any patient with significant cellulitis or evidence of deeper infection, such as abscess, perichondritis, or chondritis, should be treated with intravenous antibiotics. The infectious organism is usually a gram-positive bacterium such as *Staphylococcus* and *Streptococcus*. Infections related to burn injuries have a high incidence of *Pseudomonas*,[7] but it is not clear if this is the case for non-burn-related chondritis. Nonetheless, it would be prudent to treat all serious infections of the auricle with broad-spectrum coverage for both gram-positive and gram-negative organ-

isms until culture results can narrow the treatment regimen.

Any abscess requires incision and drainage, with placement of a drain if needed. The development of chondritis typically results in an infection that does not respond to appropriate antibiotic treatment. In these cases, a more locally invasive treatment is needed. In the past, total or near-total removal of the cartilage was performed. This procedure usually results in improved response of the infection to antibiotic therapy but it also results in severe deformity of the pinna. If the area of infected cartilage is small, a limited resection may be effective without causing significant deformity. In the past, a locally intensive treatment has been described in which fenestrated catheters are placed surgically under the skin around the cartilage of the auricle[8,9] (Fig. 17–3). Antibiotics are irrigated through these catheters. Alternatively, iontophoresis has also been described as a method to infuse the auricular cartilage with antibiotics such as gentamicin.[10] Case reports have shown that these methods have been used successfully, but controlled studies have not been performed. There is no agreed-upon standard for treatment of this condition, but it may be reasonable to attempt these less deforming treatments prior to resorting to resection of large areas of cartilage. After initial surgical treatment, a prolonged period of antibiotics and local care is required. Even with conservative treatments, it is common to have some auricular deformity as a sequela of chondritis.

TABLE 17–2 PROPHYLAXIS RECOMMENDATIONS FOR TRAUMA TREATMENTS

Procedure	Antibiotic prophylaxis (example drug)
Incision and drainage of hematoma	Oral antibiotic 5 to 7 days (cephalexin)
Repair of laceration, clean	Single dose intravenous antibiotic (cefazolin) then oral antibiotic 5 to 7 days (cephalexin)
Repair of laceration, heavily contaminated or bite injury	Intravenous antibiotics (ticarcillin/clavulanate) 3 to 4 days followed by oral antibiotics 5 to 7 days (clindamycin/levofloxacin)

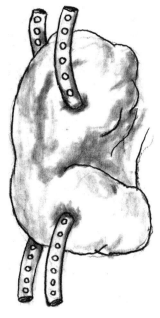

FIGURE 17–3 Irrigation catheters inserted for treatment of bacterial chondritis.

SUMMARY

Auricular trauma encompasses a variety of injury types, each requiring specific treatments for optimal results. The early initiation of appropriate treatment is the key to best outcomes. Complications related to delayed treatment can result in deformity and serious infection.

PEARLS: AURICLE TRAUMA

- Auricular hematomas should be drained within 2 weeks, to avoid the complication of "cauliflower ear."
- In general, lacerations should be closed primarily, in layers. Lacerations involving the meatus should be addressed with care, to avoid meatal stenosis.
- If the auricle is avulsed and there is a pedicle remaining, the remnant should be reattached with the pedicle intact, no matter how small the pedicle. Any tissue not surviving can be debrided later.
- The management of complete avulsion is more controversial, and reimplantation using the "pocket principle" and microvascular techniques have both been reported. Direct reattachment is not successful.
- Wound infection of the auricle requires treatment with systemic antibiotics.

REFERENCES

1. Bernstein L, Nelson RH. Replanting the severed auricle. An update. Arch Otolaryngol 1982;108: 587–590
2. Mladick RA, Carraway JH. Ear reattachment by the modified pocket principle. Case report. Plast Reconstr Surg 1973;51:584–587
3. Pribaz JJ, Crespo LD, Orgill DP, Pousti TJ, Bartlett RA. Ear replantation without microsurgery. Plast Reconstr Surg 1997;99:1868–1872
4. Turpin IM. Microsurgical replantation of the external ear. Clin Plast Surg 1990;17:397–404
5. Kind GM, Buncke GM, Placik OJ, Jansen DA, D'Amore T, Buncke HJ Jr. Total ear replantation. Plast Reconstr Surg 1997;99:1858–1867
6. Stierman KL, Lloyd KM, De Luca-Pytell DM, Phillips LG, Calhoun KH. Treatment and outcome of human bites in the head and neck. Otolaryngol Head Neck Surg 2003;128:795–801
7. Mills DC II, Roberts LW, Mason AD Jr, McManus WF, Pruitt BA Jr. Suppurative chondritis: its incidence, prevention, and treatment in burn patients. Plast Reconstr Surg 1988;82:267–276
8. Apfelberg DB, Waisbren BA, Masters FW, Robinson DW. Treatment of chondritis in the burned ear by the local instillation of antibiotics. Plast Reconstr Surg 1974;53:179–183
9. Baers HA. Otologic aspects of ear burns. Am J Otol 1981;2:235–242
10. Greminger RF, Elliott RA Jr, Rapperport A. Antibiotic iontophoresis for the management of burned ear chondritis. Plast Reconstr Surg 1980;66:356–360

Chapter 18

TEMPORAL BONE TRAUMA

John S. Oghalai

The topic of temporal bone trauma ranges from the aggressive use of a cotton-tipped applicator in the ear canal to massive traumatic injuries following motor vehicle accidents and gunshot wounds. Simple injuries may require only counseling the patient that the injury will heal spontaneously, whereas severe injuries may be associated with a comatose state, hospitalization for several months in a neurologic intensive care unit, and the need for multiple surgical procedures. Thus, the management of temporal bone trauma is complex and involves a broad spectrum of issues.

PERTINENT ANATOMY OF THE SKULL BASE

The anatomy of the skull base is the key to understanding the potential complications of temporal bone trauma (Fig. 18–1). The skull base includes the frontal bone, the sphenoid bone, the temporal bone, and the occipital bone. A fracture of the skull base (otherwise known as a basilar skull fracture) must involve at least one of these bones, and may involve all of them.

The auditory system lies within the temporal bone, and is often injured in patients who sustain temporal bone trauma. There are three segments to the auditory system: the external ear, the middle ear, and the inner ear. The external ear functions to funnel sound pressure waves to the tympanic membrane, and includes the pinna and the external auditory canal. The middle ear transmits the sound pressure waves from the air-filled outside environment to the fluid-filled inner ear, and includes the tympanic membrane and the ossicular chain. The inner ear converts the sound pressure waves into electrical signals, sending the signals to the brainstem for processing, and includes the cochlea and auditory nerve. As well, the inner ear contains the vestibular organs, which sense head position and send this information to the brainstem to help maintain balance and upright posture. Damage to the external or middle ear results in conductive hearing loss that is often repairable. Damage to the inner ear results in sensorineural hearing loss that is usually not recoverable, as well as vertigo.

All cranial nerves (CNs) exit the skull base. However, several are often involved in patients who sustain temporal bone trauma. Most importantly, the facial nerve (CN VII) exits the brainstem and courses through the temporal bone before exiting the stylomastoid foramen. It is within the temporal bone that the facial nerve is most commonly injured. The facial nerve injury is only briefly mentioned in this chapter because it is thoroughly covered in Chapter 19. The cranial nerves important for oculomotor control (CN III, IV, and VI) are also often affected in patients who sustain severe temporal bone trauma. They exit the brainstem, and course along the petrous apex and greater wing of the sphenoid bone. Fractures of the skull that affect these cranial nerves are usually associated with an initial comatose state.

The dura of the middle and posterior cranial fossa is adherent to the temporal bone. The temporal lobe lies superior and the cerebellum and brainstem lie posterior to the temporal bone. Thus, fractures that involve the intracranial surfaces of the temporal bone usually tear the dura, predisposing the patient to cerebrospinal fluid (CSF) leak and encephalocele formation.

Finally, the vascular anatomy of the temporal bone may be traumatized. Most importantly, the internal carotid artery enters the inferior aspect of the temporal bone, turns horizontally, and courses

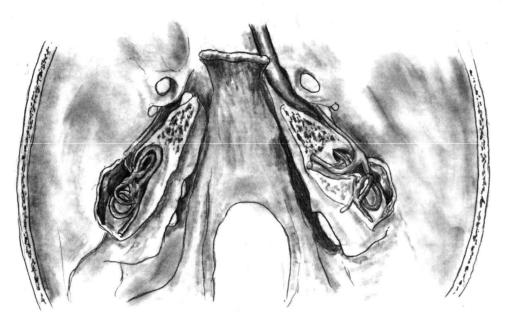

FIGURE 18–1 Top view of the skull base. The skull base consists of the occipital, temporal, sphenoid, and frontal bones. The external, middle, and inner ear lie within the temporal bone and are often affected by skull base fractures. Other structures commonly involved include the facial nerve, the internal carotid artery, and the sigmoid sinus–jugular vein system.

through the petrous portion of the temporal bone, before entering the cavernous sinus. Additionally, the middle meningeal artery, a branch of the external carotid artery, enters the cranium through the foramen spinosum and supplies the temporal lobe dura deep to the squamous portion of the temporal bone.

PATHOGENESIS OF TEMPORAL BONE TRAUMA (TABLE 18–1)

LOCAL TRAUMA

Injuries localized to the external or middle ear include auricular hematoma (covered in Chapter 17), external auditory canal abrasion or laceration, tympanic membrane perforation, and ossicular chain dislocation.[1] Local trauma to the tympanic membrane and ossicles can occur by a penetrating injury with objects such as a cotton-tipped applicator, a bobby pin, a pencil, or a hot metal slag during welding. Additionally, barotrauma, such as a slap to the ear or a blast injury, can cause a tympanic membrane perforation or ossicular chain dislocation.

BLUNT TRAUMA

Temporal bone fractures represent roughly 20% of all skull fractures. Risk factors include being male and under 21, as this population is more commonly involved in risky activities predisposing them to blunt head trauma. The most common etiologies include motor vehicle accidents, falls, bicycle accidents, seizures, and aggravated assaults. Blunt trauma to the lateral surface of the skull (the squamous portion of the temporal bone) often results in a longitudinal fracture (Fig. **18–2**).[2] Longitudinal fractures involve the squamous portion of the temporal bone, follow along the axis of the external auditory canal to the middle ear space, and then course anteriorly along the geniculate ganglion and eustachian tube, ending near the foramen lacerum. By definition, the otic capsule is spared in a longitudinal temporal bone fracture.

TABLE 18–1 CHARACTERISTICS OF TEMPORAL BONE FRACTURES

Longitudinal fracture
- Involves the external auditory canal and middle ear
- No involvement of the otic capsule
- Higher risk of conductive hearing loss
- Lower risk of sensorineural hearing loss
- Lower risk of facial nerve palsy

Transverse fracture
- Involves the foramen magnum and crosses the otic capsule
- Lower risk of conductive hearing loss
- Higher risk of sensorineural hearing loss
- Higher risk of facial nerve palsy

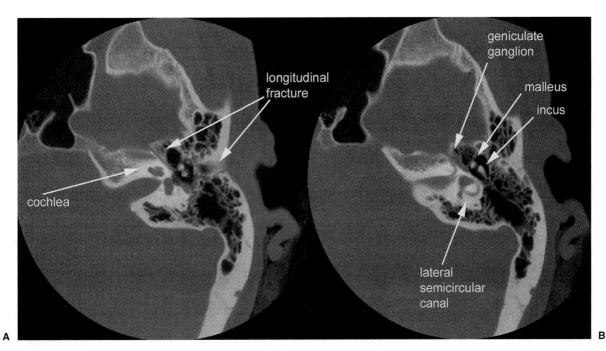

FIGURE 18–2 Axial computed tomography (CT) of a patient who sustained a longitudinal temporal bone fracture several months previously. This patient had a 60-dB conductive hearing loss with a normal tympanic membrane on physical exam. The inferior cut (A) demonstrates the line of the fracture. It coursed along the line of the external auditory canal and up to the geniculate ganglion. The patient did not have facial nerve dysfunction. The superior cut (B) shows ossicular dislocation secondary to separation of the incudomalleolar joint.

A blow to the occipital skull often goes through the foramen magnum and results in a transverse fracture of the temporal bone (Fig. **18–3**). Transverse fractures course directly across the petrous pyramid, fracturing the otic capsule, and extend anteriorly along the eustachian tube and geniculate ganglion.

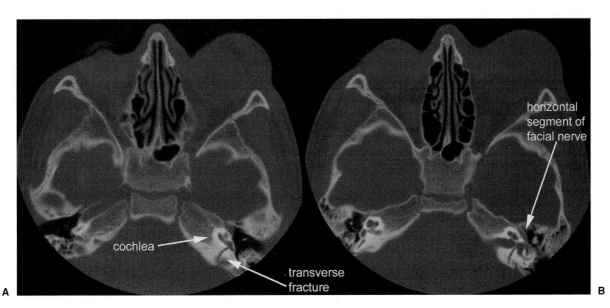

FIGURE 18–3 Axial computed tomography of an 8-year-old boy who sustained a transverse temporal bone fracture 2 weeks previously. This patient had nystagmus and a complete sensorineural hearing loss. The inferior cut (A) demonstrates the line of the fracture that extends through the dense, white bone of the otic capsule. The superior cut (B) shows that the fracture involves the canal of the horizontal segment of the facial nerve. Fortunately, the patient's facial function was normal.

Longitudinal temporal bone fractures represent 80% and transverse temporal bone fractures represent 20% of temporal bone fractures.[3]

GUNSHOT WOUNDS

Penetrating trauma to the temporal bone basically consists of gunshot wounds. They are usually much more damaging to the temporal bone than blunt trauma.[4] There is often significant injury to the external auditory canal, and it may be occluded with debris and bone chips. Soft tissue loss may be severe and require regional or free flap reconstruction. Tympanic membrane perforation, ossicular discontinuity, and labyrinthine fracture are also common entities with a gunshot wound to the temporal bone. Epithelial elements can be introduced into the mastoid or middle ear cavities and not be detected as a cholesteatoma until years later.

CLINICAL ASSESSMENT

SYMPTOMS AND SIGNS

Symptoms of temporal bone trauma depend on the location and extent of the injury. An abrasion of the ear canal or traumatic perforation of the tympanic membrane may be quite painful because of the rich innervation of these areas. However, an uncomplicated temporal bone fracture may not be associated with any symptoms. Involvement of the auditory and/or vestibular system cause hearing loss, nausea and vomiting, or vertigo.

Clinical signs of a temporal bone fracture include the Battle sign, which is a postauricular ecchymosis resulting from extravasated blood from the postauricular artery or mastoid emissary vein. Raccoon's sign (periorbital ecchymosis) is associated with basilar skull fractures that involve the middle or anterior cranial fossa. Physical exam may demonstrate an external auditory canal laceration with bony debris. A hemotympanum is almost always identified.[5] CSF otorrhea or rhinorrhea may be noted. Tuning fork tests are helpful in evaluating the extent of injury in patients with a temporal bone fracture. The Weber tuning fork test lateralizes to the fractured ear if conductive hearing loss is present and lateralizes to the contralateral ear if sensorineural hearing loss is present. Additionally, the presence of nystagmus is a clue that the inner ear may have been injured. Immediate-onset facial nerve paralysis may be present, although a patient may present with normal facial nerve function initially and then develop a delayed palsy 24 to 72 hours later.

IMAGING STUDIES

Computed tomography (CT) of the head is usually the first study done on patients with head trauma after initial resuscitation in the emergency room to rule out intracranial hemorrhage that may require urgent neurosurgical treatment. It is at this point that a temporal bone fracture may be identified. However, the large slice thickness of a head CT often makes it difficult to follow the entire course of the fracture. High-resolution CT of the temporal bone is quite valuable in delineating the extent of the fracture, but is not required unless a complication is suspected (otic capsule fracture, facial nerve injury, CSF leak, etc.).[6] Patients with a longitudinal fracture associated with hemotympanum lateralize to the affected ear on Weber tuning fork test. If there is no nystagmus, no evidence of a CSF leak, and normal facial nerve function, then typically the patient does not need a CT of the temporal bone. Angiography may be performed if there is significant hemorrhage from the skull base to rule out vascular injury, but this is uncommon.

SPECIAL TESTS

Audiometry is useful to perform on patients with a temporal bone fracture. However, this does not need to be done acutely unless the patient has signs or symptoms of inner ear dysfunction. If clinical examination is consistent with conductive hearing loss and there is no evidence of otic capsule fracture, audiometric assessment can be performed several weeks after the injury, permitting time for the hemotympanum to resolve. An audiogram that demonstrates a conductive hearing loss in a patient with a hemotympanum does not help differentiate whether or not an ossicular dislocation occurred. Hemotympanum will typically resolve spontaneously within 3 to 4 weeks of the injury with no sequelae.

Facial nerve testing should be performed if a delayed, complete facial palsy occurs. The rationale is to identify patients with >90% degeneration of the facial nerve, as those patients have poorer recovery of function and may benefit from surgical decompression (see Chapter 19).[7]

COMPLICATIONS AND MANAGEMENT OF TEMPORAL BONE TRAUMA (TABLE 18–2)

EAR CANAL INJURIES

Injuries to the external auditory canal usually occur when a patient is trying to remove earwax with a

TABLE 18–2 Complications of Temporal Bone Trauma

- External auditory canal laceration or stenosis
- Tympanic membrane perforation
- Ossicular chain dislocation
- Sensorineural hearing loss and vertigo
- Perilymphatic fistula
- Facial nerve injury
- Cerebrospinal fluid leak
- Temporal lobe encephalocele
- Vascular injury

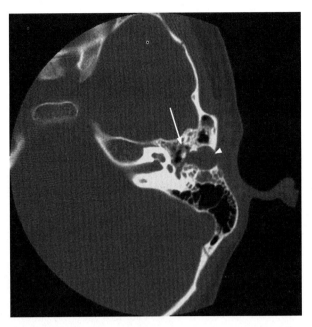

FIGURE 18–4 Acquired stenosis of the external auditory canal. This is an axial CT scan of the left temporal bone. A canal cholesteatoma has formed (arrowhead) and has eroded into the mastoid air cells posteriorly. The head of the malleus is identified (arrow).

cotton-tipped applicator or bobby pin. The injury is typically a simple abrasion or laceration. Treatment consists of using an antibiotic otic drop to prevent bacterial or fungal superinfection of the area. Alternatively, there may be a localized area of blood collection underneath the skin of the external auditory canal, called a bulla. Perforating the tense bulla with a sharp pick often helps to reduce the patient's discomfort. Patients with diabetes are at a high risk of developing external otitis from injuries to the skin of the ear canal because of their poor microcirculation. These patients need to be followed closely to verify that uncomplicated wound healing occurs.

Temporal bone fracture lines often course along the external auditory canal. This can lead to an acquired stenosis of the ear canal if there are a substantial amount of bony fragments in the canal and a soft tissue injury to the skin of the canal (Fig. 18–4). The acute management of a patient with external auditory canal trauma involves the debridement of all loose bone fragments under microscopic visualization, and stenting the canal open (an expandable sponge ear wick works nicely). This generally keeps the ear canal open while it is healing. If stenosis does occur, a canaloplasty may be required several months later.

Tympanic Membrane Perforations

A tympanic membrane perforation can occur after the use of a cotton-tipped applicator, a bobby pin, a pencil, or the entry of a hot metal slag down the ear canal during welding.[8] Also, barotrauma, such as a slap to the ear or a blast injury, can cause a perforation. In all cases, patients usually complain of pain and hearing loss, and the perforation can be diagnosed by otoscopy. It is important to note how much of the tympanic membrane has been perforated. A central perforation does not involve the annulus of the eardrum, whereas a marginal perforation does.

If no evidence of sensorineural hearing loss is found (Weber tuning fork test lateralizes to the affected ear and there is no nystagmus), no specific treatment is required because traumatic tympanic membrane perforations have an excellent chance of healing spontaneously, especially central perforations.[9] Within 1 month 68% are healed, and within 3 months 94% are healed. However, strict dry ear precautions should be followed to prevent water from getting into the ear. Instructions to the patient include no swimming and the use of a Vaseline-soaked cotton ball in the affected ear during bathing. An audiogram should be performed after 2 to 3 months to verify that hearing has returned to normal and that there is no ossicular chain discontinuity. If the perforation has not spontaneously healed by this time, either a paper patch myringoplasty in the office (for a small, dry, central perforation) or a formal tympanoplasty in the operating room can be performed (for a large central perforation or a marginal perforation).

Ossicular Chain Dislocation

Ossicular chain dislocation may occur with a temporal bone fracture, traumatic tympanic membrane perforation, or barotrauma (Fig. 18–5).[10] The tympanic membrane may or may not be perforated. Ossicular chain dislocation with an intact eardrum manifests as a maximal (60 dB) conductive hearing

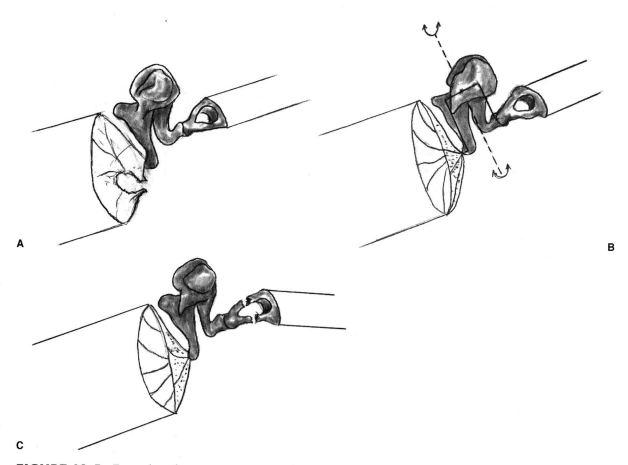

A

B

C

FIGURE 18–5 Examples of some tympanic membrane and ossicular injuries. A: Tympanic membrane perforation. B: Ossicular rotation and partial subluxation of the incudomalleolar joint. C: Fractured stapes superstructure.

loss.[11] Ossicular chain dislocation with a perforated eardrum entails lesser degrees of hearing loss. The most common form of ossicular discontinuity after temporal bone trauma is an incudostapedial joint dislocation. The second most common is incudomalleolar joint dislocation. Fracture of the stapes crura may also occur. Ossicular fixation may occur several months after the temporal bone fracture if exuberant growth of new bone at the fracture line fuses the ossicular chain. Treatment in any case is middle ear exploration and ossicular chain reconstruction.

SENSORINEURAL HEARING LOSS AND VERTIGO

Sensorineural hearing loss and vertigo may be found in patients who sustain a transverse temporal bone fracture with otic capsule involvement. Audiogram usually demonstrates a complete sensorineural hearing loss in that ear. Clinical examination also reveals the patient to have nystagmus, consistent with a unilateral vestibular deficit. Sensorineural hearing loss can also be sustained without otic capsule fracture if a labyrinthine concussion occurs.[5,12] This

is thought to involve shearing of the membranes or hair cell stereocilia due to the rapid acceleration and deceleration forces within the inner ear. Labyrinthine concussion manifests as a high-frequency hearing loss. Finally, patients exposed to traumatic noise exposure or blast injury may sustain a temporary threshold shift in their hearing. This is also thought to be representative of damage to the soft tissue structures within the inner ear, but this temporary sensorineural hearing loss resolves as these structures recover. There are no proven therapies for posttraumatic sensorineural hearing loss.

PERILYMPHATIC FISTULA

Posttraumatic perilymph fistula can occur after a fracture of the otic capsule or with stapes subluxation from the oval window. Barotrauma during scuba diving, a rapid descent in an airplane, an explosion, or a difficult childbirth may also cause perilymphatic fistula by subluxing the stapes.[13] Postsurgical perilymphatic fistula is a well-recognized entity. This can occur after stapedectomy if the oval window fails to seal appropriately or after mastoidectomy if an iatrogenic lateral canal fistula was created.

Perilymph fistula manifests as episodic fluctuating vertigo and sensorineural hearing loss. The patients may have tinnitus, hearing loss, headache, and occasionally aural fullness. Patients may state that their symptoms are least intense in the morning but that they worsen progressively during the day. Most importantly, symptoms become much worse with any type of coughing, sneezing, or straining. Occasionally, altitude change such as going up and down in an airplane or in an elevator can precipitate symptoms. Patients often complain of Tullio's phenomenon, whereby loud noises precipitate a vertiginous attack. Clinically, the fistula test can be performed by insufflating air into the external auditory canal and observing the patient for evidence of nystagmus. This test is very insensitive, and is positive in only ~50% of patients with a fistula. Additionally, it is nonspecific, because many patients without a fistula experience disequilibrium during the test.

Computed tomography is not particularly useful in the identification of a perilymphatic fistula. However, occasionally patients may have obvious symptoms of perilymphatic fistula immediately after the trauma and demonstrate a visible fracture line through the otic capsule on CT scan of the temporal bone. In other cases, no radiographic evidence of an inner ear fistula is visible and the patient's symptoms may be quite vague. In this situation, the only definitive way to make the diagnosis of perilymphatic fistula is surgical exploration with visualization of the leak.[14] Even this is not necessarily definitive, as it is quite difficult to verify that small amounts of clear fluid within the middle ear cavity represent a perilymphatic leak and not serous transudate from the middle ear mucosa. Fluid suspicious for perilymph can be sampled on a pledget and sent for β_2-transferrin testing.[15–20] β_2-transferrin is a protein found only in CSF and perilymph; it is not found in other fluids of the body. Although the test result is not immediately available, it may be useful when following these patients postoperatively.

The long-term prognosis in patients with a perilymph fistula is that fluctuating, but progressive, sensorineural or mixed hearing loss will occur. Also, these patients will have progressive disequilibrium. Because there is a fistula from the middle ear space to the inner ear, an episode of acute otitis media is worrisome, as bacteria in the middle ear can easily enter the inner ear and CSF. This situation may lead to permanent sensorineural hearing loss and/or meningitis.

FACIAL NERVE INJURY

Facial nerve palsy occurs in 20% of longitudinal temporal bone fractures and 50% of transverse temporal bone fractures. The most important clinical feature to identify is whether the facial nerve palsy was of delayed onset or immediate. Delayed palsy suggests that intraneural edema occurred, and that good facial nerve function may be anticipated when this resolves.[21–24] Immediate palsy suggests that the facial nerve was transected, and indicates the need for surgical repair. The rate of facial nerve paralysis with penetrating trauma to the temporal bone is 36%. Facial nerve injury most commonly occurs in the tympanic and mastoid segments. Essentially all penetrating injuries with facial palsy are of immediate onset and occur because of nerve transection.

CEREBROSPINAL FLUID LEAK

There is a 2% incidence of CSF leak in all skull fractures and a 20% incidence in temporal bone fractures. CSF leaks usually start within the first 48 hours of the trauma and is noted as clear fluid emanating from the ear or nose. Straining, standing up, or bending over worsens the CSF leak. Eighty percent of posttraumatic CSF leaks close spontaneously after 7 days and the risk of meningitis is quite low (3%) within this time period.[21] If the leak persists longer than 7 to 10 days, the risk of meningitis increases dramatically (23 to 55%). If clear fluid emanating from the nose or ear is suspicious for CSF, the fluid can be collected and sent for β_2-transferrin testing for verification, if desired. The site of a CSF leak from the temporal bone is usually from a fracture in the otic capsule without new bony callus formation.[12] This may be noted with a CT scan of the temporal bone. If not, injection of intrathecal contrast during CT scanning often delineates the specific site of the leak. A CSF leak may be noticed immediately after the trauma or it may not be noticed until several weeks have passed. This is usually reported by patients as water dripping from their nose every time they bend forward. This finding can be easily noted by the physician in the clinic, and is essentially diagnostic of a CSF leak.

POSTTRAUMATIC ENCEPHALOCELE

If a large bony defect in the floor of the middle cranial fossa occurs, an encephalocele may be present immediately after the trauma.[25–27] Alternatively, it may develop after several months.[28] Presumably, this situation occurs because of the constant downward force of normal intracranial pressure, which causes herniation of the dura and temporal lobe brain down into the middle ear and mastoid cavity (Fig. **18–6**). An encephalocele may be visible on otoscopic examination of the ear as a white mass with blood vessels behind the tympanic membrane. Additionally, any mass in the mastoid cavity noted during "routine" chronic ear surgery that has blood vessels along its surface should be carefully inspected to rule out an encephalocele. A CSF leak usually occurs in combination with an encephalocele.

VASCULAR INJURY

Vascular injury is rare with blunt trauma to the temporal bone. However, fracture of the squamous portion of the temporal bone may result in rupture of the middle meningeal artery. This commonly causes an epidural hematoma, which can result in a rapid decline in mental status and death.

The most important complication of penetrating trauma to the temporal bone is injury to a major vascular structure such as the internal carotid artery, internal jugular vein, or dural venous sinus.[29-31] Vascular injury is found in 32% of patients with penetrating trauma to the temporal bone; therefore, these injuries should be considered a penetrating trauma to zone III of the neck and treated accordingly. Angiography is useful in both diagnosing a vascular injury and in managing it with embolization or balloon occlusion. If the hemorrhage continues to remain uncontrolled or there is evidence of major vessel injury on angiogram, surgical exploration may be required.

SURGICAL APPROACHES AND TECHNIQUES (TABLE 18–3)

TREATMENT OF EAR CANAL INJURIES

If conservative measures, such as debriding and stenting, do not prevent ear canal stenosis, a canaloplasty may be required. This is indicated for patients with ear canals that are so stenotic that they get repeated bouts of external otitis or fill rapidly with squamous debris. Canaloplasty is usually performed through a postauricular incision. Soft tissue stenosis in the cartilaginous portion of the canal is divided superiorly and inferiorly. The skin of the ear canal is elevated as much as possible and a drill is used to enlarge the bony canal. This should be done carefully in the posterior and inferior regions as the facial nerve may be nearby. Finally, the skin flaps are laid back down over the enlarged bony opening. If a significant amount of skin is missing, a split-thickness skin graft can be used to

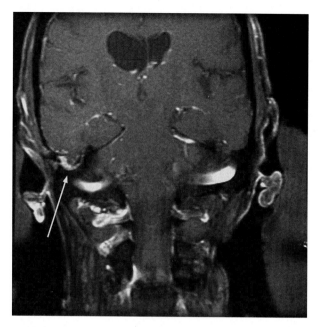

FIGURE 18–6 Coronal magnetic resonance imaging demonstrating a right temporal lobe encephalocele (arrow).

cover the canal. The postauricular incision is closed and the ear canal stented open. Close postoperative wound care is needed to reduce the amount of stenosis that naturally occurs during the healing process. Typically, the ear canal should be made ~ 50% larger than normal, to account for this.

TREATMENT OF TYMPANIC MEMBRANE perforations

A paper patch myringoplasty can be attempted in the office setting for small perforations (less than

TABLE 18–3 SURGICAL INDICATIONS AFTER TEMPORAL BONE TRAUMA

During initial hospitalization:
- Treatment of facial nerve palsy
- Treatment of cerebrospinal fluid leak unresponsive to lumbar drainage
- Vascular injury
- Repair of perilymphatic fistula

Two to 3 months after the injury:
- External auditory canal stenosis
- Persistent tympanic membrane perforation
- Ossicular chain dislocation associated with conductive hearing loss
- Repair of perilymphatic fistula
- Treatment of delayed-onset cerebrospinal fluid leak or encephalocele

25% and not involving the margins of the eardrum). Additionally, the middle ear mucosa should be dry and uninfected. The edges of the perforation are freshened with a Rosen needle and a paper patch (cigarette paper or a Steri-Strip) is placed over the perforation. If the perforation is large or has failed an attempt at paper patch myringoplasty, the patient should be taken to the operating room for a standard tympanoplasty. The ossicular chain should also be explored during this procedure to verify that it is intact. The results of tympanoplasty for uncomplicated traumatic tympanic membrane perforations are good. The rate of complete closure of the perforation is roughly 90% and the rate of hearing improvement is similar.

TREATMENT FOR OSSICULAR CHAIN DISLOCATION

A patient with a normal tympanic membrane but persistent conductive hearing loss probably has ossicular chain discontinuity. A middle ear exploration can be performed through the canal by raising a tympanomeatal flap with careful inspection and palpation of the ossicles. The specific details of ossicular chain reconstruction depend on the site of the injury.

TREATMENT FOR PERILYMPH FISTULA

Treatment of perilymph fistula is initially based on conservative therapy. Patients should be at bed rest with their head elevated for 3 to 6 weeks. They are placed on stool softeners, and serial audiograms should be obtained to follow up for evidence of disease progression. If symptoms persist or the sensorineural hearing loss worsens, surgical treatment is indicated. One option is to simply draw blood from the patient's arm and inject it through the eardrum into the middle ear space. This blood seal often helps to allow a fistula to heal. Alternatively, a middle ear exploration can be performed using a transcanal approach with elevation of the tympanomeatal flap and careful examination of the oval and round window. If a defect is noted, a graft of fascia or muscle should be laid over the defect. Many surgeons place fascia around both the oval window and the round window even if a fistula is not definitively seen, because defects are thought to be quite difficult to detect.

TREATMENT OF FACIAL NERVE PALSY

The surgical indications and techniques involved in the management of traumatic facial nerve palsy are covered in Chapter 19.

TREATMENT OF CEREBROSPINAL FLUID LEAK OR ENCEPHALOCELE

Initially, the management of posttraumatic CSF leak without encephalocele is conservative. This includes head elevation, stool softeners, and the placement of a lumbar drain. Patients with intracranial hemorrhage who have undergone craniotomy often already have an intraventricular drain in place, in which case a lumbar drain is not needed. If the leak stops within 3 or 4 days, the lumbar drain can be removed and the patient placed on acetazolamide to decrease CSF production for 2 to 3 weeks.

Short-term antibiotics have been shown to be potentially useful in preventing meningitis.[32,33] The most common organisms that cause meningitis in this situation are *Pneumococcus, Staphylococcus, Streptococcus,* and *Haemophilus influenzae*. If the CSF leak persists beyond 7 to 10 days, the risk of meningitis increases dramatically (> 20%) and surgical repair of the CSF leak should be performed. This situation is most common in patients who sustain a transverse temporal bone fracture with CSF leaking through the otic capsule. Otic capsule bone does not heal with new bone formation but by fibrous union, and this is often not strong enough to contain CSF.[34]

An encephalocele should always be surgically repaired (Fig. **18–7**). There are two methods of repairing either a persistent CSF leak or an encephalocele. If the patient has normal hearing, a hearing preservation approach is favored. This entails performing a mastoidectomy to remove the necrotic brain and dura, and a middle fossa craniotomy to lift up the temporal lobe and suture repair the dura. The bone flap can be split to provide a segment of bone to lay over the defect in the temporal floor. Also, the posterior half of the temporalis muscle can be rotated to lie between the dura and the bone segment. This brings well-vascularized tissue to the wound. In a patient with no useful hearing, obliteration of the ear with an abdominal fat graft, plugging of the eustachian tube, and closure of the ear canal can be performed through the mastoid alone.

VASCULAR INJURY

Vascular injuries following temporal bone trauma are often best managed by embolization or balloon occlusion by the interventional radiologist. However, there are occasions in which interventional radiologic techniques cannot control bleeding from the skull base. In these situations, surgical wound exploration may be necessary, and this is likely to be a bloody undertaking. Ligation of the external carotid artery or jugular vein is usually of no

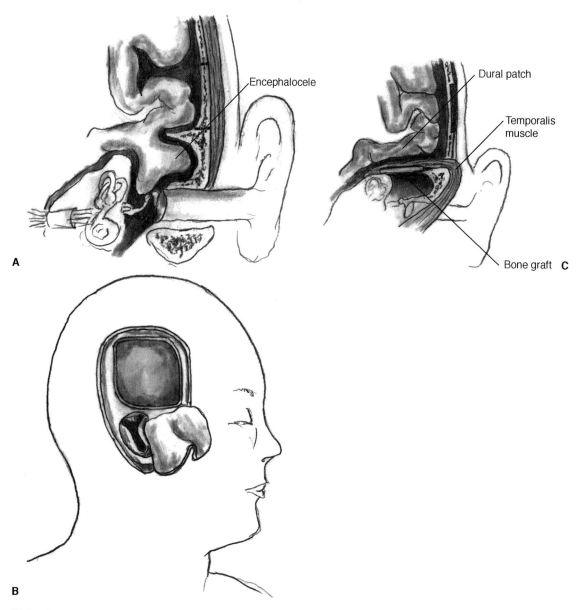

FIGURE 18–7 A: Coronal view of a temporal lobe encephalocele. B: The combined middle fossa–transmastoid approach for repairing a temporal lobe encephalocele. This is used in patients with normal hearing. C: The temporal lobe is elevated and the dural defect closed with a patch. A bone graft is place over the defect in the temporal floor. The temporalis muscle is rotated in between the bone graft and the dura.

particular consequence. The sigmoid sinus can be occluded extradurally by compression with a large sheet of surgical cellulose, or ligated by passing a suture around it intradurally. This should be done distal to the transverse-sigmoid sinus junction so as to prevent occlusion of the vein of Labbé at its entry point. If the vein of Labbé is sacrificed, a venous temporal lobe infarct may occur. In the event that internal carotid artery laceration is found, repair may be attempted by a vascular surgeon. Alternatively, the proximal stump can be ligated and a Fogarty catheter used for distal control.

PEARLS: TEMPORAL BONE TRAUMA

- There are many important structures within the temporal bone, including the ossicles, inner ear, facial nerve, carotid artery, and sigmoid sinus.
- After blunt trauma, 80% of temporal bone fractures are longitudinal, and 20% are transverse in orientation.
- Gunshot wounds to the temporal bone usually cause significantly more damage than blunt trauma.

- Thin-cut computed tomography scanning is the best imaging technique for temporal bone injuries.
- Systematic evaluation and treatment of all sequelae and injured structures is essential; this includes injuries to the tympanic membrane, ossicles, inner ear, vascular structures, and facial nerve, as well as perilymph fistula, CSF leak, and encephalocele.

References

1. Backous DD, Minor LB, Niparko JK. Trauma to the external auditory canal and temporal bone. Otolaryngol Clin North Am 1996;29:853–866

2. Dahiya R, Keller JD, Litofsky NS, Bankey PE, Bonassar LJ, Megerian CA. Temporal bone fractures: otic capsule sparing versus otic capsule violating clinical and radiographic considerations. J Trauma 1999;47:1079–1083

3. Goodwin WJ Jr. Temporal bone fractures. Otolaryngol Clin North Am 1983;16:651–659

4. Bellucci RJ. Traumatic injuries of the middle ear. Otolaryngol Clin North Am 1983;16:633–650

5. Browning GG, Swan IR, Gatehouse S. Hearing loss in minor head injury. Arch Otolaryngol 1982;108:474–477

6. Kahn JB, Stewart MG, Diaz-Marchan PJ. Acute temporal bone trauma: utility of high-resolution computed tomography. Am J Otol 2000;21:743–752

7. Fisch U. Management of intratemporal facial nerve injuries. J Laryngol Otol 1980;94:129–134

8. McGuirt WF Jr, Stool SE. Temporal bone fractures in children: a review with emphasis on long-term sequelae. Clin Pediatr (Phila) 1992;31:12–18

9. Griffin WL Jr. A retrospective study of traumatic tympanic membrane perforations in a clinical practice. Laryngoscope 1979;89:261–282

10. Meriot P, Veillon F, Garcia JF, et al. CT appearances of ossicular injuries. Radiographics 1997;17:1445–1454

11. Bellucci RJ. Traumatic injuries of the middle ear. Otolaryngol Clin North Am 1983;16:633–650

12. Lyos AT, Marsh MA, Jenkins HA, Coker NJ. Progressive hearing loss after transverse temporal bone fracture. Arch Otolaryngol Head Neck Surg 1995;121:795–799

13. Whitehead E. Sudden sensorineural hearing loss with fracture of the stapes footplate following sneezing and parturition. Clin Otolaryngol 1999;24:462–464

14. Emmet JR, Shea JJ. Traumatic perilymph fistula. Laryngoscope 1980;90:1513–1520

15. Bachmann G, Nekic M, Michel O. Traces of perilymph detected in epipharyngeal fluid: perilymphatic fistula as a cause of sudden hearing loss diagnosed with beta-trace protein (prostaglandin D synthase) immunoelectrophoresis. J Laryngol Otol 2001;115:132–135

16. Bluestone CD. Implications of beta-2 transferrin assay as a marker for perilymphatic versus cerebrospinal fluid labyrinthine fistula. Am J Otol 1999;20:701

17. Lund VJ, Savy L, Lloyd G, Howard D. Optimum imaging and diagnosis of cerebrospinal fluid rhinorrhoea. J Laryngol Otol 2000;114:988–992

18. McGuirt WF Jr, Stool SE. Cerebrospinal fluid fistula: the identification and management in pediatric temporal bone fractures. Laryngoscope 1995;105:359–364

19. Nandapalan V, Watson ID, Swift AC. Beta-2 transferrin and cerebrospinal fluid rhinorrhoea. Clin Otolaryngol 1996;21:259–264

20. Ryall RG, Peacock MK, Simpson DA. Usefulness of beta 2-transferrin assay in the detection of cerebrospinal fluid leaks following head injury. J Neurosurg 1992;77:737–739

21. Brodie HA, Thompson TC. Management of complications from 820 temporal bone fractures. Am J Otol 1997;18:188–197

22. Darrouzet V, Duclos JY, Liguoro D, Truilhe Y, De Bonfils C, Bebear JP. Management of facial paralysis resulting from temporal bone fractures: our experience in 115 cases. Otolaryngol Head Neck Surg 2001;125:77–84

23. Grobman LR, Pollak A, Fisch U. Entrapment injury of the facial nerve resulting from longitudinal fracture of the temporal bone. Otolaryngol Head Neck Surg 1989;101:404–408

24. Quaranta A, Campobasso G, Piazza F, Quaranta N, Salonna I. Facial nerve paralysis in temporal bone fractures: outcomes after late decompression surgery. Acta Otolaryngol 2001;121:652–655

25. Dedo GG, Sooy FA. Endaural encephalocele and cerebrospinal fluid otorrhea. Ann Otol Rhinol Laryngol 1970;79:168–177

26. Jones RM, Rothman MI, Gray WC, Zoarski GH, Mattox DE. Temporal lobe injury in temporal bone fractures. Arch Otolaryngol Head Neck Surg 2000;126:131–135

27. Valtonen H, Geyer C, Tarlov E, Heilman C, Poe D. Tegmental defects and cerebrospinal fluid otorrhea. ORL J Otorhinolaryngol Relat Spec 2001;63:46–52

28. Byrne JV, Britten JA, Kaar G. Chronic post-traumatic erosion of the skull base. Neuroradiology 1992;34:528–531

29. Resnick DK, Subach BR, Marion DW. The significance of carotid canal involvement in basilar cranial fracture. Neurosurgery 1997;40:1177–1181

30. Jahrsdoerfer RA, Johns ME, Cantrell RW. Penetrating wounds of the head and neck. Arch Otolaryngol 1979;105:721–725

31. Duncan NO, Coker NJ, Jenkins HA, Canalis RF. Gunshot injuries of the temporal bone. Otolaryngol Head Neck Surg 1986;94:47–55

32. Brodie HA. Prophylactic antibiotics for posttraumatic cerebrospinal fluid fistulae. A meta-analysis. Arch Otolaryngol Head Neck Surg 1997;123:749–752

33. Megerian CA, Hadlock TA. Case records of the Massachusetts General Hospital. Weekly clinicopathological exercises. Case 40–2001. An eight-year-old boy with fever, headache, and vertigo two days after aural trauma. N Engl J Med 2001;345:1901–1907

34. Oghalai JS, Favrot SR, Coker NJ. Imaging quiz case 2. Soft tissue fibrosis. Arch Otolaryngol Head Neck Surg 1996;122:1267–1269

Chapter 19

FACIAL NERVE TRAUMA

Newton J. Coker and Michael G. Stewart

Facial nerve injuries are fortunately uncommon after facial trauma, but the sequelae—weakness, synkinesis, spasm, exposure keratitis—can be significant. The facial nerve can be injured by blunt or penetrating trauma, and may be injured along its extratemporal or intratemporal course. This chapter discusses evaluation and management of facial nerve injuries according to site of injury. Chapter 18 reviews temporal bone trauma and aspects of that trauma other than injury to the facial nerve.

EXTRATEMPORAL FACIAL NERVE INJURY

From the stylomastoid foramen, the main trunk of the facial nerve courses 2 to 3 cm to enter the parotid and divides at the *pes anserinus* into an upper division and a lower division. Rarely, there is a third branch at the level of the *pes*. Beyond the two main divisions, the individual anatomy and degree of branching are quite variable, but there are usually five end branches supplying different areas of the face: the frontal, zygomatic, buccal, ramus mandibularis, and cervical branches. The nerve travels through the parotid gland between the superficial and deep lobes and exits the gland to become closer to the skin and muscles of facial expression as it courses more distally toward the midface.

The extratemporal facial nerve can be injured by blunt or penetrating trauma to the face. In blunt trauma, the nerve is usually severely compressed or stretched. In most injuries the anatomic continuity of the nerve remains intact, the motor axons regenerate, and the muscles of facial expression recover function over time, usually returning to a preinjury level of function. The major potential problem for extratemporal facial nerve recovery after blunt trauma is

synkinesis or "mass motion," which is the undesired contraction of multiple facial muscles when volitionally contracting only one specific group of muscles in a region of the face. The degree to which synkinesis may occur depends on the site of injury. If a distal branch that supplies only one subunit of the face is injured, then synkinesis will not be a problem. Severe proximal injuries along the main trunk or upper or lower divisions almost always result in some degree of synkinesis. Severe blunt injury can lead to neurotmesis with the loss of endoneurial tubules that direct the regenerating axons to their respective motor end plates, resulting in misdirected regeneration across the injury site. The clinical sequela of this abnormal regeneration is synkinesis. There is no way to definitively predict the clinical recovery that will occur after blunt injury, but electrical prognostic testing may be helpful. This is discussed in a later section.

The timing and progression of facial weakness after blunt trauma may yield some clues about the severity of nerve injury. For example, a patient who presents with intact facial function after blunt trauma, but then develops progressive weakness over several hours obviously still has nerve continuity, and may have a more mild injury than a patient who presents with significant weakness and progresses to total paralysis quickly (even though in the second case, the nerve will still be anatomically intact because there was some function initially). In contrast, a patient who presents with immediate total facial paralysis after blunt trauma has a more severe injury and a poorer prognosis. In some patients the assessment of facial nerve function is difficult because of unconsciousness or intoxication at presentation; consequently, facial weakness may not be documented for several hours or even days after injury. If, however, facial movement was clearly evident at an earlier point in time after the blunt trauma, this finding indicates that the nerve is anatomically intact, and that prognosis for return of facial function is good.

After blunt trauma, patients generally recover some level of function with no additional intervention. The potential for regeneration of the facial nerve is very good; animal studies have indicated that the nerve can actually regenerate even when a small segment is missing, that is, axons bridge the gap between the cut ends of the nerve.[1] Therefore, many researchers advocate no exploration for non-penetrating trauma to the extratemporal facial nerve, unless there is no clinical or electromyographic evidence of recovery at 6 months after injury.[2] In the unusual case of blunt trauma with evidence of severe nerve injury (immediate paralysis and evidence of complete degeneration on electrical testing), exploration may be indicated. If the nerve is anatomically intact, then regeneration should provide as good an outcome as surgical anastomosis or repair with a nerve graft. If the nerve has been transected, then surgical repair is indicated; techniques for this are discussed later. There may be a role for oral steroids in blunt injuries, if edema is presumed to be a factor in neural injury. However, use of steroids is probably more appropriate for intratemporal facial nerve injuries.

In a penetrating injury of the face with immediate onset of facial paralysis, the nerve should be assumed to be transected (>90% probability). As soon as the patient's condition permits, surgical exploration and nerve repair should be performed. The exact techniques of nerve repair are described in a later section. Often, there coexists a significant soft tissue injury that requires debridement, irrigation, or closure. Facial nerve exploration and repair can be performed at the same time as wound management. If exploration is performed within 48 hours of injury, then an electrical nerve stimulator will still elicit muscle contraction when distal branches are stimulated. Nerve stimulation can greatly assist in identification of transected nerves. This is one of the main reasons for early intervention in facial nerve repair. Loupe magnification or use of the operating microscope is also helpful in identifying nerve branches. A clinical pearl is that the midface branch of the facial nerve usually runs immediately adjacent to the parotid duct. So, if there is salivary leakage from a duct injury, then the facial branch might also be injured; similarly if there is midface weakness after penetrating trauma, then concomitant parotid duct injury should be considered. In a penetrating injury without facial paralysis, the nerve was not transected. If there is movement with weakness, then

there is likely a bruise or stretch injury, but the nerve is still anatomically intact; those injuries can be treated similar to blunt trauma.

For either penetrating or blunt trauma, the site of injury and degree of clinical dysfunction should also be considered. Injuries to the terminal branches outside the parotid gland and near their insertion into facial muscles are often not explored or repaired, because spontaneous nerve regeneration may result in reinnervation of the target muscle. Because the nerves are small and difficult to find at that level, exploration and attempted repair can potentially disrupt natural reinnervation that might otherwise occur. Also, patients have varying degrees of branching and cross-innervation of the facial muscles, and in some patients even a transection of a distal branch will not result in any clinical weakness, due to arborization and cross-innervation from other (intact) branches. Some have argued that only injuries to the periorbital branches innervating the orbicularis oculi muscle require exploration and repair. However, it has been our practice that any facial weakness is undesirable, so we recommend attempted repair for any branch weakness, assuming that the patient's condition permits. There is less reliable cross-innervation to the marginal mandibular and forehead branches; however, weaknesses in these areas may also have less cosmetic impact.

Facial nerve recovery is typically graded using the House-Brackmann scale shown in Table **19–1**. The use of this outcome scale is appropriate for patients who have had sufficient time for recovery from their injury and repair: 6 to 12 months for extratemporal trauma, and 12 to 18 months for intratemporal trauma.

INTRATEMPORAL INJURY

The facial nerve enters the temporal bone from the brainstem at the porus acusticus and travels through the internal auditory canal; the nerve enters a bony canal, the fallopian canal, at the end of the internal auditory canal (the labyrinthine segment). At the level of the geniculate ganglion, it makes a sharp turn (the "first genu") and gives off the greater superficial petrosal nerve. It then travels horizontally across the middle ear space, just superior to the oval window and stapes (tympanic segment). Just past the oval window, the nerve turns 90 degrees (the "second genu") and travels inferiorly through the mastoid cavity; this is the mastoid segment. The stapedial and chorda tympani nerves branch off the mastoid segment after the second genu. The nerve exits the temporal bone at the stylomastoid

TABLE 19–1   THE HOUSE-BRACKMANN SCALE FOR GRADING FACIAL NERVE RECOVERY AFTER INJURY

Grade	Description	Characteristics
1	Normal	Normal function in all areas
2	Mild dysfunction	Gross: Slight weakness noticeable on close inspection. May have slight synkinesis. At rest, normal symmetry and tone.
		Motion: Forehead—moderate to good function
		Eye—complete closure with minimal effort
		Mouth—slight asymmetry
3	Moderate dysfunction	Gross: Obvious but not disfiguring difference between two sides. Noticeable but not severe synkinesis, contracture or hemifacial spasm. At rest, normal symmetry and tone.
		Motion: Forehead—slight to moderate movement
		Eye—complete closure with effort
		Mouth—slightly weak with maximum effort
4	Moderately severe dysfunction	Gross: Obvious weakness and/or disfiguring asymmetry. At rest, normal symmetry and tone.
		Motion: Forehead—none
		Eye—incomplete closure
		Mouth—asymmetric with maximum effort
5	Severe dysfunction	Gross: Only barely perceptible motion. At rest, asymmetry.
		Motion: Forehead—none
		Eye—incomplete closure
		Mouth—slight movement
6	Total paralysis	No movement

foramen, just adjacent to the attachments of the digastric muscle and the styloid process.

There is a large body of literature on the topic of facial nerve injury following temporal bone trauma[1,3–6]; Chapter 18 covers other aspects of temporal bone injury. Similar to extratemporal facial nerve injury, blunt and penetrating trauma with facial weakness should be treated differently. Blunt trauma injuries, for example, closed head trauma, resulting in temporal bone fracture may injure the facial nerve, either through a stretch or compression injury, or impalement or even transection of the nerve by bony fragments at the fracture site. Patients who never develop complete paralysis clearly have anatomic continuity of the facial nerve, and should be observed for eventual recovery. Patients who develop delayed paralysis also have anatomic continuity and will likely have a good outcome, unless they exhibit progressive and complete degeneration on electrical testing. Patients with immediate paralysis may still have nerve continuity, but even in blunt trauma the possibility of transection should be considered. Computed tomography (CT) thin-cut

scanning in the axial and coronal planes can demonstrate the course of the fallopian canal, and often delineate the site of injury. Sometimes extensive injuries not identified on CT scan are noted at surgery, however. The findings from CT images can be combined with findings from electrical testing to help characterize the site and severity of nerve injury.

A large clinical review found that facial nerve dysfunction occurred in 7 to 10% of patients with temporal bone fracture[1]; other studies have shown a higher prevalence of ~25%. Facial weakness is more prevalent with transverse fractures (facial nerve injury in ~30% to 50% of fractures), but longitudinal fractures can also cause facial nerve injury (~20% of fractures). In both patterns of fracture, the nerve is most commonly injured in the area of the geniculate ganglion, with the tympanic segment being the next most commonly injured segment. Of course, the nerve can be injured in more than one segment.

In blunt injuries with anatomic continuity of the nerve, outcome should be excellent in most patients. If there is severe nerve injury, outcome is usually worse, but it is unclear how much worse the outcome will be.[1] Poor prognostic factors include immediate onset of paralysis, step-deformities in the fracture across the fallopian canal, and evidence of complete degeneration on the electrical tests. There is evidence from a nonrandomized trial that in patients with Bell's palsy and severe degeneration, there is improved outcome with surgical decompression medial to the geniculate ganglion.[7] There have been no prospective clinical trials addressing facial nerve management in patients with temporal bone fracture, but clinical experience indicates that in patients with significant nerve degeneration, surgical nerve decompression may result in improved outcomes. Again, electrical testing may help identify patients most likely to benefit from surgical exploration.

Standard otologic surgical approaches can be used to explore the facial nerve within the temporal bone. Injuries to the tympanic and mastoid segments can be examined via mastoid surgery. Injuries in the region of the geniculate ganglion often necessitate an approach through the middle cranial fossa. In patients with poor or no hearing in the ear all intratemporal segments of the facial nerve can be explored via mastoid surgery with removal of the labyrinth (translabyrinthine approach). These surgical approaches are usually chosen taking into account the CT findings, status of hearing, medical condition of the patient, and coexisting intracranial injuries.

Penetrating trauma to the temporal bone is usually due to a gunshot wound (GSW). Because the otic capsule is made up of extremely compact bone, the bullet often stops and fragments at that level, causing significant injury within the remainder of the temporal bone. Series of patients with GSW to the temporal bone have indicated that the facial nerve is injured in at least 50% of gunshot injuries.[3,4] If there is facial paralysis after a GSW, the nerve has almost invariably been transected. The most common areas of injury are the tympanic and mastoid segments. In addition, at exploration the area of nerve damage is often larger than initially suspected or shown on CT scan, because of the high-energy transfer and tissue damage caused by the missile.

Patients with a GSW to the temporal bone almost always require surgical debridement and mastoidectomy; patients with facial paralysis can have the facial nerve explored at that time. At surgery the nerve should be widely exposed, and if transected, then the edges debrided with removal of nonviable tissue. Once this has been completed, the nerve should be repaired. To achieve a tension-free repair, this may require an interpositional graft using the

greater auricular or sural nerve. The best result that can be expected following grafting with an interpositional graft in a GSW is a grade 3 House-Brackmann; the typical outcome is grade 4.[4]

ELECTRICAL AND PROGNOSTIC TESTING

It is important to remember that in partial nerve injury, the best prediction of eventual outcome is the amount of actual motor axon damage; the larger the proportion of axons damaged, the poorer prognosis for normal return of function. Therefore, if the degree of axonal damage could be assessed, then clinical outcome could be predicted. Fortunately, there are some diagnostic tests that can assist in assessment of the severity of nerve injury, and therefore identify patients who have a high probability of poor outcome. These patients should be considered for more aggressive facial nerve management.

Electrical testing is appropriate only in patients with complete paralysis; if there is any motor function at all, then there is nerve continuity and a high probability of good to excellent recovery. Available tests include the nerve excitability test, electroneuronography (or "evoked electromyography"), the maximal stimulation test, and electromyography (EMG).[8] The only test helpful early in the course of management, that is, in the first 3 days after injury, is EMG.

The following stimulation tests are most useful within 5 days to 3 weeks after injury. The nerve excitability test (NET) and maximal stimulation test (MST) both use an externally placed electrical nerve stimulator (the Hilger stimulator). In NET, the intact side is tested first and the minimum current required to stimulate the facial nerve and produce just perceptible movement is noted; then the paralyzed side is tested and the amount of current required to just stimulate the face is also noted. A difference between sides of 3.5 mA or larger is suggestive of significant nerve injury. In the MST, the stimulator is used at 10 mA on both sides, and the strength of response is compared between sides. The relative difference can predict the return of function; detailed prognostic algorithms can be found elsewhere.[8]

Electroneuronography (ENoG) is a commonly used test, in which an electrode is placed on the skin over a facial muscle to measure the peak-to-peak amplitude of the myogenic compound action potential while the main trunk of the nerve is stimulated using high current. ENoG has also been called "evoked electromyography." Compound action potentials are measured on each side of the face, and the amplitudes are compared; test results are expressed as a percentage of the intact nerve fibers. A reduction in amplitude of more than 90% (indicating less than 10% intact motor axons) on the paralyzed side is predictive of severe injury and poor outcome.

Electromyography (EMG) measures the muscle electrical activity at rest and during voluntary activity; results are expressed based on the characteristics of the potentials seen. At rest, there should be a resting potential and during contraction a voluntary motor unit potential. Fibrillation potentials indicate that the muscle's nerve supply has undergone degeneration. Polyphasic motor units and nascent motor units herald nerve regeneration. For the first 3 days after injury, the presence of volitional motor units on EMG indicates that the nerve is at least in part intact, but does not predict severity of injury. EMG is also useful in the evaluation of chronic paralysis (beyond 3 weeks) to determine evidence of complete degeneration or of regeneration.

ENoG is very useful because it gives a quantifiable (not subjective) result, and it has been shown to correlate with the degree of actual nerve damage and, therefore, prognosis.[2] In addition, Coker et al[9] showed that a NET difference of at least 3.5 mA is highly predictive of an ENoG amplitude difference of at least 85 to 90%. Because the ENoG requires specialized equipment and expertise in interpretation, but the NET requires only a Hilger stimulator, there is clearly a role for NET in early electrical evaluation of the paralyzed nerve.

NERVE GRAFT

There is no accepted ideal technique for nerve graft, but authors do agree on several principles to maximize outcome after repair. First, the nerve edges should be freshened and necrotic and fibrotic tissue removed to allow a healthy surface for nerve regeneration. Second, the edges of the nerve should be sutured under no tension. Third, the repair should be stabilized so that tension from other tissues does not disrupt the nerve anastomosis.

The optimal timing of nerve repair is not firmly established.[2,10] There is a theoretical advantage in performing repair at 21 days after injury, because that is the period of maximal physiologic activity of the regenerating axons. However, clinical studies have not indicated improved outcomes when repair is performed at that time. Others have noted improved outcomes when repair is performed within 30 days versus later than 30 days.[11] An animal study

found no significant difference in outcomes between repairs performed immediately, at 5 days, and at 21, 30, and 60 days after transection.[10] Because fibrosis and healing can hinder identification and dissection of the nerve, a reasonable recommendation is to perform repair relatively soon after injury, as soon as the patient's condition permits.

The epineurium is the denser capsule-like tissue surrounding the entire nerve; the perineurium is inside the epineurium, is thinner tissue, and surrounds individual fascicles. Although both epineurial and perineurial repair generally yield good outcomes, perineurial repair is recommended, because proliferation of epineurial tissue at the site of anastomosis can interfere with neuron regeneration.[2] The epineurium should be trimmed a few millimeters back from the suture line, and fine monofilament suture (9-0 or 10-0) is used for repair.[2] If the nerve ends are freshened and cut at an oblique angle, then there is a larger surface area for regeneration. See Fig. 19–1 for an illustration of techniques of nerve repair.

If there is a missing segment of nerve, either due to the injury or after removal of damaged tissue, or if the repair is under significant tension, then an interpositional graft should be used. For shorter defects the greater auricular nerve is a popular choice, because its caliber is similar to that of the facial nerve, and it can be accessed in the neck at the time of surgery. For longer defects, the sural nerve or the antebrachial cutaneous nerve are options. The auricular nerve can provide up to 7 cm of nerve, and the sural nerve can provide 30 cm.[2] The nerve should be reversed before repair, because of the direction of branches off the trunk of the donor nerve.

SUMMARY

Blunt trauma to the extratemporal facial nerve resulting in facial weakness or paralysis usually resolves within 6 months. Penetrating trauma to the face resulting in nerve paralysis usually means the nerve has been transected. Surgical exploration and repair should be performed. Blunt trauma to the temporal bone resulting in facial nerve injury should be treated according to the severity of the weakness. If some facial function remains, facial nerve recovery should be adequate with observation alone. In total paralysis, CT imaging to evaluate for bony impingement, and electrical testing to assess severity of degeneration should be performed. If there is evidence of severe degeneration on electrical testing, facial nerve exploration and repair should be strongly considered. If the injury does not meet criteria for severe degeneration, then recovery of

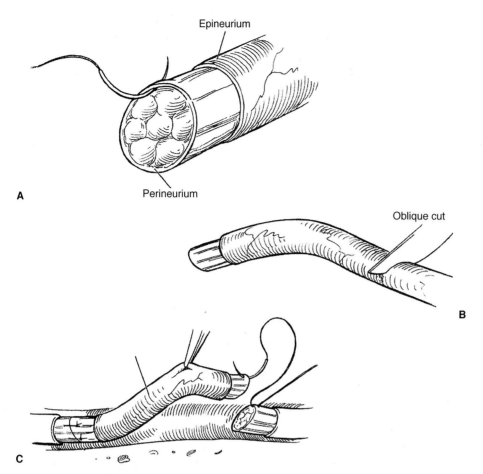

FIGURE 19–1 Techniques of facial nerve repair and grafting. A: The epineurium is trimmed back and the repair is performed using fine sutures at the perineurial level. B: The oblique cut, shown being made in an autograft nerve section. C: Placement of an interpositional graft, with epineurium trimmed back and repair at the level of the perineurium. (From Coker NJ, Jenkins HA. *Atlas of Otologic Surgery*. Philadelphia: WB Saunders, 2001, with permission.)

function should be very good. In penetrating trauma to the temporal bone, there is a high chance of facial paralysis; in effectively all cases of paralysis, the nerve has been transected, and surgical exploration and grafting will be required.

PEARLS: FACIAL NERVE INJURY

- Blunt extracranial nerve injuries usually recover good-quality facial nerve function over time.
- Penetrating facial trauma with facial nerve paralysis should be considered a nerve transection. Branches and the main trunk of the nerve should be explored and repaired if transected, except for distal small branches where cross-innervation may provide adequate facial function.
- Optimal facial nerve repair is achieved with a tension-free, perineurial closure using small monofilament suture. Optimal timing of repair is uncertain, but repair is recommended as soon as the patient's condition permits.

- Interposition nerve grafts should be used to replace missing sections of nerve; the greater auricular nerve, antebrachial cutaneous nerve, and the sural nerve are options for the donor nerve.
- Blunt trauma to the temporal bone results in facial nerve injury 10 to 20% of the time.
- Electrical testing can help predict the severity of nerve injury, which is associated with eventual functional outcome. The most useful and accurate prognostic tests are the ENoG and the NET.
- In blunt trauma to the intratemporal nerve, if there is incomplete weakness, or complete weakness with favorable electrical testing (NET difference < 3.5 mA, or ENoG evidence $< 90\%$ degeneration) observation is recommended and should result in very good functional outcome.
- In temporal bone fractures with facial paralysis and evidence of progressive degeneration (NET difference > 3.5 mA or ENoG evidence of $> 90\%$ degeneration) surgical exploration of the facial nerve should be considered. Repair may be

mediated via decompression, removal of bone fragments, or grafting, depending on the pathology. Standard otologic surgical approaches are used for nerve exploration.

• Gunshot wounds to the temporal bone have at least a 50% chance of facial paralysis. When paralysis is present, the nerve has usually been transected and surgical repair with interpositional grafts will be required.

REFERENCES

1. Chang CYJ, Cass SP. Management of facial nerve injury due to temporal bone trauma. Am J Otol 1999; 20:96–114

2. Coker NJ. Management of traumatic injuries to the facial nerve. Otolaryngol Clin North Am 1991;24: 215–227

3. Duncan NO, Coker NJ, Jenkins HA, Canalis RF. Gunshot injuries of the temporal bone. Otolaryngol Head Neck Surg 1986;94:47–55

4. Coker NJ, Kendall KA, Jenkins HA, Alford BR. Traumatic intratemporal facial nerve injury: management rationale for preservation of function. Otolaryngol Head Neck Surg 1987;97:262–269

5. Wiet RJ, Valvassori GE, Kotsanis CA, Parahy C. Temporal bone fractures: State of the art review. Am J Otol 1985;6:207–215

6. Brodie HA, Thompson TC. Management of complications from 820 temporal bone fractures. Am J Otol 1997;18:188–197

7. Gantz BJ, Rubinstein JT, Gidley P, Woodworth GG. Surgical management of Bell's palsy. Laryngoscope 1999;109:1177–1188

8. Hughes GB. Prognostic tests in acute facial palsy. Am J Otol 1989;10:304–311

9. Coker NJ, Fordice JO, Moore S. Correlation of the nerve excitability test and electroneurography in acute facial paralysis. Am J Otol 1992;13:127–133

10. Barrs DM. Facial nerve trauma: optimal timing for repair. Laryngoscope 1991;101:835–848

11. May M. Trauma to the facial nerve. Otolaryngol Clin North Am 1983;16:661–670

Chapter 20

Principles of Ballistics and Penetrating Trauma

Michael G. Stewart

In the management of penetrating trauma, knowledge about ballistics, injury patterns, and pertinent anatomy are important to the evaluating physician. As opposed to blunt trauma, in which the skin remains intact, in penetrating trauma an object enters the body through the skin, although the penetrating object may be withdrawn or may pass through the body and not be present internally at the time of evaluation. Penetrating trauma includes injuries from sharp objects such as knives or glass, or even blunt objects that penetrate, such as hard edges of an automobile, as well as projectiles fired from weapons. This chapter reviews the ballistics of projectiles, and discusses some general principles of treating penetrating trauma.

PROJECTILES

When a projectile penetrates tissue it decelerates, but as it does so, it dissipates its energy—which is in the form of *kinetic energy*—into the tissue. The amount of kinetic energy (KE) contained by the projectile is determined by this equation: $KE = 1/2\ MV^2$, where M = mass and V = velocity. Because the velocity term is squared in the equation, the speed of the projectile is the most important factor in determining its level of energy. In other words, a projectile with twice the velocity has four times the kinetic energy of the lower-velocity projectile. Because energy is ultimately conserved, the energy contained by the projectile is transmitted into the tissues impacted. Therefore, high-velocity projectiles can impart significantly larger amounts of energy into tissues. Of course, heavier projectiles impart more energy as well, but the velocity is a more important factor.

However, although the amount of kinetic energy is important, ballistics research indicates that the *efficiency* of energy *transfer* is an important factor in determining the degree of wounding of a bullet.[1,2] This energy transfer depends on the energy present in the bullet, but also on the *type* of bullet and its physical characteristics.[2-4] Most commercially available handgun and rifle bullets are made entirely of lead, which deforms, flattens, and widens as the bullet hits an object; even if bullets are not made entirely of lead, the tip is usually lead. In addition some bullet tips are designed with a "hollow" point or a blunt tip, which further ensures deformation of the bullet or even fragmentation as it penetrates tissue. This expanded bullet diameter means a larger path of damage created, and greater injury; fragmenting bullets cause even more damage as the pieces travel in different directions.

Military-grade rifles typically use a sharp-pointed, narrow, elongated bullet in which the lead center is covered by a complete shell of hard metal—a so-called "full metal jacket." This hard metal jacket resists deformation in tissue and almost never fragments into secondary projectiles. Because of their shape and characteristics, these military-type bullets often pass completely through the body; this means that they do not transfer all of their high energy into the tissues. Similarly, their lack of deformation means a potentially smaller path of tissue loss. So the highest velocity (and highest kinetic energy) bullets fired from military rifles actually can cause less injury than much lower-velocity bullets from civilian weapons (Fig. **20–1**). This is partially by design: military convention since the Hague Conference of 1899 has been to use weapons that incapacitate but do not always kill, and civilian handguns and hunting weapons are designed to kill with a single shot.

Another important factor in wounding is the instability of bullets—both in the air and in the

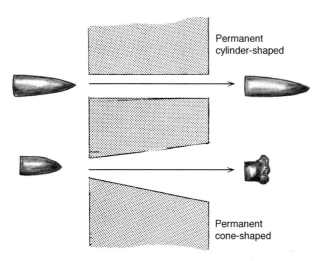

FIGURE 20–1   Differences in bullet deformation and cavity type, with different bullet characteristics.

tissue (Fig. **20–2**). The most important components of this instability are yaw and tumbling. Yaw refers to deviation of the tip of the bullet from the straight axis of flight. Most bullets fired from handguns or rifles have very little yaw while in flight: consider the symmetric round entry holes created by bullets in paper targets at shooting ranges, even at long distances. Tumbling refers to forward rotation of the bullet around the center of the mass, and bullets fired from weapons typically do not tumble while in flight. However, once inside tissue, bullets can yaw and tumble, which increases the area of tissue damage and energy deposition. Ballistic studies indicate that different types of bullets have inherently different tendencies toward yaw and tumbling, and also begin to yaw and tumble at different depths of penetration into tissue. Civilian-type bullets typically begin to yaw within 2 cm of penetration; larger bullets and bullets that deform have larger degrees of yaw. In contrast, some hard-jacketed military bullets

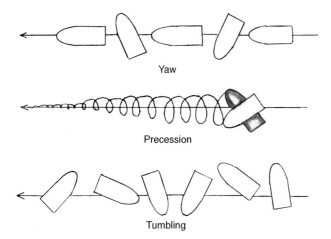

FIGURE 20–2   Rotational characteristics of bullets.

fired from powerful weapons can penetrate tissue for 60 cm without yaw, so although they contain higher energy they may cause less tissue damage along their path.

In summary, it is important for treating physicians to realize that while kinetic energy is important, it is not the only factor that determines the degree of wounding caused by a gunshot injury.

HANDGUNS AND RIFLES

Firearms are usually divided into two groups according to the speed of the bullet as it exits the muzzle: *low velocity* and *high velocity*. The boundary between low and high velocity is not standardized, but in general low velocity is considered less than 1000 ft/sec, and high velocity is considered more than 1000 ft/sec,[5,6] although some set the limit at 2000 ft/sec.[7] Another classification of guns is by size of bullet, or *caliber*. In handguns, a larger caliber bullet often means a larger and more powerful weapon, with a higher muzzle velocity. In general, most handguns are low-velocity weapons, with muzzle velocities between 500 and 800 ft/sec, although some powerful handguns such as the 0.357 Magnum have higher muzzle velocities. Many handguns available on the street are in the range of lower caliber (smaller) projectiles and muzzle velocities, such as the common 0.22 caliber pistol. Rifles are also classified by caliber, but muzzle velocity can differ significantly between weapons that use similar caliber bullets. In general, rifles are high-velocity weapons; for example, a 30–30 rifle has a muzzle velocity of ~2200 ft/sec. Some examples of weapon muzzle velocities are shown in Table **20–1**. Of course, in many circumstances, the injured patient is unable to describe the type of weapon that was used, but when that information is available, the size and muzzle velocity of the projectile can be useful clinical information.

Projectiles decelerate as they travel through the air, but only ~150 to 170 ft/sec of velocity are required to penetrate the skin,[1] so even when fired from a distance most bullets still penetrate the skin. Rifle injuries in particular retain a very high velocity even 100 or more yards from the weapon.

SHOTGUN INJURIES

A shotgun is a specialized type of weapon that has a relatively high muzzle velocity.[8–10] The difference between a shotgun and a rifle is that in a shotgun a group of pellets are fired from a *shell*. Gunpowder is ignited in the posterior part of the plastic shell,

TABLE 20–1 APPROXIMATE MUZZLE VELOCITIES OF SELECTED FIREARMS

Handguns

0.25 caliber: 800 ft/sec

0.32 caliber: 900 ft/sec

0.38 caliber: 600–850 ft/sec

0.45 caliber: 850 ft/sec

Shotguns

Most gauges: 1100–1250 ft/sec

Rifles

0.22 caliber: 1100–1200 ft/sec

0.308 Winchester: 2,900 ft/sec

AK-47: 2,300 ft/sec

M-16: 3,100 ft/sec

Partially based on Swan KG, Swan RC. Principles of ballistics applicable to the treatment of gunshot wounds. Surg Clin North Am 1991;71:221–239.

which contains some packing material and dozens or hundreds of pellets, or *shot*. These pellets are ejected from the shotgun's muzzle and travel in a grouping toward the target. There is additional material within the shell called *wadding*, which fills the dead space behind and between pellets, seals the bore to keep gas behind the pellets, and protects the powder. Wadding is usually made from paper, cardboard, felt, or composite material. The shell is usually ejected from the bottom or side of the weapon, and the wadding is expelled from the barrel and partially disintegrates, or falls to the ground.

Shotguns are typically used to hunt small moving animals that are a distance away and traveling rapidly, so that at least some of the pattern of shot will hit the moving target. Most shotgun pellets are so small that they decelerate rapidly during their travel through the air, and their small mass means each has less kinetic energy than a regular bullet. In addition, the farther the pellets travel away from the gun, the more the pellets disperse, meaning fewer might hit the intended target. The effective range for many shotguns is only 20 to 40 yards. At close range, however, shotgun pellets can impart significant kinetic energy because of their high velocity, and because the pellets are still in a close pattern and the victim is hit with multiple pellets.

Shotguns are classified by their barrel diameter, and by the type of shot used. The barrel diameter (and also the diameter of the shell used) is measured as *gauge*, which originally signified how many lead balls of that size were needed to weigh a pound. Therefore, larger gauge means smaller diameter; a 20-gauge shotgun shell is smaller than a 12-gauge shell. The size of the shot is also classified using an antiquated system, where larger numbers mean smaller pellets. "Birdshot" refers to smaller pellets (No. 6 to No. 12 shot) and "buckshot" refers to larger pellets (No. 2 and No. 1 and larger).

A landmark study evaluating shotgun injuries found that the most important aspect determining the severity of injury was the distance from the weapon to the victim.[9] Long-range injuries (type 1— more than 7 yards distance) typically caused penetration of skin or fascia only. Close range injuries (type 2— 3 to 7 yards distance) could cause perforation of deeper structures such as blood vessels and abdominal viscera, and point-blank injuries (type 3— closer than 3 yards) usually caused extensive tissue loss and damage. This classification remains in clinical use today.

MECHANISMS OF INJURY

Gunshot wounds cause tissue injury by two mechanisms: direct tissue injury and temporary *cavitation*. There is a potential third mechanism of injury— the transmission of "shock waves" into distant tissues— but the actual existence of these waves, as well as their potential for causing clinically significant damage, has been refuted by ballistics experts and remains a subject of controversy.[4] Although the impact of distant shock waves has been discussed in many medical articles and chapters, it appears there is little contemporary ballistic evidence supporting the development of distant shock waves from gunshot wounds.[3] However, ballistics research clearly confirms the creation of a temporary cavitation cavity and permanent tissue loss. In addition, ballistics research demonstrates the importance of projectile characteristics and kinetic energy in determining the characteristics and degree of tissue loss.

Cavitation refers to the creation of a pulsating temporary cavity surrounding the true path of the projectile, as shown in Fig. **20–3**. This temporary cavity lasts for only milliseconds, and its size and configuration depend on the energy and orientation of the projectile, but although it is only present briefly this temporary cavity results in potential tissue damage adjacent to the bullet path. Therefore, anatomic structures can be significantly damaged by a gunshot wound without being actually penetrated by the bullet, because of the effect of cavitation. The degree and type of damage depend on the characteristics of the tissue. Soft, compressible tissue may absorb the energy of cavitation with minimal injury, but firmer solid tissue like cartilage and bone can be

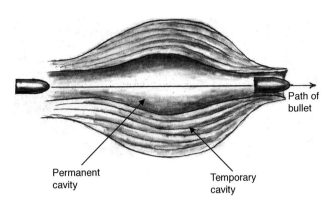

FIGURE 20–3 Typical pattern of temporary and permanent cavitation cavity caused by gunshot wound.

damaged by cavitation even a fair distance from the actual bullet path and the permanent cavity. Tissue loss caused by the projectile creates a smaller permanent cavity. This permanent cavity can take on different shapes and orientations, based on the energy and characteristics of the bullet, and the type of tissue injured. In general, higher energy projectiles create a larger temporary cavity, and the cavity expands as the bullet passes through the tissue, due to tumbling of the projectile discussed previously.

High-velocity weapons and bullets that deform can cause greater cavitation and transmission effects than low-velocity injuries. Higher velocity projectiles also penetrate deeper into tissues, or are more likely to pass completely through the body. Therefore, to oversimplify, low-velocity injuries are usually characterized by tissue *damage*, and high-velocity injuries are characterized by tissue *loss* as well as direct damage. Considering these ballistic principles, a penetrating injury where the projectile has passed through the body can be assumed to have had higher kinetic energy than a projectile that is retained, all other factors being equal. Therefore, the cavitation damage and size of the permanent cavity from projectiles that pass through the body may be greater than projectiles that do not. Of course, that is assuming that the bullets themselves are similar and that the tissue paths are otherwise identical; for example, if a bullet hits bone it is more likely to be retained even if it had very high kinetic energy.

As discussed previously, bullets have rotational characteristics that increase the possibility of an unusual and unpredictable course after impact. In addition, the rotation or tumbling of the projectile also increases the amount of direct tissue injury. If the projectile itself fragments into secondary projectiles, those have the potential for additional injury. Similarly, if impacted bone shatters, the secondary bone fragments may cause additional tissue damage.

Finally, the type of tissue penetrated influences the damage effect of a penetrating projectile injury. Tissues with very low elasticity, such as bone, tend to shatter or fragment and undergo much greater damage than more elastic tissues, such as muscle. Similarly, tissues with high density or specific gravity, such as brain or liver, tend to undergo greater damage than less dense tissue, such as lung. In the head and neck, bone, soft tissue, and air spaces are usually in close approximation, so bullets can take unpredictable paths, and bone and soft tissue are often both injured.

NONPROJECTILE PENETRATING TRAUMA

As discussed previously, nonprojectile penetrating trauma can be caused by assault with a weapon or by falls or accidents. The major difference between stab wounds or other penetrating trauma and gunshot and shotgun wounds is that in stab wounds only the tissue directly penetrated is injured.[5] There is no cavitation effect to consider in stab wounds. Nevertheless, when the size and length of the weapon are unknown, and the weapon is not left in the patient, assessment of the depth of injury can be challenging. In addition, if a knife or other sharp object is twisted or turned while inside the tissue, significant damage can result. Therefore, even a small entry wound does not rule out significant internal damage.

EVALUATION

For projectile injuries, the secondary survey is very important. Entry and exit wounds should be identified and marked; use of radiopaque markers taped or clipped to the skin adjacent to the injury is recommended, so that entry and exit sites can be seen on x-rays. Because of the effects of cavitation and bullet rotation on tissue loss, exit wounds are usually larger in size, with more missing tissue, and perhaps a more irregular border. Entry wounds are usually smaller with little irregularity. It is important to perform an independent assessment of entry and exit sites, and not just rely on secondhand accounts of events, or on the patient's reported history. In criminal cases, there may be many reasons why victims report events inaccurately to minimize their potential guilt or to attempt to blame the police or others for their injury. For example, if the patient has a small, circumscribed wound in the anterior neck and a larger, irregular wound in the posterior neck, the patient was likely shot from the front, even if he might insist that he was shot from behind.

This assessment is important, because the physician should estimate the projectile's path, which helps predict which structures might have been injured. However, projectiles often change direction after collision with tissues, so a straight path cannot be assumed. In patients with multiple injuries, particularly if shot from different directions, the assessment of bullet trajectory and entry and exit wounds can be very difficult. These patients with multiple wounds almost always require thorough investigation including surgical exploration to finally identify and repair all injured structures. After entry and exit wounds have been marked, the patient should undergo the next steps in evaluation, which may include endoscopy, radiologic evaluation, and surgical exploration.

If the patient has only an entrance wound (or wounds), then x-rays need to be taken to identify the location of the retained projectile(s). Again, assessment of the probable projectile path can guide evaluation and treatment, remembering that bullets can ricochet and change direction in the body, and also remembering that adjacent tissue can be injured by cavitation.

In shotgun wounds, shotgun pellets are easily seen on x-ray, and it is often surprising the size of the area where pellets are present. In close-range shotgun wounds, the wadding can also be impacted into the tissues, so that possibility should be considered. Retained wadding should be removed, as it is a frequent source of infection. Physical examination and radiologic evaluation are both important in the assessment of the potential extent of a shotgun injury, but the most important factor determining injury severity usually is the distance from the weapon.

Evaluation of a stab wound involves primarily assessment of its depth. This can be sometimes accomplished with gentle probing of the wound using a soft instrument such as a cotton-tip applicator. However, care should be taken to avoid removing blood clots from stab wounds, because significant bleeding from the wound can follow. Furthermore, on occasion, pain, patient cooperation, or muscle spasm does not allow the probe to be advanced very deep, which can obscure the actual depth of the wound. So, a limited evaluation of depth should not take precedence over clinical suspicion of a deep injury, and surgical exploration should be strongly considered. In addition, if there is clinical evidence of deep visceral injury, such as an expanding hematoma or subcutaneous emphysema, then surgical exploration and repair are needed.

If the weapon is still embedded in the stab injury, it should be left in place while further evaluation is performed. Under no circumstances should an embedded weapon be removed until the treating physician is prepared to treat the bleeding or fluid spillage that may ensue. Control of hemorrhage is best performed under controlled circumstances in an operating room setting, with intravenous (IV) lines, monitors, and resuscitation capacities immediately available. A weapon that is still in place in a blood vessel or tissue with high vascularity often has a tamponade effect and prevents further bleeding until it is removed.

MANAGEMENT

The individual management of penetrating trauma to specific sites is discussed in more detail in other chapters. However, there are some broad principles of penetrating trauma that are addressed here.

The management philosophies for penetrating trauma have been changing over the years, for the head and neck and other parts of the body.[11–13] In the post–World War II era, after the development of mobile surgical sites, broad-spectrum antibiotics, and advances in surgical techniques and general anesthesia, the philosophy in general was to surgically explore the area of injury in almost all penetrating trauma patients. Surgical exploration itself was safe, and if no injury was found, the patient could be observed briefly and then discharged. However, if injuries were identified, they were repaired or removed, and the surgery proceeded until all potentially injured vital structures had been explored and repaired. With that philosophy it was expected that a defined number of patients would undergo surgical exploration and no significant injury would be identified—that is, a negative exploration. Although there is some potential morbidity associated with a negative exploration, it is generally minimal, and the benefits of early identification and repair of visceral injury were felt to outweigh the disadvantages of a small number of negative explorations.

In the 1970s and 1980s, the widespread availability of endoscopic equipment as well as improved radiologic imaging, particularly the computed tomography scan and the angiogram, meant that some patients with penetrating trauma could be evaluated using nonsurgical approaches, with surgery reserved for those patients with specific injuries identified during the evaluation. Similarly, the increased role of observation rather than mandatory surgery led surgeons to realize that some injuries had a fairly benign natural history and did not always require repair.[12,13] Of course, patients with evidence of a critical injury, such as shock, airway collapse, or an expanding hematoma, still require emergency surgical evaluation and definitive treatment. However, the management of the stable patient with penetrating trauma in the modern era does not always mean mandatory surgical exploration.

In addition, recent evidence indicates that in certain patients, extensive surgery to repair all injuries may add additional risk to overall physiologic stability.[14] So a new concept of limited surgery, or "damage control" surgery, has been developed in which the patient has certain injuries repaired and others temporized, and then the surgery is interrupted and the patient is returned to the intensive care unit for further stabilization and resuscitation. As the patient can tolerate it, he or she is returned to the operating room for definitive injury repair, but, using the damage control concept, that may require several surgical procedures.

In general, all penetrating wounds are considered contaminated, and should not be closed primarily. Rather, wounds should be gently debrided and then allowed to heal by secondary intention. There is some support in the literature for more aggressive mandatory debridement of high-energy wounds, the philosophy being that the adjacent injured tissue has been devitalized and is likely to harbor bacteria, in particular dangerous organisms like clostridia. However, many times apparently devitalized tissue still survives, mainly because of better-than-expected blood supply. Thus, some authors recommend only irrigation and establishment of external drainage in penetrating injuries, with tissue removal limited to foreign bodies or obviously necrotic tissue. However, when the decision is made to explore and debride soft tissue and muscle, then a rule of thumb is to assess tissue viability using the "four C's": color, consistency, contractility (of muscle), and circulation. It is unclear which factors are most important, although a change in three of four would be a good indication of nonviable tissue.

All patients with penetrating trauma should be treated with a brief period of prophylactic antibiotics, because the skin was penetrated, and because bullets are not "sterilized" by their high heat, contrary to popular belief. If there is evidence of airway or digestive tract injury, then antibiotic coverage should be broadened to include likely pathogens, and a longer treatment course may be necessary.

LEAD POISONING

Absorption of lead from retained bullets can occur, particularly if the bullet is lodged into a joint space, bone, or an intervertebral disk. Eventual lead intoxication can present days to decades later. The presence of lead in joints in particular can lead to systemic lead absorption because lead dissolves in synovial fluid.[2] If bullets are retained in other soft tissue, the body typically forms a barrier of mature scar tissue that prevents systemic absorption of the lead.

BULLET MIGRATION

Migration of a bullet through a hollow body structure, after it has initially decelerated and come to rest, such as a blood vessel, the airway, or the digestive tract, is unusual, but has been reported in multiple instances. So that possibility should be considered if the bullet is resting in a hollow body space.

PEARLS: GENERAL PRINCIPLES OF BALLISTICS AND PENETRATING TRAUMA

- Bullets impart energy into tissue by transfer of kinetic energy, which is predominantly determined by the bullet's velocity.
- Handguns are usually low-velocity weapons and rifles are high-velocity. Shotgun pellets are usually high velocity at the muzzle, but they decelerate and disperse rapidly with travel through the air.
- High-velocity gunshot wounds have higher kinetic energy than low-velocity wounds, and tend to cause more tissue loss and secondary injuries.
- Wounding potential is not predicted by bullet velocity alone, and the composition and shape of the bullet and its movement characteristics in tissue are also important factors.
- Close-range shotgun wounds have high energy, and may cause massive tissue destruction.
- Gunshot wounds injure tissue by direct penetration and also creation of a cavitation cavity.
- Assessment of bullet trajectory and penetration are important aspects of clinical evaluation.
- Management philosophy for penetrating trauma has changed over the decades: from mandatory exploration, to endoscopic and radiologic evaluation with close observation and exploration if certain signs develop.
- Bullets and other penetrating objects are not sterile, so penetrating wounds should be irrigated and debrided and not closed primarily.

REFERENCES

1. Clasper J. The interaction of projectiles with tissues and the management of ballistic fractures. J R Army Med Corps 2001;147:52–61

2. Bartlett CS, Helfet DL, Hausman MR, Strauss E. Ballistics and gunshot wounds: effects on musculoskeletal tissues. J Am Acad Orthop Surg 2000;8:21–36

3. Fackler ML. Gunshot wound review. Ann Emerg Med 1996;28:194–203

4. Fackler ML. Civilian gunshot wounds and ballistics: dispelling the myths. Emerg Med Clin North Am 1998;16:17–28

5. Stewart MG. Penetrating face and neck trauma. In: Bailey BJ, ed. *Head and Neck Surgery—Otolaryngology*, 3rd ed. Philadelphia: Lippincott Williams & Wilkins, 2001:813–821

6. Swan KG, Swan RC. Principles of ballistics applicable to the treatment of gunshot wounds. Surg Clin North Am 1991;71:221–239

7. Bartlett CS. Clinical update: gunshot wound ballistics. Clin Orthop 2003;408:28–57

8. Goodstein WA, Stryker A, Weiner LJ. Primary treatment of shotgun injuries to the face. J Trauma 1979;19:961–964

9. Sherman RT, Parrish RA. Management of shotgun injuries: a review of 152 cases. J Trauma 1963;3:76–86

10. Ordog GJ, Wasserberger J, Balusbramaniam S. Shotgun wounds ballistics. J Trauma 1988;28:624–631

11. Chen AY, Stewart MG, Raup G. Penetrating injuries of the face. Otolaryngol Head Neck Surg 1996;115:464–470

12. Golueke PJ, Goldstein AS, Sclafani SJA, Mitchell W, Shaftan GW. Routine versus selective exploration of penetrating neck injuries: a randomized prospective study. J Trauma 1984;24:1010–1014

13. Mansour MA, Moore EE, Moore FA, Whitehill TA. Validating the selective management of penetrating neck wounds. Am J Surg 1991;162:517–521

14. Scalea T. What's new in trauma in the past 10 years. Int Anesthesiol Clin 2002;40:1–17

Chapter 21

PENETRATING TRAUMA OF THE FACE

Michael G. Stewart

Like penetrating trauma to the neck or the cranial cavity, the evaluation and treatment of penetrating trauma to the face requires a thorough understanding of anatomy, physiology, and injury patterns, and several authors have addressed the management of facial injuries. All agree that a systematic approach is essential, with careful attention to injury mechanism and area involved.

INITIAL MANAGEMENT

As discussed in Chapter 1, all patients with penetrating trauma to the face should be initially evaluated for the ABCs of trauma—airway, breathing, and circulation—and resuscitated appropriately. Potential airway compromise should be considered in all penetrating facial trauma, and this is discussed in more detail later. Assuming that patients are initially stable, the secondary survey should include a detailed evaluation of their penetrating facial injury, including type of weapon and entry zone. We have seen that patients who do not have airway compromise, major hemorrhage, or obvious intracranial penetration are often considered "lucky" and subsequently are triaged to a lower acuity level in the emergency center. This might be appropriate in some cases, but many patients with penetrating facial trauma are at risk for delayed loss of airway, occult vascular injury, intracranial penetration, and other delayed complications, so close monitoring and continued evaluation are important.

TYPES OF PENETRATING FACIAL TRAUMA

It is easiest to divide penetrating trauma into the following groups: low-velocity gunshot injury, high-velocity gunshot injury, shotgun injury, and stab injury. As discussed in Chapter 20, a too-rigid division into low velocity versus high velocity can omit important information such as the type of projectile; however, it is still a useful clinical distinction. High-velocity bullets are likely to cause a larger area of cavitation injury, a larger permanent cavity, deeper penetration, higher probability of bony fracture, and in general more tissue damage and tissue loss, as compared with low-velocity bullets. Shotgun injuries have distinct injury patterns, and are best considered as a separate category. Finally, stab wounds to the face are also considered separately, as their sequelae may be easier to predict based on the angle and depth of penetration, and there is usually less adjacent or collateral damage.

FACIAL ZONES

The first attempt to create a staging system for penetrating facial trauma was actually described in an article by Gant and Epstein in 1979, although it was first shown pictorially in 1988 by Gussack and Jurkovich.[1] This system divided the face into entry zones I, II, and III, in which zone I was superior to the supraorbital rims, zone II was from supraorbital rim to oral commissure, and zone III was below the oral commissure. The authors found that injury patterns differed in different entry zones, which was helpful in evaluation and treatment. However, that system was potentially confusing because the entry zones of the neck also use the same nomenclature of zones I, II, and III, which could make classification and distinction of combined injuries difficult. Furthermore, because zone I was superior to the supraorbital rims, those injuries are really intracranial rather than facial.

To address those issues, a new facial zoning system was subsequently developed by Dolin et al,[2] using entry zones A, B, and C. Injuries superior to the supraorbital rim were excluded for the reasons described above, and zone A represented the lateral face (zygomatic arch and mandibular ramus), zone B the anterior midface, and zone C the anterior mandible. Although that system had some advantages, the exact demarcation points between zones were unclear, and their data demonstrated that penetrating trauma entering zones A and B resulted in similar injury patterns.

Subsequently, Cole et al[3] and Chen et al[4] independently attempted to simplify facial zoning and designated two entry zones, "midface" and "mandible" (Fig. 21–1). The midface/mandible staging system has the advantage of being easy to remember, and it does not overlap with other staging systems. In the Cole series, however, no significant differences by entry site were seen; for example, gunshot wounds to the mandible zone were no more likely to have airway compromise than wounds to the maxilla zone. Those authors did find an association between vascular injury and airway compromise,

but in general noted that vascular injury, intracranial penetration, bony fracture, soft tissue loss, and airway compromise were all potentially possible regardless of entry zone. Therefore, in their series they found that entry zone was not always helpful and that in penetrating facial trauma "anything was possible," so they recommended that all patients be carefully screened for potential injuries. In contrast to those findings, other authors have found distinct differences in injury pattern by entry zone.

Gunshot Wounds to the Face

The midface/mandible zoning system is particularly applicable for gunshot injuries, because the two entry zones have distinct patterns of injury.[1,2,4] We will discuss the treatment and evaluation of gunshot wounds in the same order as all trauma cases, and begin with airway and breathing.

Airway Control

Patients with a gunshot wound to the face have a high probability of requiring airway control for several reasons, including soft tissue edema or hematoma, tissue displacement, and bleeding. Many patients require airway control in the field and arrive at the hospital intubated, and others require airway establishment at the hospital. Although some patients appear initially to have a stable airway, they can quickly decompensate and require an emergency airway. Patients with a mandible entry zone have a significantly higher chance of requiring an emergency airway than patients with a midface entry zone, although about a third of patients with midface injuries may require an emergency airway. To avoid delayed airway obstruction and emergency airway procedures, a high index of suspicion is recommended and, when indicated, early elective airway establishment. Physicians should strongly consider elective airway establishment using controlled intubation for all patients with gunshot wounds to the mandible entry zone, even if the airway appears adequate at initial presentation.

Vascular Injury

Vascular injury can occur with entry into any facial zone, although there is a trend toward a higher rate of injury with midface entry. If major vascular injury is suspected, the patient should have an angiogram—if possible with the capability for radiologic intravascular intervention. In facial injuries, angiogram is preferred over surgical exploration

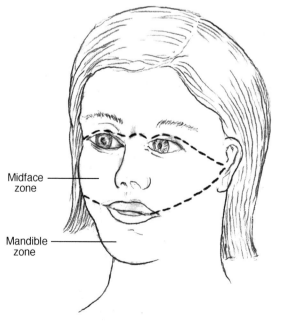

Midface
zone

Mandible
zone

FIGURE 21–1 Midface and mandible zones of the face.

because surgical access and control of major vessels near the skull base is difficult, whereas an interventional radiologist can both diagnose and potentially treat a vascular injury using stenting, occlusion, or embolization. This is the same clinical rationale behind the treatment for penetrating injuries to zone III of the neck. However, even if interventional radiology is not available, diagnostic angiography should still be performed to identify and localize vascular injuries; the surgical team can then decide on techniques for approach and repair.

The best clinical indications for angiography in penetrating facial trauma are best remembered as the two "P"s: *proximity* to a major vascular structure, and *penetration* posterior to the mandibular angle plane (MAP). The MAP[1] is an imaginary vertical coronal plane at the level of the angle of the mandible (Fig. **21–2**); penetration of a projectile posterior to this plane is an indication for angiography. Regarding proximity, if the path of a projectile is near a major vascular structure, angiogram is indicated. However, this can be difficult to assess because a projectile's path through tissue is not always predictable, and secondary projectiles that take different paths can be created. In addition, because of cavitation, the bullet may be somewhat distant from a vessel and still cause a significant injury. If the bullet is still in the patient, a lateral skull x-ray can be used to assess for penetration

posterior to the MAP. If there is an entry and exit and either is posterior to the MAP, angiogram is likely indicated. Angiography is relatively safe and very sensitive, but if suspicion of vascular injury is low, patients can be observed and only undergo angiography if new symptoms develop.

In a patient with active bleeding from deep in the wound, direct pressure with some sort of packing, or an occlusive pressure dressing should be placed, and the patient should undergo immediate angiogram with possible interventional intravascular treatment. If there is active bleeding from a wound edge, again direct pressure is recommended initially, with exploration and careful ligature of bleeding vessels when appropriate. Indiscriminate clamping or suturing of tissue in the face is to be avoided because of the risk of injury to a facial nerve branch.

ADJACENT INJURIES

After airway and vascular injuries have been evaluated, the physician should consider other potential injuries associated with facial gunshot wounds. These include intracranial penetration, globe injury, bony fracture, facial nerve injury, parotid duct injury, and penetrating neck injury. Intracranial penetration is not uncommon after facial gunshot wounds, occurring in 16% of patients in one series.[4] Bullets can reach the intracranial cavity after entry into either the midface or mandible zone. Neurosurgical consultation is obviously the next step in those cases.

Globe injury is also possible with penetrating facial trauma, and although more common in shotgun injuries, occurred in 18% of gunshot wounds in one series.[4] Again, ophthalmology consultation is essential in cases of globe injury.

BONE FRACTURES

Bone fracture is a common sequela of facial gunshot wounds. Although almost all fractures caused by gunshot wounds require some debridement and local care, not all fractures require open reduction and plate fixation. Although gunshot wounds may cause loss of bone, if the buttresses that provide midface stability are spared, then reduction and fixation may be unnecessary. Similarly, mandible injuries might involve damage only to an edge of the mandible, with sufficient stable bone above or below the injury. In that case, no reduction or fixation is necessary. Computed tomography (CT) scan with axial and coronal views is the preferred imaging study to evaluate the extent of bony injuries. In most cases, the wound should be explored, irrigated, and cleansed, and devitalized tissue, particularly bone separated from periosteum, debrided. As in all

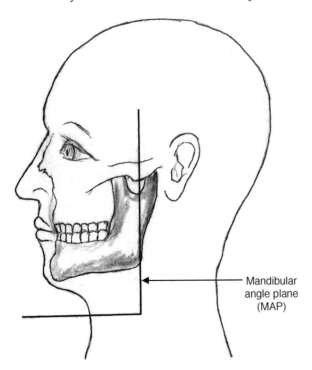

Mandibular angle plane (MAP)

FIGURE 21–2   Location of the mandibular angle plane (MAP); penetrating of a projectile posterior to the MAP is an indication for arteriogram.

gunshot wounds, the amount of damaged tissue that might survive can be surprising, so debridement should be fairly conservative. Gunshot entry and exit wounds are usually not closed, as bullets are not sterile, but are dressed and allowed to heal by secondary intention. Large or gaping soft tissue wounds can be partially approximated to facilitate healing. Local flap coverage, or even microvascular tissue transfer may eventually be necessary to close some tissue defects.

Unstable fractures should be repaired using the same plate-and-screw techniques of fracture repair as described in other chapters. If large pieces of bone are missing, consideration should be given to bone grafting, however the timing is important. If the wound is relatively clean and there is adequate surrounding blood supply, some recommend immediate bone grafting.[5] Within 48 hours, after debridement and irrigation, the wound may be ready for a bone graft, even if it does not look "clean." When there is obviously contaminated tissue, the wound should undergo progressive debridement and cleaning and the bone graft placed in a delayed fashion. However, if bone grafting must be delayed, then in all mandible fractures and most midface fractures the distance relationships between bone edges should be maintained by plating, generally using heavier plates than would normally be used for fracture repair. In the mandible, reconstruction plates are ideal for that purpose. Then, at a later date the bone graft can be affixed into the gap bridged by the plate. Because the bone graft never acquires the same strength as the original bone, the heavier plates help assume the load of the missing bone. In the mandible, in particular, if there has been tissue loss or damage in the oral cavity, the soft tissue around the mandible may be insufficient to support an immediate or early bone graft. In that case, soft tissue should be closed and placement of the bone graft delayed. Some have discussed using free tissue transfer, for example, omentum, to create a vascularized recipient bed for later bone grafting.[5] If free bone grafting is not possible, then free tissue transfer of vascularized bone, such as fibula or scapula, is another option for eventual reconstruction of a bony mandible or midface deficit.

Bone grafts placed early can heal surprisingly well, and can help maintain the position of the soft tissue overlying the bone. One problem with delaying bone grafts is that the overlying soft tissue can contract, and then when the surgeon attempts to place the bone graft, the tissue cannot be expanded back to its original size, and even if it can, it may have an unnaturally tense and stretched appearance. This can be avoided by placing bone grafts as soon as

practical, particularly in protruding visible areas like the nose, malar eminence, and orbital rim. Even if some revision is required later, the soft tissue healing is usually improved when the underlying bony projection was restored soon after injury.

The CT scan with its multiplanar images has significantly changed the management of penetrating facial injuries, and facilitates assessment of tissue damage and bullet path. Fig. **21–3** is an example of a facial scan after penetrating trauma, and demonstrates the value of CT scan in assessing the extent of injury as well as the location of bullet fragments and secondary projectiles. This assists in planning debridement as well as repair. Finally, the surgeon should keep in mind that bullets can be deflected into the tissues of the neck, particularly in mandible gunshot wounds because of the thick bone.

BULLET REMOVAL

In general, bullets should be removed from the wound, because they are a foreign body. However, that is occasionally not practical if the bullet is lodged deep in the tissues near vital structures, such that the surgical exploration necessary to expose and remove the bullet might potentially cause more injury than leaving the bullet in place. Many bullets have been left in tissues and have not caused any later problems. However, we have seen several patients with recurrent or persistent pain, infection, or foreign-body sensation from retained bullets, and after surgical removal the symptoms have resolved.

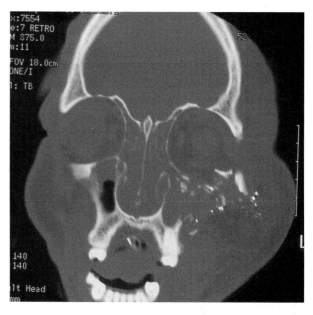

FIGURE 21–3 Computed tomography scan showing damage from a gunshot wound to the face.

SHOTGUN WOUNDS TO THE FACE

As discussed in Chapter 20, shotguns have a high muzzle velocity, and close-range shotgun injuries may impart significant energy to tissue,[6] with resultant massive tissue destruction. Most patients with shotgun wounds to the face have pellet penetration of both the midface and mandible entry zones, so the zoning system is not helpful. I recommend considering shotgun wounds as a separate category of penetrating facial trauma, and the patient should be evaluated as if both zones were entered.

The need for emergency airway establishment is uncommon in shotgun injuries to the face, although with close-range injuries involving the mandible or with significant oral cavity bleeding, the airway can be compromised. Two of 15 patients with shotgun wounds to the face required an emergency airway in one series.[4] Shotgun wounds to the face have been reported to achieve intracranial penetration as well as penetration posterior to the MAP, so careful evaluation of anterior-posterior and lateral skull x-rays is a mandatory part of evaluation. Shotgun wounds have a very high prevalence of globe injury, so all patients should undergo a careful ophthalmologic assessment. Facial bony fractures requiring reduction and fixation are unusual, even in close-range shotgun injuries. However, bony fragmentation can occur; this usually occurs along with soft tissue injury, and the bony fragments can be debrided at the same time as the soft tissue is addressed. As discussed previously, irrigation, cleansing, debridement of devitalized tissue, and removal of foreign bodies and pellets are important aspects of the early management of shotgun injuries.

STAB WOUNDS TO THE FACE

Stab wounds to the face can result in globe injury, vascular injury, unstable fracture, and even intracranial penetration. The overall management of stab wounds to the face uses the same principles of management of stab wounds elsewhere, as detailed in Chapter 20: if the weapon is still in place, assess depth of penetration using x-rays and do not attempt early removal; gently probe other wounds to assess depth; consider movement of the blade under the skin; and consider angiography to assess vascular injury. If the blade of a weapon is still impaled and there is concern about vascular injury, then diagnostic angiography can be performed prior to blade manipulation, with establishment of proximal vascular control using an inflatable balloon; in

some cases distal control can also be established. Then, with the balloon in place, the blade can be removed and if significant bleeding ensues, the balloon could be quickly inflated to stop or slow the bleeding—either as a definitive measure or to allow time for surgical exposure and an alternative means of vascular control. If interventional radiology is not available, then the surgeon could establish exposure and potential vascular control in the neck prior to blade manipulation.

Intracranial penetration and globe injury due to stab wounds require consultation with appropriate specialists. Management of facial fractures is the same as for other penetrating injuries, except that in stab wounds there is usually not a large amount of missing bone, so open reduction with internal fixation is usually adequate. Similar to bullets, the blades of penetrating weapons are not considered sterile, so stab wounds should not be closed primarily. However, there is usually little tissue loss with stab injuries, so irrigation and removal of foreign debris are usually sufficient treatment of the soft tissue injury. Other specific injuries are possible with facial stab wounds, and those are discussed in the next section.

MANAGEMENT OF SPECIFIC INJURIES

FACIAL NERVE INJURY

Patients with penetrating facial trauma and immediate paralysis of one or more branches of the facial nerve are likely to have transection of the nerve. If the wound is posterior to a vertical line drawn at the lateral canthus, these patients should undergo local exploration with primary nerve repair or nerve grafting—if their overall condition permits. Nerve injuries anterior to the lateral canthus are typically not explored because spontaneous nerve regeneration is usually adequate in that location. Although as a general principle, all patients with facial paralysis secondary to penetrating trauma should be explored and repaired; some of those injuries will recover adequate function even if completely transected because of substantial cross-innervation.[7] The areas with richest cross-innervation are the midface and zygomatic regions. In contrast, forehead and ramus mandibularis branches have poor cross-innervation, so injuries to these areas should be explored and repaired whenever possible. Gunshot wounds with immediate facial paralysis have a high probability of nerve damage beyond what is visible to the eye, so additional debridement of nerve ends and even nerve grafting should be strongly considered in gunshot injuries. Although surgical repair is the appropriate treatment, long-term functional outcomes after gunshot wounds are usually disappointing—no better than House-Brackman grade 4. This is probably due to the force and energy from the bullet that is transmitted to the facial nerve.

Severed distal facial nerve branches will retain their electrical excitability for ~48 hours, and a nerve stimulator can be used intraoperatively to identify the severed ends of nerve branches. The preferred neurorrhaphy technique is to trim back the perineurium away from the anastomosis and perform epineurial repair with 9-0 or 10-0 monofilament suture.[7] Facial nerve injuries that progress from partial to total paralysis following injury, or paresis that develops several hours after injury, are usually secondary to edema and may be treated expectantly with expected eventual resolution, similar to facial weakness following blunt trauma.

Parotid Duct Injury

Penetrating wounds to the cheek inferior to the zygomatic arch that injure the buccal branch of the facial nerve are also likely to injure the parotid duct, because that nerve branch and the duct are usually immediately adjacent. So buccal branch weakness should raise a high level of suspicion for parotid duct injury. Parotid duct injuries do not usually heal spontaneously or recanalize, so exploration and surgical repair are almost invariably required. If there is no buccal branch facial injury, but parotid duct injury is still suspected (i.e., clear saliva draining from a penetrating cheek wound, or sialocele formation), the wound should be explored. If injured, the duct should be primarily repaired over a hollow stent to allow saliva to continue to flow from the gland. Small monofilament suture is used for duct repair, and the stent can be fashioned from the tubing of a butterfly-type phlebotomy needle or a neonatal pediatric feeding tube. The stent is brought out through Stensen's duct into the lateral aspect of the mouth, and can be sutured to the buccal mucosa. The stent is usually removed after a few weeks.

Delayed Complications of Penetrating Facial Trauma

Even after successful initial stabilization and treatment, there are several potential delayed sequelae of penetrating facial injuries, which can occur in up to 35% of patients.[3,4] These include blindness, visual loss, diplopia, facial nerve weakness or paralysis, cerebrospinal fluid leak, soft tissue loss, bony malunion, malocclusion, trismus, orbital or periorbital cellulitis, sinusitis, oral-antral fistula, nasal obstruction or stenosis, and choanal stenosis. Although some of these complications can be directly caused by the injury and therefore cannot be avoided, many complications are potentially preventable with early recognition and aggressive management. In particular, nasal obstruction and stenosis, sinusitis, and choanal stenosis can be prevented or minimized with intranasal debridement and irrigation, placement of nasal stents, and using the techniques of functional endoscopic sinus surgery to restore adequate sinus drainage.

In addition, ophthalmologic complications such as diplopia and orbital infections may be prevented with careful reconstruction of the orbital floor to restore orbital anatomy and isolate the maxillary sinus from the orbit. Of course, when an orbital wall fracture causes globe displacement and diplopia, then surgical reconstruction is needed. However, even in cases of near-blindness or enucleation (where diplopia or globe position are not an issue), reconstruction of the orbital floor is still important to prevent communication between the maxillary sinus and orbit. We have seen cases of serious orbital infection, requiring removal of an orbital prosthesis, that were due to maxillary sinusitis and inadequate repair of the orbital floor, which allowed communication between the sinus and orbit.

Trismus and temporomandibular joint fibrosis can be prevented with early mobilization and stretching of the temporomandibular joint. Having the patient stack tongue depressors and place progressively larger stacks between the incisors to stretch the mouth open is a useful maneuver to prevent trismus.

Malocclusion is usually caused by inadequate open reduction and internal fixation of mandible or midface fractures, or by inadequate use of intermaxillary fixation at the time of fracture repair. That complication, therefore, is best avoided by careful attention to occlusion during fracture repair.

Pearls: Penetrating Facial Trauma

- Patients with penetrating trauma to the face should be evaluated using the trauma ABCs, followed by the secondary survey for associated injuries.
- The face is divided into two zones of entry: midface zone and mandible zone.
- Gunshot wounds to the mandible zone have a high chance of requiring emergency airway establishment.

- Gunshot wounds to the midface may cause injury to the globe or major vascular structures, or achieve intracranial penetration.
- The indications for arteriogram in penetrating facial wounds are proximity to a major vascular structure, or penetration posterior to the mandibular angle plane.
- Shotgun wounds to the face have a high prevalence of globe injury.
- Shotgun wounds can achieve intracranial penetration or cause deep vascular injury.
- When bone is missing after a gunshot wound, bone grafts should be placed relatively early if possible.
- Stab wounds can achieve significant depth of penetration.
- Facial nerve weakness after penetrating trauma is usually due to nerve transection; the wound should be explored and the nerve ends reapproximated.

REFERENCES

1. Gussack GS, Jurkovich GJ. Penetrating facial trauma: a management plan. South Med J 1988;81:297–302
2. Dolin J, Scalea T, Mannor L, et al. The management of gunshot wounds to the face. J Trauma 1992;33:508–515
3. Cole RD, Browne JD, Phipps CD. Gunshot wounds to the mandible and midface: evaluation, treatment, and avoidance of complications. Otolaryngol Head Neck Surg 1994;111:739–745
4. Chen AY, Stewart MG, Raup G. Penetrating injuries of the face. Otolaryngol Head Neck Surg 1996;115:464–470
5. Thorne CH. Gunshot wounds to the face: current concepts. Clin Plast Surg 1992;19:233–244
6. Goodstein WA, Stryker A, Weiner LJ. Primary treatment of shotgun injuries to the face. J Trauma 1979;19:961–964
7. Coker NJ. Management of traumatic injuries to the facial nerve. Otolaryngol Clin North Am 1991;24:215–227

Chapter 22

APPROACH TO PENETRATING INJURIES OF THE NECK

Bradford G. Scott

The initial approach to all trauma patients, including penetrating injury to the neck, should be assessment of the airway. If patients can talk coherently, then they have a patent airway. Signs of impending airway loss are incoherent or garbled speech, excessive bleeding from the oropharynx, extreme agitation as the patient struggles for air, stridor, and frank hypoxia. If the airway is not patent, then the physician's first duty is to secure one prior to any other procedure. Techniques are discussed elsewhere in the text.

With the establishment of a patent airway and adequate ventilation, the attention should turn to assessment of the circulatory status. Blood pressure, heart rate, respiratory rate, and oxygen saturation will dictate the immediate course of the patient. A hypotensive and tachycardic patient should be handled differently from a normotensive patient. A hemorrhagic source should be considered first with the hypotensive patient. Inspection of the wound for ongoing hemorrhage that would necessitate immediate operative intervention is the first step. There should be no delay for resuscitation in this case.[1] If there is no ongoing external hemorrhage, a quick evaluation with a chest x-ray assesses internal hemorrhage; if present, it is typically managed with placement of a tube thoracostomy. If external blood loss continues out of the wound or oropharynx, the patient may require an emergent procedure to stop the bleeding. In some cases, venous bleeding subsides with direct pressure, but arterial bleeding usually requires surgical control or an endovascular procedure.

After assessment of the circulatory status, next comes a quick neurologic exam and complete exposure of the patient. The neurologic exam should determine if the spinal cord, brachial plexus, or spinal accessory nerve (cranial nerve XI) has been injured. Simply asking patients to move their feet, hands, and arms and to shrug their shoulders will answer these questions. This information helps the surgeon determine the path of penetration, and documentation of neurologic status at presentation is important. Finally, exposure of the patient is a key maneuver. A rapid but thorough search for entrance, exit, and concomitant injuries helps plan the workup and operative management of the patient's injuries.

ENTRY ZONES

The entry zone and path of the penetrating injury determine the next steps in the patient's care. The neck has been divided into three zones of entry (Fig. 22–1). From the chest up, zone I extends from the clavicles and sternal notch up to the inferior border of the cricoid cartilage; zone II extends from the cricoid border up to the angle of the mandible, and zone III is from the angle of the mandible to the base of the skull. Evaluation and treatment patterns are unique for each zone of entry.[2]

DECISION FOR EXPLORATION

Patients with active hemorrhage, airway compromise, impending or active shock, expanding hematoma, subcutaneous emphysema, or other obvious signs of injury or instability, are taken for urgent definitive treatment—either surgical exploration, or perhaps endovascular management. In a normotensive patients without ongoing external blood loss or other hard signs of injury, however, the decision for surgical exploration is based on the zone of injury and the philosophy of the surgeon and the hospital

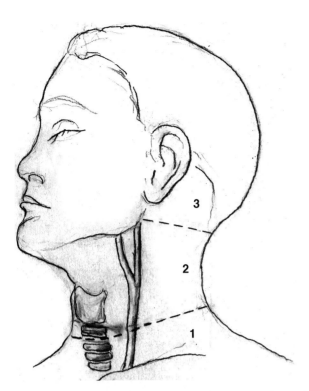

FIGURE 22–1 Zones of the neck: zone I, from the clavicles to the inferior border of the cricoid cartilage; zone II, from the cricoid to the angle of the mandible; and zone III, from the angle of the mandible to the base of the skull.

or trauma center. Each zone is discussed in more detail below.

ZONE III INJURIES

For zone III injuries, the upper aerodigestive tract, large blood vessels, the cervical spine, and the cranial cavity are the potential structures that can be injured. An examination of the oropharynx looking for penetration or bleeding, a computed tomography (CT) scan of the brain and neck, and an arteriogram of the carotid arteries identify all potentially significant injuries. Surgical exploration of zone III can be very difficult because of the presence of the mandible, the skull base, and several critical neurovascular structures. For that reason, in vascular injuries of zone III endovascular techniques such as stenting or balloon occlusion are often used; therefore, the angiogram can be both diagnostic and therapeutic in some cases.

Severe external hemorrhage coming from zone III of the neck can be temporarily occluded by inserting a 30-cc Foley catheter into the entrance wound and inflating the balloon for tamponade of the bleeding vessel. This can convert an emergent situation to an urgent one. If the balloon tamponade does stop the bleeding, then the next step is usually angiography.

Several views of the internal carotid artery should be obtained to determine the extent of injury. Also helpful is assessment of the presence of circulation to the affected side of the brain from the noninjured side of the brain. This helps the treating team in deciding if simple ligation or embolization of the injury is the best option. If bleeding continues, an anterior neck exploration is required. If a carotid injury is encountered at this location, often the only solution is ligation. This is tolerated well in young victims, but can cause cerebrovascular insufficiency in older patients. Complex vascular repairs at the base of the skull require either division or dislocation of the mandible, which is quite time consuming, and even after that is completed, access is limited in that narrow anatomic area. Any venous injury in the neck can be treated with ligation or attempted repair with little or no sequelae.

ZONE II INJURIES

For zone II injuries, all the visceral structures of the neck as well as the spinal column can be potentially injured. For the asymptomatic patient, there are two options for evaluation. Nonoperative investigation consists of arteriogram of the carotid arteries and its branches, bronchoscopy of the trachea, and evaluation of the pharynx and esophagus with endoscopy and/or contrast swallow study. However, surgical investigation (i.e., mandatory neck exploration) for zone II injuries is equally or perhaps more sensitive for diagnosis of injury than nonoperative investigation. In the opinion of many authors, when comparing the operative to the nonoperative approach for zone II injuries, the operative approach is less time-consuming and uses fewer resources, and therefore is more cost-effective, and mandatory surgical exploration of any zone II injury that penetrates the platysma can be justified.[3] Other authors recommend a nonoperative approach for evaluation of zone II injuries in the asymptomatic patient. If that approach is used, the results of diagnostic studies should be known as soon as possible. If the studies do not show a vascular or aerodigestive injury, then the patient should be observed for 24 hours from the time of the injury. This observation period helps reduce the possibility of a missed injury from the radiographic or endoscopic studies. If an injury is detected on diagnostic evaluation, then prompt operative intervention is warranted.

After exploration of a zone II penetrating injury, the wound is usually drained; some authors recommend the use of an external drain only if there was an injury to the aerodigestive tract. A drain is essential for aerodigestive injuries because if a repair suture line leaks, then that contamination will be appropriately controlled. Also, in the case of diffuse coagulopathy a drain placed deep to the platysma may prevent hematoma formation.

Zone I Injuries

For zone I injuries, the aerodigestive tract including the esophagus and the aortic arch and great vessels should be evaluated for potential injury. An arteriogram of the arch and great vessels, and evaluation of the trachea and esophagus are required to rule out injury. The trachea is best evaluated with endoscopy (tracheobronchoscopy). The esophagus can be evaluated with either endoscopy or a contrast swallow study. The choices of contrast and benefits and risks of different techniques are discussed in more detail in Chapters 24 and 25. However in summary, barium swallow alone is fairly sensitive at detection of an esophageal injury, but when esophagoscopy is added the sensitivity increases to nearly 100%.[4] Therefore, many authors advocate use of both a contrast swallow and endoscopy in all patients.

Zone I injuries should be considered with great trepidation. If the patient is hypotensive and has ongoing external blood loss, then balloon tamponade, as described for zone III injuries, should be attempted first. Because zone I injures often involve structures in the difficult-to-access thoracic inlet area, gaining a large amount of information about the injury helps plan the operation. Therefore, angiography, endoscopy, and contrast swallow studies should proceed if the patient is stable. If temporary measures fail to arrest the bleeding, however, then emergent operation should start without delay.

Positioning and prepping of the patient are keys to success. The patient should be prepped supine with a generous shoulder roll to extend the neck. Arms should be out and prepped to the elbow. The preparation should include the chin to well below the xiphoid and the lateral chest all the way to the table. This allows access for all potentially necessary approaches.

If the injury is on the left side of the patient in the medial half of the clavicle, the subclavian vein and artery should be considered as the injured vessels. Proximal control of the subclavian artery is best gained through a left anterior-lateral thoracotomy incision at the fourth intercostal space. The artery should be clamped at its origin from the aorta. Repair of the artery can then be attempted from a supraclavicular incision, and the proximal clamp removed to restore circulation once repair is complete. Often, resection of the medial one third

of the clavicle opens the space for inspection and repair. Common carotid injuries at the thoracic inlet are also approached in the same manner. If the thoracotomy does not allow access to the origin of the common carotid, a median sternotomy facilitates exposure.

For injury to the lateral areas of the subclavian artery and vein, a supraclavicular incision allows access to the site of injury. However, when using that approach alone, achieving proximal and distal control of the vessels can be more difficult.

If the injury is on the right side of the neck, then the most helpful exposure begins with a median sternotomy. Access to the common carotid and subclavian arteries at their origin from the aortic arch allows control prior to tackling the injured artery. Often resection of the medial head of the clavicle allows identification and repair of the injury.

Once exposed and after proximal control is achieved, zone I vascular injuries can be repaired primarily, with a patch or bypass graft. If repair cannot be achieved, then ligation of the injured vessel can be used. In young patients, common carotid ligation may not cause cerebrovascular insufficiency, but in older patients there is a much higher risk of stroke. Ligation of the subclavian artery can have mixed results in any age group. Some patients have immediate ischemia of the arm, whereas others may have a delayed presentation of claudication of the arm and forearm. The more proximal the ligation, the lower the likelihood of limb ischemia. If ischemia occurs with ligation, then several options are available. If primary revascularization through the wound is not possible, then a carotid to the more distal subclavian bypass is the best option. This places the graft through noncontaminated, noninjured anatomy and can be performed after the injury site is closed and both ends of the injured subclavian have been ligated at the injury site. As always, if the surgeon does not feel up to the task of approaching a complex repair, then a shunt can be placed for transfer to a higher level of care. Standard Argyle endarterectomy shunts are too small for the subclavian and common carotid arteries. In those cases, shunts have been fashioned from small chest tubes, and sterile proctoscopy or bronchoscopy suction tubing.[5]

If the patient with a zone I injury is stable and an injury to the great vessels is discovered on angiography, endovascular exclusion is possible using covered stent grafts. The lesion must be in an accessible area that a stent graft can span. The most common sites of repairs of this type are the proximal subclavian and carotid arteries.[6]

OTHER DIAGNOSTIC APPROACHES

Computed tomography of the neck is usually of little benefit in penetrating injuries.[7] It might help determine the trajectory of penetration but is not usually helpful in identifying injuries, even when CT angiography is employed. Simple observation of selected patients with asymptomatic penetrating injuries has also been employed. Most often the patients are not injured and are discharged the next day after eating a morning meal. When patients have an aerodigestive injury, the delay in treatment has had a detrimental effect on outcome.[8] One drawback to this approach is the low probability of any follow-up in trauma patients; therefore, the long-term sequelae of this approach are potentially unknown.

INJURIES CROSSING THE MIDLINE

Penetrating injuries that traverse the midline should be treated as a special case. The best way to approach these injuries is to consider each side of the neck separately and determine each zone of injury. This gives the clearest picture of the trajectory of penetration and the workup required. In the normotensive patient without ongoing hemorrhage, the nonoperative workup should include the elements for the zones of the neck that were traversed. For example, a missile that enters zone I and exits zone III would require an oropharyngeal examination looking for penetration, a CT of the brain, and an arteriogram of the carotid arteries, plus an arteriogram of the arch and great vessels, bronchoscopy of the trachea, and esophagoscopy with esophageal barium swallow. Another example would be a missile that traverses the midline from zone II to zone III. This could be approached with the nonoperative workup of both injuries or with a bilateral exploration including zone III on the affected side. Potential incisions for use in neck exploration are shown in Fig. 22–2.

SURGICAL MANAGEMENT OF VASCULAR INJURY

Zone II injuries are amenable to surgical intervention because all of the critical structures can be easily exposed. If a patient has hemorrhage from this area, temporary balloon tamponade can be tried but often with less success than in zone I and III. If direct pressure or balloon occlusion does not control hemorrhage, then immediate anterior neck exploration should be performed. The exploration should

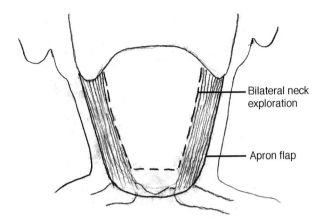

FIGURE 22–2 Incisions for neck exploration. Two options are shown: an "apron" flap, and bilateral sternocleidomastoid mastoid with a connecting "collar" incision.

include complete dissection of the carotid sheath and the external veins. A commonly injured vessel that causes considerable bleeding is the external jugular vein, which can be ligated safely and easily. When hemorrhage is discovered within the carotid sheath complete dissection of the sheath is mandated. Initial exploration of the carotid sheath should begin proximal to the injury. Once proximal control is gained, then the hematoma can be entered to gain distal control. As with all traumatic vascular injuries the hematoma has often done much of the dissection of tissue planes; all the surgeon needs to do is evacuate the hematoma and the vascular injury will present itself. Injuries of the jugular vein can be easily repaired with permanent suture, or the vein can be ligated if the injury is complex or large. Complex repairs of the jugular vein are not warranted, and if undertaken will most likely result in thrombosis of the entire vein.[9] Ligation of the vein can usually be accomplished at the site of injury.

Repairs of the carotid artery from stab wounds or very low velocity bullets are usually simple and require only primary repair. High-velocity gunshot wounds can cause extensive damage and might require more complex reconstruction. Therefore, with gunshot injuries care should be taken to debride the edges of the blast injury back to healthy artery. This will lessen the chance of immediate leak and/or pseudoaneurysm formation. After the debridement is completed, an assessment of the damage facilitates planning for reconstruction. The common carotid artery can easily be reanastomosed in an end-to-end fashion; the same is true for the internal carotid artery. The external carotid artery can be repaired, or it can be ligated with impunity. The most complex injuries are those to the bulb of the carotid. They may be handled with reimplantation of the internal carotid onto the common carotid. If this cannot be easily done, then the surgeon should consider an external-internal carotid artery switch. This is performed by ligation of the distal end of the external carotid artery at its trunk, and then using the open proximal stump of the external branch to reach to the internal in an end-to-end fashion.

For partial injuries of the carotid from a gunshot wound, primary closure can be attempted. However, if primary closure seems to narrow the lumen, then patch angioplasty should be employed. Multiple types of synthetic patches are available off the shelf, and most have been employed successfully in a trauma setting. If a concomitant aerodigestive injury occurs, use of a synthetic patch, with the chance for contamination and infection, is best avoided, so a vein patch can be employed; these are typically harvested from the neck or from the greater saphenous vein.

Bypass grafting is an option if complete destruction of the bulb is encountered. If the surgeon facing such a complex repair is not experienced in those techniques, then complete ligation is an option in young patients. If the patient is older, a carotid shunt, like those used in endarterectomy procedures, can be placed as a temporary measure to facilitate transfer to a higher level of care, with no increase in mortality.[10]

OTHER INJURIES

Injuries to the spinal column are not discussed in this text. Injuries to the upper aerodigestive tract are discussed in Chapters 24 and 25.

PEARLS: APPROACH TO PENETRATING INJURIES OF THE NECK

- The neck is divided into three zones (I, II, and III); injury to each zone results in typically different injury patterns and therefore different diagnostic and treatment protocols are used.
- Patients with obvious signs of vascular or airway injury and patients who are unstable should be taken for emergency treatment—either surgical or endovascular.

- Patients with zone II penetration who are stable and without obvious injury can be evaluated using diagnostic tests and close observation. Other surgeons recommend mandatory surgical exploration for all zone II injuries.
- Vascular injuries should be approached with caution. For arterial injuries, proximal control should be achieved first, and then the injury explored and repaired. Standard vascular surgical techniques are typically used.

REFERENCES

1. Bickell WH, Wall MJ Jr, Pepe PE, et al. Immediate versus delayed fluid resuscitation for hypotensive patients with penetrating torso injuries. N Engl J Med 1994;331:1105–1109
2. Jurkovich GJ, Zingarelli W, Wallace J, Curreri PW. Penetrating neck trauma: diagnostic studies in the asymptomatic patient. J Trauma 1985;25:819–822
3. Thal ER, Meyer DM. Penetrating neck trauma. Curr Probl Surg 1992;29:1–56
4. Armstrong WB, Detar TR, Stanley RB. Diagnosis and management of external penetrating cervical esophageal injuries. Ann Otol Rhinol Laryngol 1994;103:863–871
5. Husain AK, Khandeparker JMS, Tendolkar AG, Magotra RA, Parulkar GB. Temporary intravascular shunts for peripheral vascular trauma. J Postgrad Med 1992;38:68–69
6. du Toit DF, Strauss DC, Blaszczyk M, de Villiers R, Warren BL. Endovascular treatment of penetrating thoracic outlet arterial injuries. Eur J Vasc Endovasc Surg 2000;19:489–495
7. Gonzalez RP, Falimirski M, Holevar MR, Turk B. Penetrating zone II neck injury: does dynamic computed tomographic scan contribute to the diagnostic sensitivity of physical examination for surgically significant injury? A prospective blinded study. J Trauma 2003;54:61–64
8. Velmahos GC, Souter I, Degiannis E, Mokoena T, Saadia R. Selective surgical management in penetrating neck injuries. Can J Surg 1994;37:487–491
9. Nair R, Robbs JV, Muckart DJ. Management of penetrating cervicomediastinal venous trauma. Eur J Vasc Endovasc Surg 2000;19:65–69
10. Demetriades D, Skalkides J, Sofianos C, Melissas J, Franklin J. Carotid artery injuries: experience with 124 cases. J Trauma 1989;29:91–94

Chapter 23

LARYNGEAL TRAUMA

Steven D. Schaefer

External laryngeal injuries are rare, accounting for only one in 30,000 emergency room visits.[1] Early and careful management of these injuries has a profound consequence on the immediate probability of survival of patients and their long-term quality-of-life. Our approach to these injuries has been to apply basic principles of laryngeal mechanics to repeated observation, and to refine the medical and surgical treatment over the past 25 years (Fig. 23–1).[2]

LARYNGEAL ANATOMY AND RELEVANT PHYSIOLOGY

The human larynx is a highly evolved respiratory sphincter. As complex social and verbal animals, modern humans have benefited from the caudal descent of the larynx into the middle neck, permitting development of oral language. To this end, the phylogenetic primitive larynx of the lungfish contrasts with the complex cartilaginous skeleton joined together by muscles and ligament, and covered by mucous membrane in modern humans.

The laryngeal skeleton is a second through sixth branchial arch derivative, and consists of the hyoid bone, three single cartilages, and three paired cartilages. These are the thyroid, cricoid, and epiglottic cartilages, and the paired arytenoids, corniculate, and cuneiform cartilages. The cartilages are tethered together by fibrous ligaments and membranes. Three of these fibrous structures are the quadrangular membrane, conus elasticus (or triangular membrane), and the vocal ligament. The quadrangular membrane inserts anteriorly along the lateral border of the epiglottic cartilage and extends posteriorly to attach on the arytenoids cartilage. The superior free margin of this membrane forms the aryepiglottic fold, and the inferior border is the false vocal fold. The conus elasticus forms a triangle in which the base attaches to the midline of the cricoid and superiorly to thyroid cartilages. The apex of this membrane inserts on the vocal process of the arytenoids cartilage, and the free margin forms the vocal ligament. Both membranes are reacted directly, or indirectly as is the case of conus elasticus through its insertion on the arytenoid cartilages, by the intrinsic laryngeal muscles. Although all of the intrinsic laryngeal muscles are important, the vocal function of the larynx is particularly dependent on the thyroarytenoid muscle to form the bulk of the true vocal fold and those muscles associated primarily with rotation of the arytenoids, which are the interarytenoid, lateral cricoarytenoid, and posterior cricoarytenoid muscles. All of these muscles are innervated by the recurrent laryngeal nerve, and with the exception of the posterior cricoarytenoid, these muscles serve the sphincteric, or closure, and vocal functions of the larynx. The posterior cricoarytenoid is the only laryngeal abductor, and bilateral denervation is life threatening. The extrinsic laryngeal muscles can be defined as consisting of the cricothyroid and strap muscles, or as only the cricothyroid, in which case the strap muscles are considered accessory laryngeal muscles. In either classification, the cricothyroid is classically regarded as a tensor of the vocal folds. We believe that there is a measured contribution of intrinsic, extrinsic, and accessory muscles to the range of human phonation, swallowing, and respiration.[3-6]

Phonation is the product of chest compression of subglottic air overcoming the elastic and muscular forces of vocal fold closure. Acting as a sound source, the larynx cycles between these two forces to produce a tone that is modulated by the vocal tract (broadly, the vocal tract can be defined as extending

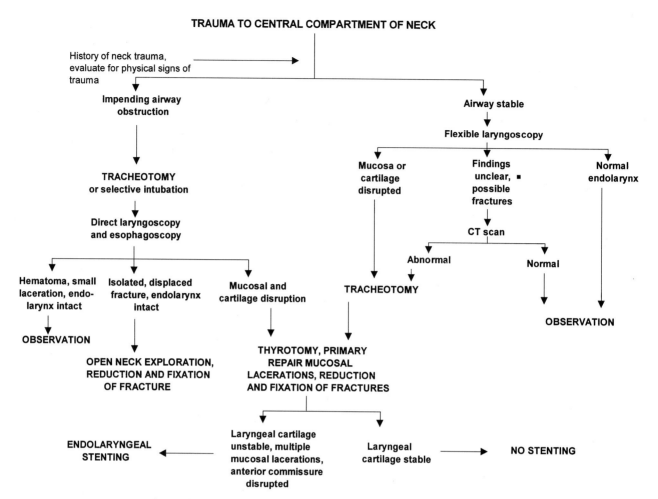

FIGURE 23-1 Management protocol for the acutely injured larynx. (Modified from Schaefer SD. The treatment of acute external laryngeal injuries. Arch Otolaryngol 1991;117:35.)

from the diaphragm to the lips). The complex interaction between vocal fold tension, mass, length, mucosal covering, and subglottic air pressure is best described by the myoelastic-aerodynamic theory.[7,8] as one seeks to repair the traumatized larynx, we must employ an understanding of laryngeal anatomy and physiology to guide us in deciding between medical and surgical management, and the extent of surgical treatment.

LARYNGEAL WOUNDING

External laryngeal injuries are now uncommonly seen in most emergency departments for several reasons. First, the overall incidence of neck trauma adjusted for the population as compared with the early 1990s has declined, reflecting regulatory and design changes in automobiles, and the decreasing violent crime rate in the United States. Second, the most severely injured patients often die at the scene of the accident or assault, and are not counted in estimates of laryngeal trauma.[2] Third, the larynx is

afforded partial protection by its position in the neck. Anteriorly, the inferior projection of the mandible partially shields the larynx from direct trauma. Posteriorly, the rigid cervical spine protects the larynx. Nonetheless, injuries occur, and the resultant damage to the larynx is usually characteristic of the mechanism of injury. The mechanisms of external laryngeal injury can be divided into blunt trauma (including clothesline, crushing, and strangulation injuries) and penetrating trauma.

Anterior blunt injuries are most commonly the result of motor vehicle accidents (Fig. 23-2).[8-11] The incidence of this type of injury is declining, presumably because of mandatory seat belt laws, reengineering the driver and passenger compartments, lower speed limits, and better education regarding drunken driving. The use of front seat air bags most likely reduces the incidence even further. If no seat belt is worn or if only a lap belt is used, the driver is thrust forward during rapid deceleration, with the neck hyperextended. This position removes the bony protection of the mandible, exposing the

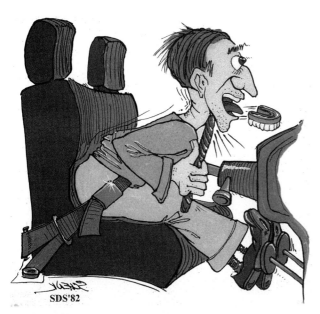

SDS'82

FIGURE 23–2 With a lap belt and without a shoulder harness, the neck is extended, removing protection that the mandible affords the neck. The larynx is crushed between the steering wheel and cervical spine. This drawing also illustrates the need to be aware of associated problems and injuries, such as aspiration of teeth or dentures and cervical spine fractures.

larynx to anterior crushing forces. If the larynx then strikes the steering wheel or dashboard, it may be compressed between these objects and the cervical spine.[10,11]

Clothesline injuries occur when the rider of a vehicle, such as a motorcycle or snowmobile encounters a fixed horizontal object, such as a clothesline at neck level. This type of injury imparts the full momentum of the rider and the vehicle over the relatively small anterior neck, resulting in massive trauma.[12] Many of these injuries lead to immediate death resulting from a crushed larynx or separation of the cricoid from the larynx or trachea. The latter injuries are frequently accompanied by disruption of one or both recurrent laryngeal nerves. A perhaps less devastating variation of this injury is a fist or object blow to the anterior neck.

Strangulation injuries occur from manual compression, from assaults with strangulation by a soft object, and from attempted suicides by hanging. Typically, the initial finding may be hoarseness or abrasions on the skin of the overlying neck. However, these injuries may later (in 12 to 24 hours) be associated with marked edema of the larynx and resultant loss of airway.[13] The magnitude of the force sustained to the anterior neck should be considered in the management of such patients to avoid subsequent potential loss of the airway.[2] Overall in blunt trauma to the anterior neck, fractures of the thyroid

cartilage occur more frequently than all other airway cartilages combined.[12]

Civilian penetrating trauma had been increasing because of the rise in personal assaults (Fig. 23–3).[2,14] For example, in a review of 148 cases of penetrating neck trauma, injury to the larynx or trachea was noted in 12 cases.[15] We believe that this form of laryngeal trauma is now most likely decreasing as violent crime has declined over the past decade. However, this is only an opinion and we do not have recent data to support this supposition. Injury from gunshot wounds depends on the type of weapon used, the effective range of the weapon, and the ammunition. Gunshots at close range impart intense energy to the soft tissues and are usually fatal. Low-velocity handguns (commonly used in domestic assaults) generally have only a moderate blast effect on surrounding tissue. These injuries may be misleading on initial examination because of the bullet's erratic course in soft tissues. High-velocity weapons, such as hunting rifles and military assault weapons, impart a significant amount of kinetic energy to the tissues.[16] In these injuries, tissue viability is widely compromised and initial impressions as to the extent of wounding are frequently inadequate. Knife injuries do not destroy tissue distant to the path of injury, and their course may be accurately estimated from the entrance and exit wounds.

The pediatric larynx is injured less often than the adult larynx. Situated higher in the neck than the adult larynx, the child's larynx is afforded greater protection by the caudal projection of the mandible. However, the pattern of injury reflects a dynamic between the loose attachments of the overlying mucous membranes and ligaments, and the increased elasticity of the cartilaginous framework. Further, the cross-sectional area of the pediatric larynx compared with that of the adult larynx is decreased. The combination of potentially increased soft tissue injury and edema and decreased cross-sectional area make the pediatric airway especially vulnerable to injury. These injuries may be difficult to recognize due the lack of obvious cartilaginous fractures.

INITIAL MANAGEMENT

In a neck injury patient who presents to the emergency department, the first priority is to establish an airway. This may be very difficult and often requires emergent tracheotomy or cricothyroidotomy. Care should be taken to avoid manipulation of the neck. Until a cervical spine injury has been excluded, no extension of the neck should be allowed during

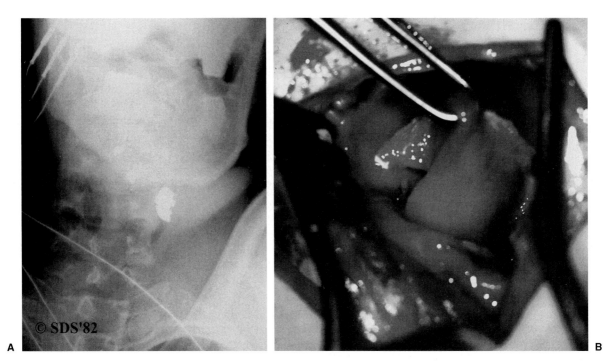

FIGURE 23–3 A: Anteroposterior (AP) radiograph showing a 0.357 magnum bullet in central compartment of neck. B: Intubation of this patient was attempted in the emergency department, resulting in compromise of the airway. Emergency tracheotomy established an airway, and the patient underwent neck exploration. This intraoperative photograph shows that the passage of the endotracheal tube had created a false passage between the right thyroid cartilage and the endolaryngeal mucous membrane.

either orotracheal intubation or tracheotomy. After the airway is secured, venous access should be obtained with at least two large-bore cannulas. Isotonic fluids are administered as needed to maintain circulation. The patient is then disrobed and examined for other injuries. If the patient is unstable after these measures, immediate surgery is needed. If the patient is relatively stable after these measures, however, diagnostic assessment may proceed. The minimum radiographic evaluation consists of a cervical spine series and a chest radiograph. Subplatysmal penetrating injuries in the area of the carotid arteries should be evaluated with arteriography. After full assessment of all injuries, the various physicians involved should determine the order of management and proceed accordingly.

DIAGNOSIS

The presentation of external laryngeal trauma varies from obvious open fractures to subtle aberrations of laryngeal function. A comprehensive and timely evaluation of the patient is essential to an optimal outcome.

HISTORY

Understanding the mechanism of wounding is important in predicting the immediate course of treatment and the potential injuries. A patient arriving in the emergency department after striking the steering wheel with the anterior neck may appear stable within the first minutes of the accident. Within the next hours the initially normal-appearing patient, including at laryngoscopy, may evolve into life-threatening endolaryngeal edema and hematomas. In such an example, the history of significant energy being imparted to the neck should alert the physician to the potentially evolving catastrophic event.[1] In contrast, a low-energy accidental fist or other less intense blow to the larynx can result in a displaced thyroid cartilage fracture (Fig. **23–4**). In penetrating trauma, the type of weapon and ammunition used, the range at which the injury occurred, and the anatomic site of the wound must all be considered. Having seen all of these events, we advocate that any patient with a history of trauma to the central compartment of the neck be considered to have a potential airway injury until proven otherwise.

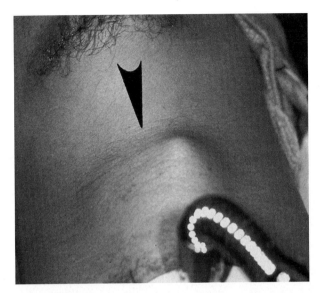

FIGURE 23–4 Following a single fist blow to the neck, this patient presented with a paramedian fracture of the thyroid cartilage. Visualization examination shows obvious displacement of the thyroid cartilage from the midline (arrow). As the endolarynx was uninjured, this patient was treated by open reduction and fixation of the fracture without performing a thyrotomy.

PHYSICAL EXAMINATION

In our experience, and much to our surprise, only respiratory distress seems to correlate with the severity of blunt injury (Table **23–1**). Visual examination of the neck may reveal an open fracture or laryngocutaneous fistula, or more often nothing in the case of blunt trauma (Fig. **23–4**). The larynx should be palpated for crepitus. Tenderness to palpation, although not specific, is often present in significant injury.[2] The skin of the neck may reveal contusions or abrasions from blunt trauma or a line pattern indicative of a strangulation injury.[17,18] Penetrating injuries are examined for an entrance and exit wound, and the most likely path of travel of the projectile should be determined. Open wounds are not explored with instruments, nor are they probed to avoid dislodging a hematoma and initiating further bleeding. The cervical spine should be palpated for any bony step-off fractures, dislocations, or tenderness. Hemoptysis may reveal an injury to the upper aerodigestive system, but it is often difficult to differentiate from bleeding from associated facial trauma.

External laryngeal injuries are often associated with a change in voice.[13] In severe trauma, the patient may be entirely aphonic. More commonly, dysphonic voice is present secondary to alterations in the larynx, or the voice is muffled secondary to supraglottic or upper vocal tract injury. Hematomas

of the true vocal folds add mass to this vibratory unit and lower the fundamental frequency of vibration. Paresis of the vocal fold from damage to the recurrent laryngeal nerve or from mechanical dislocation of the cricoarytenoid joint may cause a weak, breathy voice. Finally, any injury to the larynx that changes the airflow patterns has the potential to alter the voice.

Among the most serious alterations of laryngeal function is the abnormal flow of air through the upper airway. In instances of cricotracheal separation, the partially transected airway may be maintained solely by a bridge of mucous membrane between the cricoid and trachea. In gunshot wounds, the path of the missile serves as a laryngocutaneous fistula and allows respiration despite obstruction at the glottic or supraglottic level.[19] In this instance, airflow from the wound will be obvious, and no attempt should be made to cover, compress, or otherwise manipulate such a wound until the surgeon is ready to secure the airway. Stridor may occur from bilateral vocal fold paresis or disruption or may result from any combination of unilateral immobility and subglottic, glottic, or supraglottic edema or hematoma. If severe enough, edema alone with healthy vocal fold movement may cause stridor. As discussed above, in some patients the evolution of the edema or hematoma can be over a few hours, which may permit recognition of subglottic, glottic, or supraglottic airway compromise. In many other patients, the airway compromise is too rapid to permit distinction among inspiratory, expiratory, and mixed stridor. Another, more subtle form of laryngeal dysfunction is aspiration, which is usually caused by immobility of one or both vocal folds. Although not immediately clinically apparent postinjury, aspiration may present later as pneumonia.

After the initial examination and securing of the airway, examination of the endolaryngeal anatomy is attempted. In the past, this was only possible in the awake patient using the indirect mirror examination and was problematic in the severely injured patient. Since the 1980s flexible fiberoptic laryngoscopic examination facilitates improved nonoperative evaluation of the injured larynx.[2,20] Care should be taken in the examination of the nonintubated patient, because the minor trauma associated with insertion of the fiberoptic laryngoscope may precipitate an airway emergency. After insertion of this instrument through the nares, the oropharynx and hypopharynx are examined for injury. The larynx is examined for hematomas and lacerations, and their size and location are noted. The arytenoids are evaluated for full range of motion during phonation and respiration.[21] Partial limitation of range of

TABLE 23–1 Presenting Symptoms of 68 Patients with Laryngeal Trauma*

	Presenting symptom							Type of injury		
Group	Hoarseness	Pain/Tenderness	Hemoptysis	Dysphagia	Subcutaneous Emphysema	Impaired Respiration	Hematoma	MVA	Blunt	Penetrating
I	8	7	1	1	1	1	0	7	3	1
II	10	2	2	2	5	18	3	7	9	19
III	4	1	1	1	5	8	1	2	2	8
IV	3	0	0	1	2	6	0	2	2	6

*Groups I to IV refer to the form of management and are discussed in Table 23–2. The severity of injury, group IV being the most severe, did not correlate with the presenting symptoms. From Schaefer SD. Acute management of laryngeal trauma. Update. Ann Otol Rhinol Laryngol 1989;98:98.

motion indicates a structural deformity or dislocation of the arytenoids, whereas complete immobility is more suggestive of recurrent nerve injury.[22] Failure of the true vocal folds to meet in the same horizontal plane may also be present, indicating a structural change in the laryngeal framework or superior laryngeal nerve injury. In minor injuries with sufficient glottic closure to trigger the strobe, video stroboscopic laryngoscopy is helpful to reveal small alterations secondary to either muscle or mucosal injuries. Finally, exposed cartilage is recorded along with the integrity of the surrounding mucous membrane.

LARYNGEAL IMAGING

The role of preoperative radiographic evaluation of the injured larynx has changed dramatically with the widespread availability of computed tomography (CT).[17,23–25] Before CT scanning, soft tissue radiograms of the neck, contrast laryngography, and tomography were available to assess the soft tissues of the larynx. Frequently, these studies added little information about the integrity of the larynx to that obtained by fiberoptic laryngoscopy. Plain films might identify gross fractures but are limited to a two-dimensional image of the relevant anatomy. Application of a laryngeal lumen contrast agent in laryngography is both difficult and dangerous in the acutely injured patient because of potential airway compromise. Tomography lacks the three-dimensional analysis and clarity of CT. Magnetic resonance imaging offers superior soft tissue definition, and limited visualization of laryngeal hard tissue. In contrast, CT imaging permits evaluation of the laryngeal skeletal and soft tissue in a noninvasive manner (Fig. **23–5**). Optimal CT imaging is performed using spiral technique with millisecond scan times, particularly when employing two-dimensional sections for multiple projections or three-dimensional reconstructions.[26] *Computed tomographic scanning is employed selectively.* In patients with clinically observable fractures, exposed laryngeal cartilage, or significant mucosal lacerations, the clinical examination should suggest the need for surgical treatment, and CT adds little to the preoperative and surgical examination of the larynx.[17]

We recommend reserving CT scanning for patients in whom laryngeal trauma is suspected because of the history, but the extent of injury is not obvious on physical examination. Such patients are those who have only one sign or symptom of laryngeal trauma, such as hoarseness, and minimal physical findings suggestive of laryngeal injury. In this instance, CT scanning may allow the surgeon to confirm the lack of injury in a noninvasive manner without direct, operative laryngoscopy and the concomitant need for general anesthesia. CT might also be used to identify the patient with minimally displaced midline or lateral thyroid cartilage fractures that are otherwise unremarkable and minimally symptomatic. Such unrepaired lateral displacement of the thyroid cartilage impairs phonation by disrupting complete vocal fold closure or laryngeal valving.[27] In a relatively small number of patients with massive edema or hematomas without lacerations, direct laryngoscopy has been insufficient to visualize the laryngeal framework. In these patients, CT is employed to search for laryngeal fractures. If none are detected, the patient undergoes a tracheotomy to preserve the airway, and is observed, thus avoiding open exploration.

MANAGEMENT

Management of injuries to the larynx is based on the mechanism and extent of injury found during the initial assessment. The first priority is always securing the airway.[28] The long-term priority is restoration of a normal laryngeal function. To meet these goals, initial management can be encompassed in four questions. First, does the patient need an artificial airway? Given the propensity for trauma to the central compartment of the neck to compromise the laryngeal skeleton, this question should be cautiously answered. Second, how can the extent of injury best be evaluated? These options can include fiberoptic laryngoscopy, CT scanning, or direct laryngoscopy. Third, after satisfying the first two questions, is the injury likely to spontaneously heal with a result equal to or better than surgical intervention? Fourth, if the outcome of the injury is in doubt or so severe as to require surgical treatment, which procedures are indicated? The answers to the last two questions require a through knowledge of laryngeal mechanics and experience (Fig. **23–1**). But there is little experience because of the rarity of these injuries.

NONSURGICAL SURGICAL MANAGEMENT

The purpose of a careful physical examination and selective CT scanning is to identify potential injuries, and to decide between medical and surgical treatment.[2,17,20,29] Medical management assumes the patient does not require a tracheotomy and has an otherwise stable airway. We recommend close observation in the first 24 hours of injury and elevation of the head of the bed in patients who have only the following injuries: (1) minor endolaryngeal mucosal

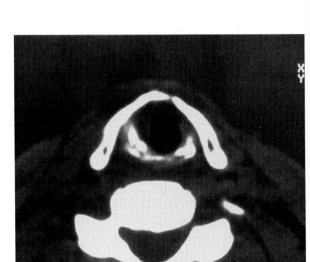
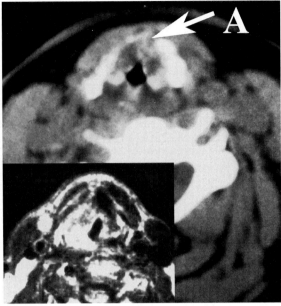

FIGURE 23–5 A: Axial computed tomography (CT) scan showing a single nondisplaced thyroid cartilage fracture (arrow). This patient was managed by observation only. B: Axial CT scan showing a displaced thyroid fracture with mild subcutaneous emphysema. An axial magnetic resonance imaging (MRI) of another patient with early glottic carcinoma appears in the lower half of the photograph to illustrate the contrast between CT and MRI. The former is preferential for showing the laryngeal skeleton, whereas the latter is superior for imaging soft tissue.

lacerations without involvement of the anterior commissure or free margin of the true vocal fold; (2) single nondisplaced, nonangulated fractures of the thyroid cartilage without overlying mucosal lacerations or exposed cartilage; (3) nonobstructing endolaryngeal edema; and (4) small, stable hematomas that are not causing respiratory embarrassment. Corticosteroids may be useful if given early after injury.

SURGICAL MANAGEMENT

Surgical treatment is indicated in injuries that do not spontaneous recover, and therefore require surgical restoration of the traumatized larynx. These are injuries (1) involving the anterior commissure or free margin of the true vocal fold; (2) resulting in exposed cartilage; (3) leading to multiple or displaced fractures of the thyroid cartilage or any fracture of the cricoid cartilage; (4) causing vocal fold paralysis or sufficient airway compromise to require intubation or tracheotomy; (5) resulting in glottic or transglottic lacerations; and (6) associated with trauma to another area of the neck that requires surgical intervention (Fig. **23–6** through Fig. **23–10**).[2] Repair of the larynx should be coordinated with all surgical teams involved and with the anesthesiologist. The person responsible for the airway at each stage of the procedure should be designated before bringing the patient to the operating room. Plans for

emergently obtaining an airway and the instruments required for surgery should also be established.

The most conservative, reliable method of securing an airway in a patient with laryngeal injury is local tracheotomy while the patient is awake. Endotracheal intubation may further damage the larynx, be exceedingly difficult, interfere with subsequent examination and repair of the larynx, and convert an urgent procedure to an emergent one (Fig. **23–3**). Endotracheal intubation is acceptable when (1) the endolaryngeal mucous membrane is intact; (2) the laryngeal skeleton is minimally displaced; and (3) the intubation is performed by one highly skilled in such procedures.

After local tracheotomy or selective use of intubation, general anesthesia is induced followed by operative, direct laryngoscopy. The larynx is examined for exposed cartilage, hematomas, lacerations, and range of motion of the true vocal folds. The subglottis is evaluated for injury to the cricoid and trachea. Rigid esophagoscopy is performed to rule out injury to the esophagus.[8]

Management of the traumatized pediatric airway presents special problems. Endotracheal intubation in the injured pediatric larynx has all of the same risks outlined above for the adult. The option of local tracheotomy is not feasible in a frightened, injured child. The time margin of error is also less because the arterial oxygen saturation drops more rapidly than in an adult. In this instance, rigid bronchoscopy

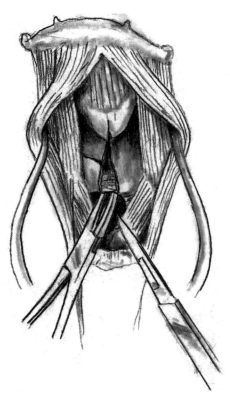

FIGURE 23–6 Exploration of the larynx is performed via a midline thyrotomy or via a paramedian vertical thyroid cartilage fracture.

is performed to secure the airway under direct visualization. A tracheotomy may then be performed over the bronchoscope.

After obtaining an airway and endoscopy, and following review of the CT findings, the need for open exploration and repair is reevaluated. Microlaryngoscopy should also be considered, particularly in evaluating lesser injuries.[21] In patients with edema, hematomas, nondisplaced fractures of the thyroid cartilage, healthy true vocal fold motion, and no injury to the anterior commissure or free margin of the true vocal fold, no further surgery is usually indicated.[2,29,30] Anesthesia is discontinued, the head of the bed is elevated, and the patient is observed carefully. Serial flexible fiberoptic laryngoscopic examinations are performed to ensure proper healing, and the tracheotomy tube is removed as soon as tolerated.

In patients with more severe injuries, surgical exploration is performed. In the past, controversy existed as to the optimal time for repair.[14,16,31,32] Some authors had advocated delay of repair for 3 to 5 days to allow edema to subside and for easier identification of mucosal lacerations. However, the best results have been obtained with early repair, avoiding the morbidity of leaving open wounds in a contaminated field.[2,21,31,33] Surgical exploration

begins with elevation of a subplatysmal apron flap to the hyoid bone. The strap muscles are separated in the midline and retracted laterally. A midline thyrotomy is used to enter the larynx (Fig. 23–6). All mucosal lacerations are meticulously repaired using 5-0 or 6-0 absorbable sutures. Dislocated arytenoids are reduced and avulsed. In most injuries, wounds can be closed using adjacent mucosa. In cases involving military weapons or other instances in which the loss of tissue is large, regional mucosal flaps or skin grafts may be used to complete the lining of the larynx. After repair of the injured mucous membrane and muscle, the anterior commissure is reconstituted by suturing the anterior margin of the true vocal fold to the outer perichondrium. Regardless of the need for stenting as is discussed below, reconstituting the anterior commissure is essential to maintain the scaphoid shape of this site and to preserve a normal voice (Fig. 23–8). The thyrotomy is closed using permanent sutures, wire, or fixation plates.

Laryngeal skeletal fractures are frequently repaired using wire or nonabsorbable suture. To avoid further damage to the laryngeal mucosa and skeleton, no fracture site sutures are tightened until all fractures have been reduced. Simple nondisplaced fractures may be repaired by suturing the outer perichondrium with nonabsorbable sutures. An alternative to wire is internal fixation using absorbable or nonabsorbable plates.[34,35] For such plating to be effective the screws must be well anchored in the laryngeal skeleton, and this can be problematic in younger patients with minimal calcification of their larynx.

The indications for stenting in laryngeal injuries are controversial.[2,9,29,36] The advantages of using a stent should be weighed against additional damage to the mucosa. Stents are recommended for injuries involving the anterior commissure, massive lacerations, comminuted fractures of the thyroid cartilage, and in cases in which the architecture of the larynx is not maintained by open fixation of the fractures (Fig. 23–7 and Fig. 23–8). The advantages of stenting in these instances are decreased web formation at the anterior commissure, decreased synechia from extensive lacerations and better support of the laryngeal architecture during healing. This additional support may be useful in light of the movement of the larynx with phonation and swallowing during the healing process. Placement of an endolaryngeal stent without open reduction with internal fixation of fractures and closure of lacerations is unsatisfactory because both these injuries and the larynx are too complex to benefit from placement of a lumen keeper. Following repair of the laryngeal wounds,

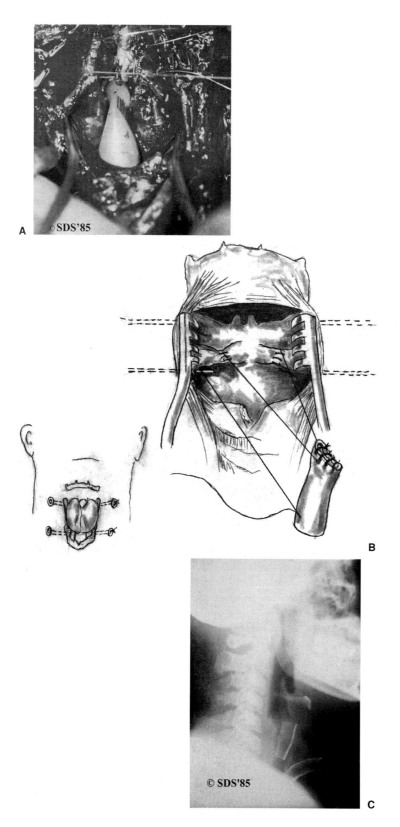

FIGURE 23–7 A: A Portex endotracheal tube stent in the larynx following closure of multiple laryngeal lacerations. B: The upper end of the modeled stent should be placed at the level of the aryepiglottic folds, and the lower limit of the stent should rest at the first tracheal ring. The stent is held in place by 0 Prolene or Mersilene sutures, which are passed through the laryngeal ventricle and cricothyroid membrane using an 18-gauge spinal needle. The sutures are held in place using skin buttons. (From Schaefer SD. Acute surgical treatment of the fractured larynx, Op Tech Otolaryngol Head Neck Surg 1990;1:65.) C: Lateral soft tissue x-ray of neck showing Portex endotracheal tube stent in larynx.

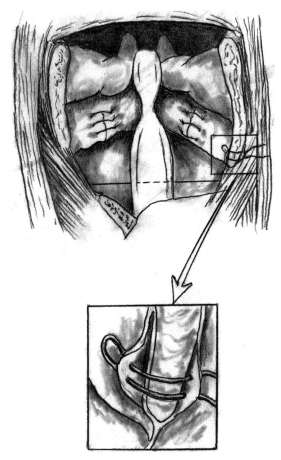

FIGURE 23–8 After endolaryngeal surgery is complete, *with or without stenting*, the scaphoid shape of the anterior commissure should be restored by suturing the most anterior aspect of the vocal folds to the outer perichondrium of the thyroid cartilage (see enlargement). This maneuver often avoids the need for stenting as long as the anterior commissure was intact before surgical exploration and no lacerations involve this site. (From Schaefer SD. Acute surgical treatment of the fractured larynx, Op Tech Otolaryngol Head Neck Surg 1990;1:66.)

the strap muscles are reapproximated, and the wound is closed over a drain.

The choice of stents range from finger cots filled with foam rubber to commercially manufactured polymeric silicone stents (Fig. **23–9**). All should be roughly in the shape of the larynx and made of soft material to avoid further mucosal damage. The stent should extend from the false vocal fold to the first tracheal ring to add stability and prevent endolaryngeal adhesions. Ideally, the stent should be secured in such a manner as to be easily remoe employed for years an easily available stent made from a 3.5-cm length of Portex endotracheal tubing (Fig. **23–9**).[37] The superior end of the tube is sewn tightly closed to prevent aspiration, and smooth clamps are placed to approximate the true and false vocal folds. The stent is then autoclaved to 82°C,

thereby reforming the tube to the desired shape. The stent is secured by two monofilament sutures through the laryngeal ventricle and cricothyroid membrane and tied to skin buttons (Fig. **23–7**).

Various other injuries may also be encountered during surgery. As much as one third of the anterior cricoid or trachea can be repaired using the sternohyoid muscle and its overlying fascia (Fig. **23–10**). Loss of the anterior third of the thyroid cartilage or hemiglottis can be repaired by closure of mucosal lacerations over a stent. If the recurrent laryngeal nerve is severed by the injury, a neurorrhaphy of the severed ends should be performed. Although the intricate abductor-adductor functions of the larynx will not likely return, reinnervation may help maintain muscle tone and therefore voice quality. If open reduction and internal fixation with stenting are unsuccessful in restoring the laryngeal architecture because of massive tissue loss, partial or total laryngectomy may be necessary. The decision for partial or total laryngectomy should be based on the defect, using the same guidelines used in oncologic reconstruction.[19] However, total laryngectomy has not been necessary in large series of laryngeal trauma and is more likely to be considered acceptable management for military wounds.[2]

POSTOPERATIVE CARE

We prescribe postoperative antibiotics for 5 to 7 days in an effort to reduce infection and granulation tissue. However, we are unaware of published verification of this practice. The head of the bed should be elevated, as tolerated, to minimize edema. The patient should be encouraged to ambulate as soon as tolerated. If a tracheotomy is present, routine care is provided. Stents placed at the time of surgery should be removed as soon as possible to prevent further mucosal damage, usually 10 to 14 days after surgery. Decannulation may be performed as soon as the stent is removed. Follow-up examinations should be scheduled for at least 1 year to assess true vocal fold function return and to monitor the development of subglottic stenosis. Antacids and H_2-blockers should be routinely used to prevent reflux, which may cause increased scarring of laryngeal tissues. When possible, nasogastric tubes are avoided to reduce reflux and prevent erosion of the posterior cricoid mucosa associated with their use.

COMPLICATIONS

Complications after repair of external laryngeal trauma include impaired vocalization, respiration, and deglutition. Postoperative granulation tissue

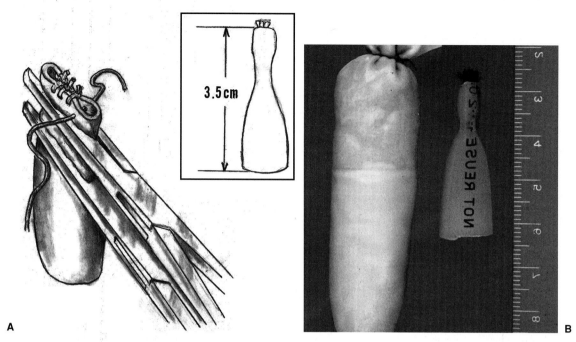

FIGURE 23-9 A: A laryngeal stent can be fabricated from a Portex endotracheal tube by using a 3.5- to 4-cm straight segment of the endotracheal tube that is cross-clamped with two parallel straight clamps. The first clamp is placed within 2 to 3 mm of the upper end of the tube, and the second clamp is positioned ~ 0.5 cm below the first clamp. The upper end of the tube is closed with 2-0 silk suture. The clamped tube is placed within a steam autoclave that is manually raised to 180°F and immediately decompressed. B: Portex endotracheal tube and finger cot stents.

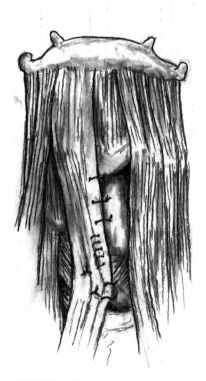

FIGURE 23-10 Anterior defects of the cricoid ring are repaired by mobilizing the sternohyoid muscle over the cricoid defect. The muscle is then sutured to the adjacent remnants of the cricoid cartilage and cricothyroid membrane.

may be seen after removal of the stent. This is best managed by prevention with meticulous closure of all mucosal lacerations at the time of surgery. Postoperative antibiotics and early removal of the stent may reduce the amount of granulation tissue. Profuse granulation tissue that persists may be debulked using endoscopy.

Unilateral vocal fold immobility may cause a weak or breathy voice. Bilateral immobility leads to aphonia, aspiration, or possible compromised respiration. Unless the recurrent laryngeal nerve was known to be severed at the time of surgery, medialization procedures should be delayed for at least 6 months to permit delayed recovery. If after 6 months no mobility is present, electromyography is recommended. This permits differentiated between laryngeal denervation and arytenoids fixation. At 6 to 12 months in the unilateral denervated larynx, a medialization procedure may be performed to strengthen the voice or prevent aspiration. Laryngeal electromyography is particularly useful in distinguishing vocal fold immobility due to cricoarytenoid fixation from that due to laryngeal denervation. If bilateral paralysis is present and the patient desires an attempt at decannulation, an arytenoidectomy or cordotomy may be performed. However, immobility secondary to cricoarytenoid joint fixation should be excluded by palpation of the arytenoid cartilages at direct laryngoscopy before considering these other procedures.[10] Subglottic stenosis may also be present and prevent decannulation (Fig. **23–11**). Again, no repair of the stenosis should be undertaken for 6 to 12 months to allow for scar maturation. After this time, direct laryngoscopy and bronchoscopy should be used to examine the lesion and plan the repair. If a short segment of tracheal stenosis is found with a healthy airway below, then an excision of the stenotic segment and primary reanastomosis may be performed, using a release of the suprahyoid suspensory system to gain further mobilization.[18] Additionally, mediastinal tracheal dissection and incision of the annular ligaments of the trachea may be used in combination with suprahyoid release to allow for excision and primary reanastomosis of lesions up to 12.5 cm in the adult.[38] Longer stenotic segments can be repaired with anterior and, if needed, posterior cricotracheal cartilage grafts as

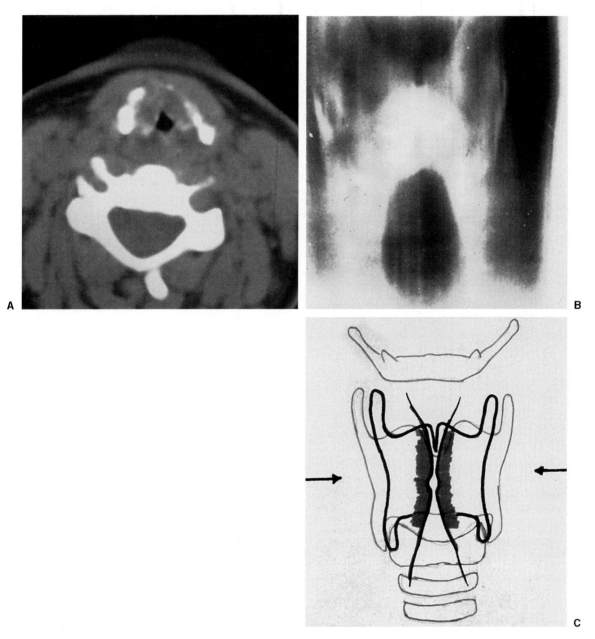

A   B   C

FIGURE 23–11   A: Computed tomography of initially unrecognized laryngeal fractures in a 23-year-old woman shows fixated arytenoid cartilages and fracture of thyroid cartilage. The patient remained aphonic and tracheotomy-dependent for 4 years until the larynx was reconstructed. B: Tomogram of larynx taken following untreated trauma to the central compartment of the neck. C: Drawing showing extent of laryngeal stenosis following a previously unrecognized blunt laryngeal injury. (Parts B and C are courtesy of Byron J. Bailey, MD.)

TABLE 23–2 VOICE AND AIRWAY RESULTS OF EVALUATED PATIENTS BY TREATMENT GROUPS*

Group	Voice			Airway			Total (n = 115)
	Good	Fair	Poor	Good	Fair	Poor	
I	20	0	0	20	0	0	20
II	38	3	0	40	1	0	41
III	18	3	0	21	0	0	21
IV	22	10	0	31	0	2	33

*Group I patients had no airway compromise and were judged to have reversible injuries. They were managed by observation only. Group II patients had airway compromise and were considered to have reversible injuries. They were managed by tracheotomy, direct laryngoscopy, esophagoscopy, and observation. Group III patients were judged to have irreversible laryngeal fractures or lacerations that required management by open reduction and fixation of disrupted cartilage or mucous membrane. Group IV patients had more severe injuries as discussed, and management differed from group III in that endolaryngeal stents were used.
From Schaefer SD. The acute management of external laryngeal trauma: A 27 year experience. Arch Otolaryngol Head Neck Surg 1992;118:598.

popularized in the repair of subglottic stenosis in children.[39]

OUTCOME

The outcome after laryngeal trauma depends on the extent of the original injury and the quality of subsequent repairs. In patients who do not require operative intervention, the prognosis for full return of function is excellent.[2,21,36] Patients requiring surgical intervention have an excellent chance of eventual decannulation with an adequate to good voice.[2,21,25] Long-term complications after repair are uncommon. In our series of 139 patients with acute laryngeal trauma managed as presented in this chapter, only two patients were left with a poor airway, as defined by the inability to decannulate (Table 23–2). Time to decannulation in those patients undergoing tracheotomy along with exploration ranged from 14 to 35 days, whereas those with stents (usually reserved for more severe injuries) needed 35 to 100 days to decannulation. All but 13 of the 115 evaluated patients achieved a good voice; those 13 were classified as having a fair voice.[2] In sum, the goal of the acute treatment of laryngeal injuries is the preservation of the airway and maintenance of laryngeal function.

PEARLS: LARYNGEAL TRAUMA

- A patient with blunt or penetrating laryngeal trauma may appear stable on first presentation, but development of edema or bleeding can result in rapid airway compromise.

- The best radiologic evaluation of the larynx is the computed tomography (CT) scan. However, the CT scan should be used selectively; for example, in a patient with obvious laryngeal injury on external and/or fiberoptic examination, the CT scan may add little to the evaluation.

- The first priorities in the patient with laryngeal trauma are evaluating and securing the airway; this can be accomplished with tracheotomy under local anesthesia, or careful endotracheal intubation by an expert.

- The following injuries may be treated conservatively, with close observation and/or corticosteroids: minor mucosal laceration not involving the free edge of the vocal fold, nondisplaced cartilage fracture, nonobstructive laryngeal edema, and small stable hematoma.

- Surgical repair is usually required for the following injuries: laceration of the anterior commissure or free margin of vocal fold, displaced thyroid or cricoid cartilage fracture, exposed endolaryngeal cartilage, and potential or actual airway compromise. If indicated, early surgical repair of laryngeal injuries is preferred.

- An external incision with midline thyrotomy (laryngofissure) is the optimal approach to the injured larynx. Mucosal injuries are repaired directly, or mucosal flaps or mucosal or skin grafts can be used.

- Laryngeal fractures are repaired using wire, nonabsorbable suture, or small plates and screws.

- Endolaryngeal stenting is controversial, but can be used for injuries of the anterior commissure, massive lacerations, comminuted fractures, or an unstable larynx.

- Complications of laryngeal injury include impaired vocalization, respiration, or swallowing.

REFERENCES

1. Schaefer SD, Close LG. Acute management of laryngeal trauma. Ann Otol Rhinol Laryngol 1989;98:98–104

2. Schaefer SD. Acute management of external laryngeal trauma: a 27 year experience. Arch Otolaryngol 1992; 118:598–604

3. Fink R. *The Human Larynx: A Functional Study.* Cambridge, MA: Raven Press, 1995

4. Sant'Ambrogio FB. Laryngeal influences of breathing pattern and posterior cricoarytenoid muscle activity. J Appl Physiol 1985;58:1298–1304

5. Schaefer SD, Roark R, Watson B, et al. Multichannel electromyographic observations in spasmodic dysphonic patients and normal control subjects. Ann Otol Rhinol Laryngol 1992;101:67–75

6. Woodson GE. Effects of cricothyroid muscle contraction on laryngeal resistance and glottis area. Ann Otol Rhinol Laryngol 1989;98:119–124

7. Hirano M. Morphological structure of the vocal cord as a vibrator and its variations. Folia Phoniatr (Basel) 1974;26:89–94

8. Van de Berg J. Myoelastic theory of voice production. J Speech Hear Res 1958;1:227–244

9. Nahum AM. Immediate care of acute blunt laryngeal trauma. J Trauma 1969;9:112–125

10. Nahum AM, Siegel AW. Biodynamics of injury to the larynx in automobile collisions. Ann Otol Rhinol Laryngol 1967;76:781–785

11. Pennington CL. External trauma of the larynx and trachea. Ann Otol Rhinol Laryngol 1972;81:546–554

12. Close DM. Traumatic avulsion of the larynx. J Laryngol Otol 1981;95:1157–1158

13. Stanley RB, Hanson DG. Manual strangulation injuries of the larynx. Arch Otolaryngol 1983;109: 344–347

14. Olson NR. Surgical treatment of acute blunt laryngeal injuries. Ann Otol Rhinol Laryngol 1978;87:716–721

15. Saletta JD, Lowe RJ, Lim LT, Thornton J, Delf S, Moss GS. Penetrating trauma of the neck. J Trauma 1976;16:579–587

16. Lemay SR. Penetrating wounds of the larynx and cervical trachea. Arch Otolaryngol 1971;94:558–565

17. Schaefer SD, Brown OE. Selective application of CT in the management of laryngeal trauma. Laryngoscope 1983;93:1473–1475

18. Williams MW. Suprahyoid release for tracheal anastomosis. Arch Otolaryngol 1974;99:255–260

19. Harrison DFN. Bullet wounds of the larynx and trachea. Arch Otolaryngol 1984;110:203–205

20. Schaefer SD. Primary management of laryngeal trauma. Ann Otol Rhinol Laryngol 1982;91:399–402

21. Kleinsasser NH, Priemer FG, Schulze W, Kleinsasser OF. External trauma to the larynx: classification, diagnosis, therapy. Eur Arch Otorhinolaryngol 2000; 257:439–444

22. Close LG, Schaefer SD, Merkel M, Watson D. Cricoarytenoid subluxation, computed tomography, and electromyography findings. Head Neck Surg 1987; 9:341–348

23. Friedman WH, Archer CR, Yeager VL, Katsantonis GP. Computed tomography vs. laryngography: a comparison of relative diagnostic value. Otolaryngol Head Neck Surg 1981;89:579–586

24. Maceri DR, Mancuso AA, Canalis RF. Value of computed axial tomography in severe laryngeal injury. Arch Otolaryngol 1982;108:449–451

25. Mancuso AA, Hanafee WN. Computed tomography of the injured larynx. Radiology 1979;133:139–144

26. Lupetin AR, Hollander M, Rao VM. CT evaluation of laryngeal trauma. Semin Musculoskelet Radiol 1998; 2:105–116

27. Stanley RB, Cooper DS, Florman SH. Phonatory effects of thyroid cartilage fractures. Ann Otol Rhinol Laryngol 1987;96:493–496

28. Krekorian EA. Laryngopharyngeal injuries. Laryngoscope 1975;85:2069–2086

29. Trone TH, Schaefer SC, Carder HM. Blunt and penetrating laryngeal trauma: a 13-year review. Otolaryngol Head Neck Surg 1980;88:257

30. Miller LH. Laryngotracheal trauma in combat casualties. Ann Otol Rhinol Laryngol 1970;79:1088–1090

31. Harris H, Tobin HA. Acute injuries of the larynx and trachea in 49 patients. Laryngoscope 1970;86: 1376–1384

32. Miles WK, Olson NR, Rodriguez A. Acute treatment of experimental laryngeal fractures. Ann Otol Rhinol Laryngol 1971;80:710–720

33. Olson NR, Miles WK. Treatment of acute blunt laryngeal injuries. Ann Otol Rhinol Laryngol 1971; 80:704–709

34. Bhanot S, Alex JC, Lowlicht RA, et al. The efficacy of resorbable plates in head and neck reconstruction. Laryngoscope 2002;112:890–898

35. de Mello-Filho FV, Carrau R. The management of laryngeal fractures using internal fixation Laryngoscope 2000;110:2143–2146

36. Leopold DA. Laryngeal trauma. Arch Otolaryngol 1983;109:106–112

37. Schaefer SD, Carder HM. Fabrication of a simple laryngeal stent. Laryngoscope 1980;40:1561–1563

38. Grillo HC. Circumferential resection and reconstruction of the mediastinal and cervical trachea Ann Surg 1965;162:374–388

39. Whited RE. A prospective study of laryngotracheal sequelae in long term intubation Laryngoscope 1984; 94:367–377

Chapter 24

PHARYNGEAL TRAUMA

Michael G. Stewart

Penetrating injuries to the pharynx have been given little attention in the literature, although they are usually discussed in articles concerning penetrating neck trauma, the aerodigestive tract, or laryngopharyngeal injuries. In addition, some authors studying esophageal trauma have considered the cervical esophagus to include most of the digestive tract present in the neck, including the pharynx, which makes the distinction of the pharynx even more difficult. However, pharyngeal injuries are truly unique, and it is useful to discuss them separately. Therefore, this chapter discusses injuries to the pharynx. Larynx and esophagus injuries are addressed elsewhere in this text.

ANATOMY

The pharynx is a complicated structure that makes up portions of the upper airway and upper digestive tract, before forming a separate structure behind the larynx that finally empties into the cervical portion of the esophagus. The superior boundary of the pharynx is the skull base and the inferior boundary is the cricopharyngeus portion of the inferior constrictor muscle, which is usually at the level of the C6 vertebrae. The pharynx is ~ 15 cm in length and roughly funnel shaped; its widest point is near the hyoid bone, and it narrows inferiorly as it nears the esophagus. Pharyngeal anatomy is shown in Fig. **24–1**.

The pharynx is divided into three segments from superior to inferior: the nasopharynx, oropharynx, and hypopharynx (which some anatomists call the "laryngopharynx"). The inferior border of the nasopharynx is the inferior edge of the soft palate, and the oropharynx extends from the soft palate to the tip of the epiglottis. The hypopharynx is the portion of the pharynx that is behind the larynx, and it extends inferiorly to the esophageal inlet. The hypopharynx includes the pyriform sinuses, which are pouches of mucosa lateral to the aryepiglottic folds of the larynx.

The pharyngeal wall has five layers. The innermost layer is mucosa, the next layer is submucosa, and next is a fibrous layer—the pharyngobasilar fascia—that attaches to the base of the skull. Next is a muscular layer, which is composed of the superior, middle, and inferior constrictor muscles; these muscles overlap each other, and their sequential contraction and relaxation creates pharyngeal peristalsis. The inferior-most portion of the inferior constrictor is thickened muscular tissue that is often called the "cricopharyngeus muscle," although it is not actually a distinct muscle but rather a specialized part of the inferior constrictor with a sphincter function that prevents air from entering the esophagus. The pharyngeal constrictors are attached to structures anteriorly, such as the pterygoid plate, the hyoid bone, and the thyroid and cricoid cartilages, and they meet in a median raphe in the posterior midline of the pharynx. The outermost layer of the pharyngeal wall is thin areolar tissue that creates the buccopharyngeal fascia.

The pharynx and aerodigestive tract are centrally located in the neck and are surrounded by several other structures. Because of this, the pharynx is not commonly injured by penetrating external trauma. One large registry study of 1,560 patients with neck trauma (blunt or penetrating) from Los Angeles County found that 4.9% of all patients had aerodigestive tract injury: 10.2% of gunshot wounds, 4.6% of stab wounds, and 1.2% of blunt trauma.[1] Pharyngeal injuries are typically a smaller proportion of that total. Because external penetrating trauma to the pharynx can involve the potential for

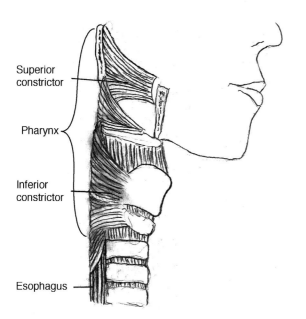

FIGURE 24–1 Anatomy of the pharynx.

injury to other key anatomic structures, the management of the pharynx is often not performed in isolation. Blunt trauma to the neck, however, can potentially cause an isolated pharyngeal injury.

CLINICAL ASSESSMENT

Some authors have considered the hypopharynx and the cervical esophagus to be identical, for the purpose of diagnostic evaluation and surgical treatment.[2] However, other studies have found clinical significance in the localization of injury site to either the hypopharynx or cervical esophagus. Our clinical results have supported that distinction, and we recommend that the hypopharynx be evaluated and treated as a distinct injury site, rather than applying the principles of esophageal injury to those cases.

CLINICAL SIGNS AND SYMPTOMS

The use of signs and symptoms alone (such as dysphagia or subcutaneous emphysema) as predictive factors for pharyngeal or esophageal injury is controversial. One study of patients with *esophageal* injury found a specificity of 64% and a sensitivity of 80% for predicting actual injury, using the presence of any positive signs or symptoms as a predictive factor.[3] That study found clinical evaluation to be somewhat *less* accurate than a prior report that cited specificity of 93% and sensitivity of 69%. However, both reports found several patients with false-positive or -negative findings, using only clinical signs or symptoms. Others studying *aerodigestive*

tract injuries as a group have found that signs and symptoms are more helpful, and one study reported that no asymptomatic patient had a significant injury[1]; in other words there were no false negatives, meaning a sensitivity of 100%. The differences in those reports were likely due to the fact that the groups of patients studied were heterogeneous, and included different injury patterns. However, it seems reasonable to draw the conclusion that while cervical esophageal or pharyngeal injury can be difficult to detect using signs and symptoms alone, laryngeal or airway injury is much easier to predict.

Along those same lines, the clinical presentation of a pharyngeal injury can be relatively silent when combined with a laryngeal or tracheal injury. So, in a patient with laryngeal trauma and rapid onset of subcutaneous air, the possibility of simultaneous pharyngeal injury should always be considered during evaluation and exploration. Similarly, patients with vascular or spine injury can also present with dramatic physical findings that will initially obscure the presence of a concomitant pharyngeal injury.

IMAGING

The ideal imaging test for the pharynx is somewhat controversial, and the options include the contrast esophagram using barium or Gastrografin, or the computed tomography (CT) scan. For the contrast esophagram, the question is: Which contrast medium is best? Barium-based contrast is thicker, and if there is a penetrating injury, the barium may be more likely to demonstrate it. However if the barium gets into the soft tissues of the neck, there is significant potential risk for infection. Gastrografin (meglumine diatrizoate) is a thinner material, and if it leaks into the neck is less likely to promote infection. However, if Gastrografin is aspirated into the lungs, it will cause a more severe inflammatory pneumonitis than barium. In addition, many feel that Gastrografin is a poorer contrast agent because smaller injuries can be missed.

There are a few studies of the sensitivity and specificity of radiologic tests to detect pharyngeal or esophageal injury. In a group of patients with potential *esophageal* injury, using mandatory neck exploration with rigid esophagoscopy to definitively identify injuries, one study calculated that barium esophagram had a specificity of 100% and sensitivity of 89%.[3] The authors did not perform Gastrografin swallow studies, because the radiologists at their institution considered it less reliable. Another study of esophageal injuries found that Gastrografin swallow studies identified perforations only 50% of the time.[4] Another study limited to *cervical esophageal* injuries found that contrast esophagrams (either Gastrografin or barium) identified only 62% of actual perforations.[5]

A study of *hypopharynx* injuries found that of six patients who underwent a contrast swallow study prior to surgery, the injury was identified in only three (50%) of those patients.[6] A different study of hypopharynx injuries found that a contrast swallow was successful in identifying the injury in all five patients in whom it was used.[7] In that study, patients were not randomized and the decision for evaluation (endoscopy versus contrast swallow) was made by the availability of ancillary personnel. Their protocol for contrast studies was first use Gastrografin, and if negative, then dilute barium was used.

One group also studied different types of endoscopy as well as swallowing studies, and although none of the tests was 100% accurate, in each patient with a penetrating injury, at least *one* of the diagnostic tests—rigid or flexible esophagoscopy, or barium swallow—demonstrated the injury.[3] So the authors concluded that a combination of those tests should not miss any injuries.

Another option for assessment is the CT scan.[1,8] CT scans were found to be very helpful in determining the path of the projectile (using the tract of air bubbles, damaged tissue or projectile particles), which then helped guide decision making for further evaluation and treatment.

One report identified three patients with penetrating injuries of the posterior oropharynx, none of whom had any external neck signs of perforation, but all of whom had retropharyngeal air on a lateral neck x-ray.[9] All of those injuries were in children and were caused by rigid objects that had been held in the mouth, and all resolved without surgical intervention. Other studies have found that lateral neck x-rays demonstrate retropharyngeal air in both internal perforating and external penetrating pharyngeal injuries as well.[6,10,11] So the lateral neck x-ray may play a role in suspected pharyngeal perforation.

ENDOSCOPY

The options for endoscopic evaluation include flexible fiberoptic endoscopy and rigid endoscopy. Flexible fiberoptic examination of the larynx and pharynx can be performed fairly easily in the awake patient. Flexible endoscopic examination of the esophagus can also be performed in the awake patient, but requires additional cooperation of the patient, an endoscope with insufflation capabilities, perhaps additional sedation, and additional skills by the endoscopist. Rigid endoscopic evaluation of the larynx, pharynx, or esophagus usually requires general anesthesia, and some would argue that if patients are going to undergo general anesthesia, then they should simply undergo open neck exploration. However, if rigid endoscopy were very accurate and could prevent an open exploration, that would be preferable.

In a group of patients with potential *esophageal* injury, using mandatory neck exploration to definitively identify injuries, rigid esophagoscopy alone had a specificity of 95% and sensitivity of 89%, and flexible esophagoscopy had a specificity of 99% but a sensitivity of only 38%.[3] Another study of injuries to the short *cervical esophagus* found that rigid endoscopy identified 100% of injuries.[5]

A study of *hypopharynx* injuries found that awake flexible fiberoptic laryngopharyngoscopy was very helpful, identifying blood in the larynx or pharynx in *all* patients with injury, and actually visualizing the site of perforation in a large proportion.[6] Not all patients in that study underwent fiberoptic endoscopy, however, so sensitivity or specificity could not be identified. Rigid endoscopy of the pharynx and esophagus was also performed in the operating room in several cases, and all injuries were identified using rigid endoscopy. Another study of hypopharyngeal injuries found that rigid endoscopy was successful in identifying injuries in all nine patients in whom it was used.[7]

OVERALL EVALUATION

In summary, it appears that the anatomy of the pharynx and the relative ease of fiberoptic examination in the awake patient make that evaluation the first option, because it does not require transporting the patient to another area such as radiology and does not require general anesthesia. In addition to its ease of use, fiberoptic laryngopharyngoscopy seems to be very accurate in the evaluation of penetrating pharyngeal trauma. If the patient requires general anesthesia anyway, or the flexible examination cannot be performed prior to surgery, then rigid endoscopy is also very accurate in the diagnosis of pharyngeal injury. Contrast swallowing studies appear to be less helpful as a primary test, although if performed for another reason they can potentially identify pharyngeal injuries as well.

SURGICAL INDICATIONS

Many authors have divided the surgical indications for neck exploration into "hard" and "soft" indications, but most of those reports considered *all* potential injuries, and not only aerodigestive tract injuries. However, some authors have considered indications for surgical exploration concerning aerodigestive injuries only[1,12] (Table 24–1). In general, "hard" signs call for mandatory neck exploration, and "soft" signs call for further diagnostic evaluation, such as endoscopy or a contrast swallow study. Of course, in many patients with penetrating neck trauma and potential pharyngeal injury, the decision about whether or not to undergo surgical exploration is based on other potential injuries, such as suspected vascular injury or obvious airway injury.

BLUNT TRAUMA

Pharyngeal perforation resulting from blunt trauma is rare, but the few reports on that subject have found that nonsurgical management—intravenous antibiotics, no oral intake for several days, and close observation—can result in good outcomes.[8,11,13] However, if injuries are missed initially, and patients are allowed to eat or are not treated with antibiotics, then salivary leak and infection can occur, and eventual surgical exploration with external drainage and possible surgical repair may be necessary.[11,13] A high level of clinical suspicion is important, because the signs of pharyngeal perforation may not be present initially. The mechanism of perforation from blunt trauma is not entirely clear, but probably results from some combination of barotrauma, distention, and shear forces. For example, if a patient suffers blunt force trauma to the anterior neck, the hyoid bone or thyroid cartilage can be driven backward against the spine, closing the airway, while at the same time there is a rapid increase in intrathoracic pressure; this pressure cannot escape and the resulting sudden barotrauma to the pharynx can

TABLE 24–1 INDICATIONS FOR EXPLORATION OF PENETRATING NECK TRAUMA, DUE TO AERODIGESTIVE TRACT INJURY

"Hard" signs

- Airway obstruction
- Air escaping from neck wound
- Major hemoptysis

"Soft" signs

- Dyspnea
- Hoarseness
- Subcutaneous emphysema
- Odynophagia
- Rare hemoptysis

result in distention and perforation. Similarly, since the larynx, pharynx, and their surrounding muscles are attached to adjacent structures, then deceleration trauma can result in significant traction or shear forces, which can tear the pharyngeal wall.

PERFORATING TRAUMA

A similar logic can also be applied to pharyngeal perforation resulting from iatrogenic injuries (such as intubation, endoscopy or other instrumentation) and swallowed foreign bodies.[8,10,13] Early suspicion and identification, along with restriction of oral intake, intravenous antibiotics, and close observation, may allow adequate healing without complication. If, during the period of observation, the patient develops signs of infection or ongoing salivary leak, further evaluation and possibly surgical exploration should be undertaken promptly.

PENETRATING TRAUMA

Years of experience with penetrating trauma have demonstrated that if injuries to the cervical and thoracic esophagus were missed, then serious and often fatal complications would usually result.[2,3,14] In fact, delay in exploration and repair beyond 12 or 24 hours after esophageal injury was linked in many studies to markedly higher complication rates and lower survival. Therefore, surgical teaching held that all potential esophageal injuries should be explored and primarily repaired.

For many years, the hypopharynx was considered to be similar to the cervical esophagus, and open exploration and repair were recommended. However, oropharyngeal penetrating injuries were usually not explored or surgically closed, and those injuries usually did well with close observation, antibiotics and limited oral intake. In addition, evidence began to emerge that perforation of the hypopharynx did not always require exploration and closure.[1,6,7] Therefore, hypopharynx injuries are best considered as distinct from the cervical esophagus.

Considering the anatomy of the hypopharynx, because the upper portion of the hypopharynx has a low intraluminal pressure, large lumen, and thick muscular wall—like the oropharynx—the edges of an injury could potentially coapt together and heal without surgical closure. Equally important, saliva does not tend to pool in the upper and middle pharynx, so even if a defect is present, saliva may not leak into the neck. The esophagus, in contrast, has a small lumen, high intraluminal pressure, and a thinner muscular wall, so there is a higher likelihood of salivary leak. Also, the inferior portion of the hypopharynx—near the cervical esophagus—is anatomically more similar to the esophagus than the upper hypopharynx. In addition, in the lower hypopharynx some pooling of saliva is common, and if a wall defect is present the saliva can more easily leak into the neck.

A group from Los Angeles County–University of Southern California Hospital reviewed their experience with externally penetrating hypopharynx injuries and noted that injuries that were closer to the esophagus tended to have more complications, specifically infection and fistula formation, than injuries that were located more cephalad.[6] They noted that a reasonable line of demarcation was at the top of the arytenoid cartilage, as demonstrated in Fig. 24–2. Injuries below that level, such as in the base of the pyriform sinus, were classified as "low" hypopharynx. Injuries above the top of the arytenoid were classified as "high" hypopharynx. The study was a retrospective review of patients that had been treated in a nonrandomized fashion, nevertheless in the data and outcome analysis, some important trends emerged. First, whether treated with surgical repair or observation, high hypopharynx injuries tended to do well. Second, if low hypopharynx injuries were treated with observation alone, there was a higher complication rate. Also, larger size injuries, usually caused by gunshot wounds rather than stab wounds, tended to have a higher complica-

tion rate. There was a single small (ice pick) injury to the lower pyriform sinus, and that patient did well with medical management only. Therefore, based on their review, surgical exploration with repair and external drainage was recommended for the following types of hypopharynx injuries: low hypopharynx injuries (low pyriform sinus and below the level of the arytenoids), large injuries (greater than 2 cm, or involving more than one hypopharynx subsite), and gunshot wounds through the pharynx that also involved the cervical spine. Other penetrating hypopharynx injuries—high hypopharynx injuries and small injuries—could be safely observed and treated medically.

Another report from the same authors explored further the distinctions between the cervical esophagus and the low hypopharynx.[5] That retrospective study found that cervical esophageal injuries usually required surgical repair or at least external drainage, and that low hypopharyngeal injuries or large complicated hypopharyngeal injuries had similar outcomes as esophageal injuries. So those data supported previous recommendations that low hypopharynx injuries be treated with exploration, repair, and drainage.

Another series of 14 patients with hypopharyngeal injury—11 gunshot wounds, one shotgun wound, and two stab wounds—found that medical management and observation without surgical exploration or repair yielded good outcomes overall.[7] There was a single case of neck abscess, but that abscess was successfully drained, and no fistula or other complication developed subsequently. The authors did not distinguish between hypopharyngeal subsites in their treatment protocol.

In the author's personal experience, we have managed all penetrating pharyngeal injuries at Ben Taub General Hospital in Houston since 1995 using the following philosophy. We perform open exploration, closure, and external drainage for low hypopharynx and cervical esophageal injuries, and use nonsurgical treatment (close observation, intravenous antibiotics, and no oral intake for seven days) for upper hypopharynx injuries, unless those injuries are very large. If the neck has already been opened for another reason such as a laryngeal injury, and an upper hypopharyngeal injury is identified, we close the injury if technically possible, and place an external drain. Practically speaking, we have found that there are very few "large" hypopharynx injuries that do not require open exploration for some other reason, so the decision making for a high hypopharynx lesion rarely hinges on the size of the lesion alone. Oropharynx injuries are also not closed,

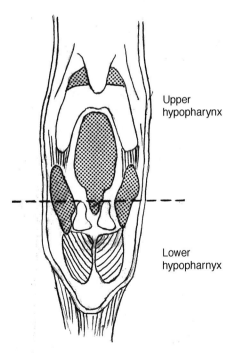

FIGURE 24–2 Anatomy of the hypopharynx, with the line of demarcation at the top of the arytenoid cartilages.

but are treated similarly to upper hypopharynx injuries.

Finally, repair of nasopharynx injuries is not discussed in the literature, because mucosal repair is not required, and those injuries are adjacent to critical structures such as the skull base and major vascular structures, which take precedence in evaluation and treatment. Assuming there is no other major injury, then nasopharynx injuries can be treated with antibiotics and close observation.

In summary, *nasopharynx* and *oropharynx* injuries are treated with antibiotics, no oral intake for several days, and close observation. Surgical exploration and repair are almost never required. For both blunt and penetrating injuries resulting in perforation, *hypopharynx* injuries are explored, repaired, and drained if they are large, or if they involve the lower portion of the hypopharynx (below the top of the arytenoid cartilage). Smaller injuries involving the upper hypopharynx can be treated with antibiotics, no oral intake, and close observation.

SURGICAL APPROACH

To explore and repair the pharynx, the surgeon should choose the external incision most appropriate for the case, remembering that many penetrating pharyngeal injuries will also have some other injury, such as a larynx injury, vertebral injury, or vascular injury. Therefore, incisions that allow wide exposure and possible extension to the opposite side are preferred, such as an extended apron-type incision, or bilateral vertical incisions anterior to the sternocleidomastoid muscle. If a unilateral apron incision is made on one side, then if the opposite side must be opened, the incision can easily be extended across the midline to create a symmetric tissue flap for elevation.

The sternocleidomastoid muscle needs to be retracted laterally, and the strap muscles and larynx rotated medially to allow access to the pharynx. Placement of a soft bougie or an esophageal tube of some kind can facilitate identification of the pharynx and esophagus. The retropharyngeal tissue plane anterior to the cervical spine can be easily dissected in a blunt fashion, and if both sides are exposed, a retractor or a Penrose drain can be passed through and used as a retractor to rotate the pharynx and expose the posterior wall. Of course the recurrent laryngeal nerves travel in the tracheoesophageal groove, so sharp dissection should be avoided in that area; similarly, the area of the thyrohyoid membrane should also be avoided because of the proximity of the internal branch of the superior laryngeal nerve.

The pharynx should be carefully inspected circumferentially to identify potential injuries. Injury identification can be facilitated by rigid endoscopy; this can also be performed simultaneously by another surgeon. Another useful technique is to use a large bulb syringe filled with water or saline and have a member of the surgical team scrub out (or ask the anesthesiologist to assist) and irrigate into the oropharynx with some force, while the surgeon visually inspects the exposed pharynx. Leakage of fluid into the neck will help identify the site of injury.

SURGICAL TECHNIQUES

Surgical repair of a pharyngeal injury is fairly straightforward. Most authors recommend a two-layer closure if possible, reapproximating the mucosa and the muscular layer. However, a single-layer closure has not been shown to result in a higher fistula rate.[2,6] Similarly, use of different suture materials does not affect fistula rate. The use of muscle flaps or other techniques to bolster closure sites in the pharynx has not been shown to improve the success rate in pharyngeal repair, although it is still recommended by several authors. Finally, studies indicate that the use of external drainage does reduce complications, but the type of drain used—open versus closed suction—does not seem to be an important factor. The author's preferences are two-layer closure and closed-suction drainage. I use absorbable suture material to close the mucosa, and interrupted sutures of permanent material (such as silk) for closure of the muscular layer. Closed-suction drainage is preferred because it prevents leakage of fluids onto the neck skin, and allows more precise assessment of drainage volume.

Regardless of technique, achieving a *watertight* closure seems to be important whenever possible. In some larger injuries and gunshot wounds, however, the surgeon should recognize that a watertight seal might not be possible, and even if achieved might result in excessive luminal narrowing with resultant dysphagia, which can be a difficult problem to manage. In those cases, close reapproximation (but not watertight closure) and adequate external drainage should be performed. The perforation still might heal without complication even if the initial closure was not entirely watertight. However, if it does not, then the external drain helps create a controlled salivary fistula; this avoids an uncontrolled saliva leak that can track along fascial planes and cause a serious deep neck or mediastinal infection. An appropriately directed cutaneous fistula is not necessarily a bad outcome in patients with a significant injury, because eventually the fistula almost invariably closes and the patient will usually have adequate swallowing function.

In massive injuries with a large amount of tissue loss, some type of pharyngeal diversion can be performed—either a cervical lateral pharyngostomy, or for lower injuries involving the esophagus, a complete pharyngeal/esophageal end-diversion. These diversions prevent saliva from bathing the injury site, and therefore facilitate healing and prevent development of deep neck infections. Either technique can be closed eventually; however, the complete diversion with subsequent reanastomosis has been associated with a higher level of eventual swallowing dysfunction. Therefore, a proximal pharyngostomy with attempted primary repair of the injury and adequate external drainage should be adequate, even for severe injuries. However, external diversion is usually not needed even in large injuries if exploration and repair are accomplished within 24 hours after injury.

When a cervical vertebral body is injured by a transpharyngeal bullet, there is some controversy about the need for additional surgical exploration and debridement of the spine itself. Of course, neurosurgical consultation is essential in these cases. There are reports of osteomyelitis and other infectious complications if the cervical vertebrae are not debrided and foreign bodies removed, so that possibility should be considered in clinical decision making. In addition, the cervical spine injury can mean that evaluation of the pharyngeal injury might be delayed or not performed (for example, if rigid esophagoscopy cannot be safely performed), which can also increase the chance of a missed pharyngeal injury.

COMPLICATIONS

The most common complications of penetrating trauma to the pharynx are salivary leak and subsequent neck abscess, deep neck infection, or pharyngocutaneous fistula formation. Neck infections can lead to mediastinal infection or fasciitis. As discussed above, these complications should be rare in upper pharyngeal injuries. However, in the cervical esophagus and lower hypopharynx, even when repair is performed immediately and using standard surgical techniques, a fistula rate of 9 to 20% can be expected.[2,6] Almost all pharyngocutaneous fistulas eventually close without additional surgical management, as long as patients are treated with restricted oral intake, adequate drainage, and antibiotics. Swallowing function is usually adequate

after the fistula closes. Fistulas are more common after gunshot wounds than stab wounds, probably because of the additional tissue injury caused by the energy of a bullet. In esophageal injuries (and by extension, low hypopharyngeal injuries), the rate of fistula formation has been reported to double if surgical repair is delayed by 24 hours or more, or if antibiotics are not started by 12 hours after the injury.

Other complications of pharyngeal injury result from the associated nearby structures, such as the cervical spine and larynx; these injuries are best avoided by careful systematic evaluation and initial treatment.

PEARLS: KEY CLINICAL POINTS IN PHARYNGEAL TRAUMA

- Because of its central location in the neck, isolated pharynx injuries are uncommon in penetrating trauma.
- Signs and symptoms of pharyngeal injury are not always accurate predictors of actual injury.
- Rigid endoscopy and flexible fiberoptic endoscopy are the best diagnostic tests to identify injury; contrast swallowing studies are less accurate but can be helpful in many cases.
- Blunt trauma can rarely result in pharyngeal perforation.
- Penetrating trauma of the hypopharynx should be treated differently from penetrating trauma of the cervical esophagus.
- Upper hypopharynx injuries (above the top of the arytenoid) can be treated conservatively, with antibiotics, no oral intake, and close observation.
- Lower hypopharynx injuries (below the top of the arytenoid) should be treated with open exploration, surgical repair, and external drainage.
- Penetrating nasopharynx and oropharynx injuries can be treated like upper hypopharynx injuries.
- Early identification and treatment of pharyngeal injuries lowers the rate of complication.

REFERENCES

1. Vassiliu P, Baker J, Henderson S, Alo K, Velmahos G, Demetriades D. Aerodigestive injuries of the neck. Am Surg 2001;67:75–79
2. Winter RP, Weigelt JA. Cervical esophageal trauma: incidence and cause of esophageal fistulas. Arch Surg 1990;125:849–852

3. Weigelt JA, Thal ER, Snyder WH, Fry RE, Meier DE, Kilman WJ. Diagnosis of penetrating cervical esophageal injuries. Am J Surg 1987;154:619–622

4. Yap RG, Yap AG, Obeid FN, Horan DP. Traumatic esophageal injuries: 12-year experience at Henry Ford Hospital. J Trauma 1984;24:623–625

5. Armstrong WB, Detar TR, Stanley RB. Diagnosis and management of external penetrating cervical esophageal injuries. Ann Otol Rhinol Laryngol 1994; 103: 863–871

6. Fetterman BL, Shindo ML, Stanley RB, Armstrong WB, Rice DH. Management of traumatic hypopharyngeal injuries. Laryngoscope 1995;105:8–13

7. Yugueros P, Sarmiento JM, Garcia AF, Ferrada R. Conservative management of penetrating hypopharyngeal wounds. J Trauma 1996;40:267–269

8. Dolgin SR, Kumar NR, Wykoff TW, Maniglia AJ. Conservative medical management of traumatic pharyngoesophageal perforations. Ann Otol Rhinol Laryngol 1992;101:209–215

9. Smyth DA, Fenton J, Timon C, McShane DP. Occult pharyngeal perforation secondary to "pencil injury." J Laryngol Otol 1996;110:901–903

10. Shockley WW, Tate JL, Stucker FJ. Management of perforations of the hypopharynx and cervical esophagus. Laryngoscope 1985;95:939–941

11. Hagan WE. Pharyngoesophageal perforations after blunt trauma to the neck. Otolaryngol Head Neck Surg 1983;91:620–626

12. Back MR, Baumgartner FJ, Klein SR. Detection and evaluation of aerodigestive tract injuries caused by cervical and transmediastinal gunshot wounds. J Trauma 1997;42:680–686

13. Jacobs I, Niknejad G, Kelly K, Pawar J, Jones C. Hypopharyngeal perforation after blunt neck trauma: case report and review of the literature. J Trauma 1999;46:957–958

14. Sheely CH, Mattox KL, Beall AC, DeBakey ME. Penetrating wounds of the cervical esophagus. Am J Surg 1975;130:707–711

Chapter 25

TRACHEA AND ESOPHAGUS TRAUMA

Matthew J. Wall, Jr. and Anthony J. Ascioti

Injuries to the trachea or esophagus are uncommon. Traversing the central area in the neck, both the trachea and esophagus are relatively protected. Tracheal injuries may be immediately life threatening from either penetrating trauma or direct blunt force crush of the trachea. Esophageal injuries alternatively can be extremely difficult to diagnose. Esophageal injuries may also be iatrogenic with increased utilization of endoscopic diagnostic and treatment modalities. These injuries periodically occur secondary to devices utilized to resuscitate patients such as blocker airways inserted into the esophagus. A high index of suspicion for these injuries is helpful in diagnosis of these injuries.

PREHOSPITAL ISSUES

Esophageal injuries are not immediately life threatening, but any injury to the trachea can rapidly cause death. Seventy-five percent of patients with acute blunt tracheal trauma die prior to arrival at the hospital.[1] The trachea may suffer a crush injury due to direct force on the anterior trachea. This can occur during "clothesline" injuries, in which motorcycle or bicycle riders get stopped by an unseen rope or wire across their path. Avulsion injuries occur commonly at points of fixation, such as the cricoid or carina.[2] Blunt injuries can also occur from collision with the steering wheel or dashboard of a vehicle. Tracheal and esophageal injuries have also occurred from inexperienced operators attempting to achieve a surgical airway with many of the various devices used in the field. Penetrating neck injuries involve the trachea in 3 to 6% of patients.[3,4]

Due to its accessible location, the cervical trachea is the more commonly injured portion of the trachea, making up three fourths of penetrating tracheal trauma.[5] These injuries often result in combined vascular, tracheal, and esophageal injuries that can be extremely difficult to manage. In one series, 28% of patients with a tracheal injury had an associated esophageal injury and 8% had a recurrent laryngeal nerve injury.[6]

The key to managing these injuries in the prehospital arena is establishing an airway. A penetrating injury to the neck, subcutaneous emphysema, hemoptysis, hoarseness, or dysphonia such as a high-pitched voice may suggest the possibility of a tracheal injury. For massive tracheal injuries, passage of an endotracheal tube through the vocal cords may not ensure that the tube is ventilating the distal trachea, because the endotracheal tube may pass through the injury to outside the trachea. Rapid transport to an appropriate facility for airway establishment may be the only treatment possible in this dire situation. Cricothyroidotomy in the field has similar limitations to endotracheal intubation in that while the tube may go into the proximal trachea it may not communicate with the more distal trachea. In large anterior neck injuries some enterprising medics have passed an endotracheal tube through the injury into the distal trachea securing an airway. Many patients with injuries this severe do not survive even until emergency medical services personnel arrive.[7]

EMERGENCY DEPARTMENT ISSUES

Patients are commonly initially evaluated and managed using the Advanced Trauma Life Support (ATLS) protocols.[8] The primary survey of the ATLS course identifies the reversible, immediately life-threatening injuries. The airway is the first element of the primary survey, indicating its importance.

Respiratory distress is seen in three fourths of patients with tracheal injuries.[6] Injury to the recurrent laryngeal nerves may also result in proximal airway obstruction.

Associated injuries to major vascular structures in the neck and mediastinum can cause an expanding hematoma, further complicating management. An expanding hematoma can make the achievement of a surgical airway extremely difficult, and establishment of a surgical airway through an expanding hematoma due to a thoracic outlet gunshot wound can potentially release contained bleeding from intrathoracic vessels, resulting in exsanguinating hemorrhage.[9] Thus other specialty airway maneuvers should be considered.

For injuries such as from a stab wound or a small-caliber gunshot wound, where tracheal continuity is likely to remain, endotracheal intubation with passage of a cuffed tube past the injury will control the airway. For dire situations with a large anterior wound where the tracheal defect can be palpated through the wound, an endotracheal tube can sometimes be passed directly into the intrathoracic trachea securing the airway.[3,10] Many patients present in a sitting position, as it is the only way they can keep their airway clear of the massive bleeding that is occurring. A fiberoptic endotracheal intubation either in the operating room or the emergency center by qualified personnel can be a lifesaving intervention.[5] It is often safest to bring these patients directly to the operating room, where a team approach can include anesthesia and surgery. As the surgeon or anesthesiologist passes the fiberoptic bronchoscope beyond the cords, the trachea can be rapidly inspected for injuries to facilitate operative planning. In extreme cases the rigid bronchoscope may be required to locate the distal end of the injured trachea and ventilate the patient until a more definitive airway can be obtained.[11]

Acutely, cricothyroidotomy for massive injuries has the same limitations as endotracheal intubation as one cannot be sure of the status of the distal trachea. Emergent formal tracheostomy is periodically required. However, it can be technically demanding in the emergency department. If an operating room is readily available, it may be beneficial to move the patient directly to the operating room for airway control, and then move the patient again for other diagnostic tests if needed. It is helpful to anticipate the anatomic relationship between where the trachea will be entered surgically and the anticipated area of tracheal injury.

After establishing an airway, the primary and secondary surveys of the ATLS protocol are completed. A chest x-ray can be useful to determine the presence of hemopneumothorax, aspiration of foreign bodies, or aspiration of blood.

Imaging

Plain films such as a lateral cervical spine film may be obtained to look for retropharyngeal air or widening of the retropharyngeal stripe. Computed tomography (CT) is not routinely obtained for the diagnosis of cervical tracheal/esophageal trauma, although the CT is useful in the evaluation of laryngeal trauma. CT scans of the neck have been used by some to try to determine missile trajectory in the stable patient who is not likely to have an injury.

Contrast esophageal swallow studies demonstrate many but not all esophageal injuries. In our practice barium is the contrast agent of choice, as water-soluble contrast poses a risk if aspirated. Contrast swallow studies can be difficult to obtain in intubated patients.

Diagnostic Maneuvers

Endoscopy is one of the most common modalities used to diagnose tracheal and esophageal injuries. As previously mentioned, it can be helpful if the operating surgeon is available during fiberoptic intubation to allow visualization of the upper trachea that is normally obscured once the endotracheal tube is in place. In the already-intubated patient, the endotracheal tube can be pulled back along the bronchoscope to examine the proximal trachea. Flexible esophagoscopy can visualize the cervical esophagus, though it is often difficult to intubate the esophagus in the patient with significant neck swelling. In the intubated, paralyzed patient it may be useful to insert the scope, guiding it digitally with gloved fingers placed in the mouth. For examination of the trachea and esophagus, the endoscopes are passed distally, and then each structure is examined while slowly withdrawing the scope. It is important to remember that many of these injuries are relatively subtle and may manifest only as a bruise or a collection of blood that cannot be removed with irrigation or suction. These should raise significant suspicion for injury and consideration for exploration. Rigid endoscopy either with a rigid bronchoscope or the rigid esophagoscope provides excellent visualization of the trachea and esophagus. The ability of the rigid bronchoscope not only to visualize the airway but also to provide ventilation in an emergency can be extremely helpful.[11] The patient with massive amounts of blood in the tracheal/bronchial tree can also be much easier to manage with the rigid bronchoscope. Its use is limited by operator experience as well as the need to position the patient and manipulate the neck of the patient during endoscopy. In many patients, there is concern for cervical spine injury, so the neck cannot be manipulated. Thus, rigid bronchoscopy or esophagoscopy often cannot be used.

As mentioned earlier, the yield for contrast swallow or endoscopy alone is not 100% for esophageal injuries. However, the use of both modalities increases the sensitivity for detecting injury, and should be considered when there is a high index of suspicion.

OPERATIVE PREPARATION

When injuries are limited to the neck, the patient is typically placed supine with the arms tucked and the head extended if possible. A shoulder roll can be placed to get further head extension so that the entire neck can be accessible; however, if there is concern for a possible cervical spine injury, the neck cannot be extended. In those cases the patient is placed supine with the neck neutral and the head secured to the operating room table. Although this approach is suboptimal due to its limitation of operative exposure, it may be the only way to accomplish exploration. A CT scan of the cervical spine may help rule out an osseous injury, although it may not rule out a ligamentous injury.

Airway and esophageal injuries often need to be addressed in a patient who also has several injuries to multiple cavities. Thus, two or three surgical teams may be needed to approach the neck, extremity, chest, or abdomen, and patient position may need to be a compromise. In general the supine position offers the most flexibility, particularly if vascular access can be placed in the arms so they can be tucked prior to operation. Cardiopulmonary bypass is seldom needed, and is infrequently utilized even for intrathoracic tracheal injuries. Unfortunately, many of the patients who require cardiopulmonary bypass have massive injuries and later succumb to multiorgan failure.

INCISIONS

There are a variety of incisions available to manage elective head and neck procedures. However, the two most common incisions utilized to manage cervical trauma are the lateral incision anterior to the sternocleidomastoid muscle and the bilateral apron flap incision (Fig. 25–1). In a patient with cervical vascular trauma, the vessels are usually exposed through the lateral incision similar to the exposure for carotid endarterectomy.[12] This exposure provides excellent proximal and distal control for the midcervical carotid and jugular vessels. Further exploration may then reveal the presence of a tracheal or esophageal injury. For injuries limited to the operative side, extending the incision further toward the sternal notch may allow adequate visualization of the trachea or esophagus to accomplish repair. The incision may also be extended toward the midline raising flaps for better exposure.

A more versatile incision for either bilateral injuries or through-and-through injuries to the trachea and esophagus may be the apron flap incision.[13] This is a U-shaped incision traversing low across the midline of the neck. Subplatysmal flaps are raised and this allows access to the cervical vasculature laterally, the trachea and esophagus laterally from both sides, as well as the trachea anteriorly by splitting the strap muscles and dividing the isthmus of the thyroid. In addition, the larynx is readily available, and there are several options for muscle flaps to buttress repairs. The upper sternum may also be split to gain exposure to the middle trachea.

CONDUCT OF OPERATION

There are two scenarios in which tracheal and esophageal injuries are managed. One scenario develops when the patient is brought emergently to the operating room for a life-threatening vascular injury and a tracheal and esophageal injury is noted after the bleeding is controlled. In this scenario the neck is often opened via a lateral incision, so the carotid or jugular injury can be addressed. Assessment of trajectory might then suggest extension to the esophagus or trachea. At this point it is often useful to extend the incision to the opposite side to gain further exposure.

Sometimes on opening the neck an unanticipated tracheal injury is noted. If possible, the endotracheal tube can be advanced beyond the injury allowing ventilation. The patient sometimes has had a nasotracheal intubation with a short endotracheal tube. Although this approach is suboptimal, we have found that using a connector for cardiopulmonary bypass tubing facilitates placing an extension on an endotracheal tube so that it can be advanced further down the trachea or perhaps into the right main stem bronchus.

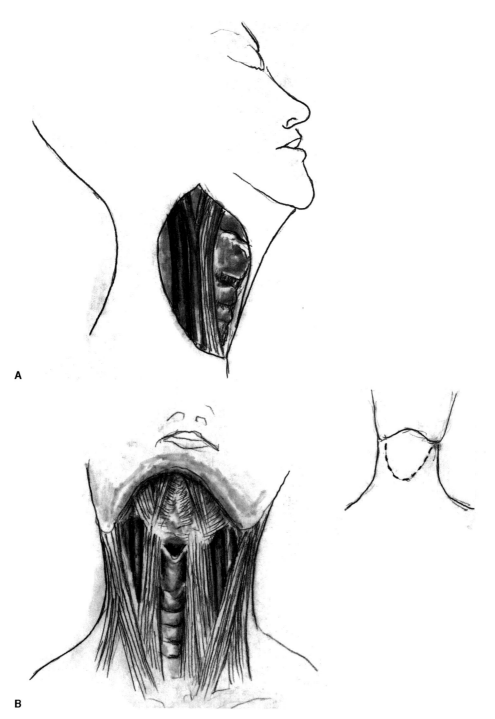

FIGURE 25–1 A: The neck is often opened via a lateral incision for access to vascular injuries. After the vascular injuries are controlled, the trachea and esophagus can be examined for injury by extending the incision inferiorly and anteriorly. B: When operating on a known tracheal/esophageal injury, the bilateral apron flap incision can be a more useful incision. This can be extended inferiorly into an upper sternotomy to expose the middle third of the trachea.

Diagnostic maneuvers can be performed in a stable patient, enabling a planned approach when injuries to the trachea and esophagus have been identified. If possible, surgeons should try to fully understand the trajectory of the missile or knife to prevent missed injuries.[14]

REPAIR OF TRACHEAL INJURY

Once identified, limited tracheal injuries are repaired primarily with an interrupted fine (such as 3-0) absorbable suture such as polyglycolic acid. More extensive injuries such as near-transection may require debridement followed by an end-to-end anastomosis with an absorbable suture. For straightforward injuries tracheostomy is often not needed. For massive injuries a tracheostomy can be performed, and an anterior tracheal wound can be converted into a formal tracheostomy after the posterior injury is repaired. If possible, the recurrent laryngeal nerves should be identified intraoperatively; it is particularly helpful to have assessed bilateral vocal cord function preoperatively. Even if anatomically intact, the recurrent nerves may suffer stretch or blast injury.

Massive injuries with loss of tracheal substance may require mobilization of the trachea to achieve primary closure. The blood supply of the trachea comes from the lateral direction: the upper trachea is supplied by the inferior thyroid arteries and the lower trachea is supplied by the bronchial arteries.[15] Thus, dissection in these areas should be minimized. The anterior tracheal plane into the chest can be readily developed similarly to the dissection for mediastinoscopy. The posterior tracheal plane can be developed in a similar manner. Several supralaryngeal or suprahyoid releases have been described to decrease tension and oppose the ends of the trachea.[16,17] For rare extreme cases, some authors have described opening the chest and dissecting the hilum of the lung to allow further mobilization of the distal trachea.[18] In general, however, the most common maneuvers are laryngeal release and flexing the neck to allow the two ends of the trachea to appose for repair. In some cases, a stitch from the chin to the presternal fascia to maintain the neck in flexion can be placed at the end of the case. Anastomosis of the trachea is performed using 3-0 absorbable sutures with the knots tied on the outside. Polypropylene sutures and other permanent suture material is usually avoided for primary mucosal closure in the nonirradiated neck as the knots can migrate inside the trachea and form granuloma.

REPAIR OF ESOPHAGEAL INJURY

The esophagus is immediately posterior to the trachea and anterior to the vertebral column. Lying slightly to the left of the trachea in the cervical region, the esophagus is often identified via a low lateral neck incision. By dividing the facial vein and dissecting medial to the carotid sheath, the esophagus can be identified behind the trachea and followed to the thoracic outlet. A nasogastric tube placed intraoperatively can assist in identification of the esophagus. The planes anterior and posterior to the esophagus can be developed, and the esophagus looped with a soft drain aiding mobilization; care should be taken to identify and preserve the recurrent laryngeal nerves. For combined tracheal and esophageal injuries the esophagus may be exposed via transection of the trachea through the injury.

Injuries to the esophagus are commonly closed in two layers. The muscular injury may need to be extended and opened to achieve adequate visualization of the mucosal defect. Our institutional preference is to close the mucosal injury with a fine absorbable suture followed by a second layer of interrupted silk on the esophageal musculature. For bilateral or through-and-through injuries, access from both sides of the neck may be required. In rare cases of a high esophageal injury, particularly from iatrogenic causes such as endoscopy, it may not be possible to specifically identify a small posterior injury and perform direct repair. Generous use of drains in this area to manage the esophageal leak as a fistula may be the best option.

We recommend routine drainage of an esophageal injury. For an esophageal injury with a concomitant vascular injury, it may be preferable to bring the drain out the opposite side of the neck, thus avoiding the vascular repair. Either closed suction or soft drains can be used.

Esophageal diversion is often discussed in the management of esophageal trauma. Diversion of the proximal esophagus is most useful for devastating middle to distal esophageal injuries that may have an extremely tenuous repair.[19] The short segment of injured cervical esophagus is not amenable to proximal diversion unless a massive injury is present. In this case, for a patient in extremis with loss of esophageal continuity, the proximal esophagus can be brought out as an end fistula. However, this is needed only in extremely rare cases. When diversion for an intrathoracic esophageal injury is needed, the esophagus is looped with a Penrose drain and brought up to the wound. The esophagus is opened and sewn to the skin. This is not always easily performed and is perhaps better described as bringing the skin down into the esophagus as a loop esophagostomy. For this reason some authors recommend placing a nasogastric tube through the wound into the esophagus or into the pharynx via the pyriform sinus. However, esophageal diversion is seldom needed for cervical injuries.

Muscle flaps can be extremely useful in the management of combined tracheal, esophageal, and vascular injuries. The strap muscles can be mobilized, detached, and brought to the area of injury. It can be helpful to place a muscle with its good blood supply between an esophageal and tracheal injury (Fig. **25–2** and Fig. **25–3**).[20,21] Combined esophageal and vascular injuries can be extremely treacherous. Muscle flaps can be placed on the esophageal repair in an attempt to separate it from the vascular repair. Some devastating results have occurred when a small esophageal leak develops in the area of the vascular repair. This often presents as exsanguination from dehiscence of the vascular repair. Thus, if possible, the esophageal drain should be routed to an area distant from the vascular repair.[20]

POSTOPERATIVE MANAGEMENT

When the patient's condition permits, the patient is extubated, so that the tracheal repair is under negative pressure. Thus, if possible, the anesthesia is planned so that the patient can be extubated at the end of the procedure. Postoperatively patients need aggressive pulmonary toilet. They often benefit from routine therapeutic flexible bronchoscopy to help manage secretions. For a massive tracheal injury, where a tracheostomy is placed, the patient can be removed from mechanical ventilation when appropriate and the tracheostomy left in place. Later the cuffed tube can be replaced with a large metal tracheal cannula. The tracheostomy may act as a pressure relief valve preventing the development of high pressure within the trachea against a closed glottis. If the patient's condition permits, the tracheostomy can be downsized over a week until it is eventually removed. Difficulty in downsizing the tracheostomy tube may be due to an undiagnosed recurrent laryngeal nerve injury.

Postoperatively patients may develop some degree of tracheal narrowing at the site of repair. Stenosis or granuloma formation at the suture line can often be managed endoscopically with laser ablation.[22] Circumferential stenosis of the repair may also be amenable to dilatation and stent placement. Postoperative tracheal stenosis may require reoperation and re-resection.[23] In some severe injuries, the safest course may be permanent tracheostomy.

For esophageal repairs, an important aspect of postoperative care is maintaining adequate nutrition. A soft feeding tube passed into the duodenum can be extremely helpful in maintaining early enteral nutrition. Hard nasogastric tubes when combined with a cuffed tracheostomy can exert pressure on the esophagus through the membranous trachea and cause further injury if left for long periods of time. If external drain output increases during early feeding, a thoracic duct leak unrelated to the esophageal repair should be considered (Table **25–1**). This can be confirmed by sending the fluid for a triglyceride level. These leaks can usually be managed conservatively with total parenteral nutrition, giving the thoracic duct a chance to heal. In extreme circumstances of long-term leak, direct operative repair may be required to ligate the thoracic duct.[24]

Approximately 7 days post-repair a contrast swallow is obtained to evaluate the esophageal repair. If no leak is demonstrated, the patient's diet is advanced over several days while observing drain output. Large increases in drain output should prompt repeat contrast study. If a leak is demonstrated on repeat contrast study, feeding is stopped and the patient maintained on some other form of nutrition until a repeat contrast swallow is obtained

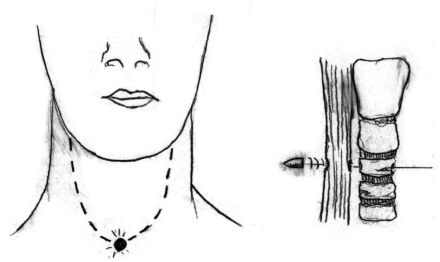

FIGURE 25–2 Gunshot wound to the neck/thoracic outlet. The projectile caused a through-and-through injury to the trachea and a lateral injury to the esophagus. The injury was managed via an apron flap incision with primary repair of the tracheal and esophageal injuries.

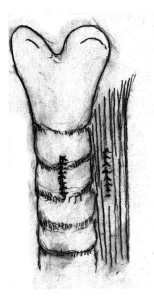
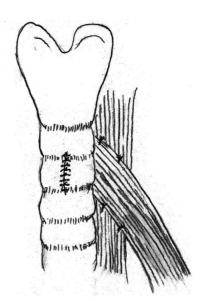

FIGURE 25–3 Following repair of the tracheal and esophageal injuries, a muscle flap was fashioned by dividing the strap muscle inferior attachments and rotating it between the tracheal and esophageal repair. A drain was placed in the area of the esophageal repair.

in a week. If the patient tolerates advancing diet with no leak after 10 to 14 days, the cervical drain can be removed.

PEARLS: TRACHEA AND ESOPHAGUS TRAUMA

- Tracheal injuries can be immediately life threatening. Improvement in emergency medical systems has resulted in more of these patients reaching the hospital alive. Specialty airway maneuvers such as flexible bronchoscopy or tracheostomy via the anterior wound can be extremely useful for establishing an airway.
- The trachea is repaired using an interrupted 3-0 absorbable suture.
- Tracheostomy is not routinely performed after tracheal repair, although tracheostomy may be an adjunct for massive tracheal injuries.
- The esophagus is typically repaired in two layers.
- Esophageal leak is not uncommon postrepair, and the liberal use of drains is encouraged.

TABLE 25–1 DIAGNOSIS OF CHYLOUS LEAK

Triglycerides > 110 mg/100 mL

Positive Sudan red stain for fat

Lymphocytosis > 500 lymphocytes/mL

Chylomicrons present

Cholesterol/triglyceride ratio < 1

- The strap muscles can be extremely useful to buttress a tracheal or esophageal repair. They are also helpful to separate tracheal, esophageal, and vascular repairs.
- If possible, vocal cord function should be assessed preoperatively. Injury to the recurrent laryngeal nerves is often not recognized until after the operation.
- Lymphatic leak is a common associated injury. The majority of these can be managed conservatively with drainage.

REFERENCES

1. Bertelsen S, Howitz P. Injuries of the trachea and bronchi. Thorax 1972;27:188–194
2. Mathisen DJ, Grillo HC. Laryngotracheal trauma. Ann Thorac Surg 1987;43:254–262
3. Flynn AE, Thomas AN, Schecter WP. Acute tracheobronchial injury. J Trauma 1989;29:1326–1330
4. Lee RB. Traumatic injury of the cervico-thoracic trachea and major bronchi. Chest Surg Clin N Am 1997;7:285–304
5. Mulder DS, Ratnani S. Tracheobronchial trauma. In: Pearson FG, Deslauriers J, Ginsberg RJ, et al, eds. Thoracic Surgery. New York: Churchill Livingstone, 1995:1543–1554
6. Kelly JP, Webb WR, Moulder PV, et al. Management of airway trauma: I. Tracheobronchial Injuries. Ann Thorac Surg 1985;40:551–555
7. Chagnon FP, Mulder DS. Laryngotracheal trauma. Chest Surg Clin N Am 1996;6:733–748
8. Committee on Trauma. American College of Surgeons: Advanced Trauma Life Support Program for

Doctors. Chicago: American College of Surgeons, 1997

9. Wall MJ Jr, Granchi T, Liscum K, Mattox KL. Penetrating thoracic vascular injuries. Surg Clin North Am 1996;76:749–761

10. Edwards WH Jr, Morris JA Jr, Delozier JB III, Adkins RB Jr. Airway injuries: the first priority in trauma. Am Surg 1987;53:192–197

11. Barmada H, Gibbons JR. Tracheobronchial injury in blunt and penetrating chest trauma. Chest 1994; 106 :74–78

12. Britt LD, Peyser MB. Penetrating and blunt neck trauma. In: Mattox KL, Feliciano DV, Moore EE, eds. Trauma, 4th ed. New York: McGraw-Hill, 2000: 437–450

13. Hirshberg A, Wall MJ Jr, Johnston RJ Jr, Burch JM, Mattox KL. Transcervical gunshot injuries. Am J Surg 1994;167:309–312

14. Hirshberg A, Wall MJ Jr, Allen MK, Mattox KL. Causes and patterns of missed injuries in trauma. Am J Surg 1994;168:299–303

15. Salassa JR, Peerson BW, Payne WS. Gross and microscopic blood supply of the trachea. Ann Thorac Surg 1977;24:100–107

16. Dedo H, Fishman NH. Laryngeal release and sleeve resection for tracheal stenosis. Ann Otol Rhinol Laryngol 1969;78:285–296

17. Montgomery WW. Suprahyoid release for tracheal anastomosis. Arch Otolaryngol 1974;99:255–260

18. Heitmiller RF. Tracheal release maneuvers. Chest Surg Clin N Am 1996;6:675–682

19. Popovsky J, Lee YC, Berk JL. Gunshot wounds of the esophagus. J Thorac Cardiovasc Surg 1976;72:609–612

20. Feliciano DV, Bitondo CG, Mattox KL. Combined tracheoesophageal injuries. Am J Surg 1985;150: 710–715

21. Symbas PN, Hatcher CR, Boehm GA. Acute penetrating tracheal trauma. Ann Thorac Surg 1976;22: 473–477

22. Beamis JF, Vergos K, Rebeiz E, Shapstay S. Endoscopic laser therapy for obstructing tracheobronchial lesions. Ann Otol Rhinol Laryngol 1991;100:413–419

23. Sulek M, Miller RH, Mattox KL. The management of gunshot and stab injuries of the trachea. Arch Otolaryngol 1983;109:56–59

24. Nussenbaum B, Liu JH. Systematic management of chyle fistula. Otolaryngol Head Neck Surg 2000;122: 31–38

Page numbers in italics indicate figures; those followed by t indicate tables.